The New Complete
MEDICAL
and HEALTH
ENCYCLOPEDIA

The New Complete
MEDICAL
and HEALTH
ENCYCLOPEDIA

EDITED BY
Richard J. Wagman, M.D., F.A.C.P.
Assistant Clinical Professor of Medicine
Downstate Medical Center
New York, New York

AND BY
the J. G. Ferguson Editorial Staff

Volume 1

J. G. FERGUSON PUBLISHING COMPANY / CHICAGO

Acknowledgments

Grateful acknowledgment is made of the courtesy of the following organization:

Holt, Rinehart and Winston, Inc., New York, New York, for permission to reprint art and caption material from *Field & Stream Guide to Physical Fitness*, with illustrations by Alex Orr.

Portions of *The New Complete Medical and Health Encyclopedia* have been previously published under the title of *The Complete Illustrated Book of Better Health* and *The Illustrated Encyclopedia of Better Health*, edited by Richard J. Wagman, M.D.

Contributors to
The New Complete Medical and Health Encyclopedia

Editor
RICHARD J. WAGMAN, M.D., F.A.C.P.
Assistant Clinical Professor of Medicine
Downstate Medical Center
New York, New York

Consultant in Surgery
N. HENRY MOSS, M.D., F.A.C.S.
Associate Clinical Professor of Surgery
Temple University Health Sciences Center
and Albert Einstein Medical Center;
Past President, American Medical Writers Association;
Past President, New York Academy of Sciences

Consultant in Gynecology
DOUGLASS S. THOMPSON, M.D.
Clinical Professor of Obstetrics and Gynecology
and Clinical Associate Professor of Community Medicine
University of Pittsburgh School of Medicine
Pittsburgh, Pennsylvania

Consultant in Pediatrics
CHARLES H. BAUER, M.D.
Clinical Associate Professor of Pediatrics
and Chief of Pediatric Gastroenterology
The New York Hospital-Cornell Medical Center
New York, New York

Consultants in Psychiatry
JULIAN J. CLARK, M.D.
Assistant Professor of Psychiatry
and
RITA W. CLARK, M.D.
Clinical Assistant Professor of Psychiatry
Downstate Medical Center
New York, New York

Consulting Editor
KENNETH N. ANDERSON
Formerly Editor
Today's Health

BRUCE O. BERG, M.D.
Associate Professor
Departments of Neurology
  and Pediatrics
Director, Child Neurology
University of California
San Francisco, California

D. JEANNE COLLINS
Assistant Professor
College of Allied Health
  Professions
University of Kentucky
Lexington, Kentucky

ANTHONY A. DAVIS
Vice President and
  Education Consultant
Metropolitan X-Ray and
  Medical Sales, Inc.
Olney, Maryland

PETER A. DICKINSON
Editor Emeritus
Harvest Years/Retirement
  Living

GORDON K. FARLEY, M.D.
Associate Professor of Child Psychiatry
Director, Day Care Center
University of Colorado Medical Center
Denver, Colorado

ARTHUR FISHER
Group Editor
Science and Engineering
Popular Science

EDMUND H. HARVEY, JR.
Editor
Science World

HELENE MACLEAN
Medical writer

BEN PATRUSKY
Science writer

STANLEY E. WEISS, M.D.
Assistant Attending Physician,
  Renal Service
Beth Israel Hospital and Medical
  Center
New York, New York

JEFFREY S. WILLNER, M.D.
Attending Radiologist
Southampton Hospital
Southampton, New York

Contents

Volume 3

Color Illustrations

Diagrams of Systems and Organs of the Body

Introduction

Many questions may run through your mind when you or a family member are ill. Even if you see a physician, you still have a lot of questions afterward. The doctor was very busy and didn't take time to discuss all the aspects of your condition that you would like to discuss. Or, you did have a good talk with your doctor, but he or she used several terms you didn't understand. You didn't get the details of the diagnosis; surgery was mentioned—what does this kind of operation involve?

The NEW COMPLETE MEDICAL AND HEALTH ENCYCLOPEDIA is designed to give you clear, accurate answers to your questions about health care. Thorough discussions of major diseases like cancer and heart problems are included, along with facts about many other less serious diseases and physical problems and how they are treated.

Many people today have adopted a consumerist point of view and want to take an active part in their own treatment. This usually takes the form of asking your doctor to present the treatment options available to you, then making a decision about which course to follow. Let's assume that your physician is in tune with this approach and willing to relinquish some of the authority doctors traditionally have assumed to tell patients what to do. Still, you need information to ask intelligent questions and to understand the alternatives being discussed.

Fortunately, research in medicine is continually advancing. The NEW COMPLETE MEDICAL AND HEALTH ENCYCLOPEDIA has been revised in this edition to include material on some recent developments—like the portable insulin pump for diabetics—that you may have heard about. In line with the idea of treatment options, the editors have also included information on the many types of surgery now used for breast cancer patients—no longer is the total mastectomy the treatment of choice for that disease.

Generic drugs have been in the spotlight increasingly in recent years. For your convenience in sorting out which drug is equivalent to which, the editors have included a new chapter on 100 commonly prescribed generic drugs. The chapter includes information on brand names, the action that each drug has in the body, and possible side effects.

Becoming ill and being treated are only part of the picture in health care today. More and more, professionals and lay people are putting the emphasis on preventive medicine, doing everything you possibly can to stay well and healthy. To help you and your family keep in the best possible condition, the editors have included detailed information on food and nutrition, dieting, care of skin and hair, dental health, exercises, and physical fitness. (The section on exercises includes not only detailed instructions, but also diagrams of how to perform each exercise.) A new section on jogging has been added for this edition, to outline the prospects and possible problems of the millions who run regularly to keep fit.

Families often have questions about children's health. Parents, stepparents, and grandparents want to know what is normal and expected from a child at various ages in terms of physical, mental, and emotional development. Therefore, the editors have included two chapters, one on younger children, and the other on teenagers, that discuss everything from the common cold to stuttering, from creativity to sexual maturation.

Older people, too, have special health concerns. Senior citizens or their families will want to read the information on diet, daily habits, mental health, activities to pursue during retirement, nursing homes, and retirement homes for the aging.

These are just a few of the subjects covered in this encyclopedia. How can you make the best possible use of these books? First and foremost, do *not* use this information to treat yourself or anyone else except temporarily in an emergency. If any symptom of disease is present, no one can take the place of a trained professional.

Use the NEW COMPLETE MEDICAL AND HEALTH ENCYCLOPEDIA for background information on a host of topics, as a handy guide to first aid, and as a reference on where to get further information. Throughout these volumes, the editors have included the names and addresses of organizations that deal with health-related matters, places you can write for further information.

Get acquainted with these books by looking through the table of contents in each volume. Then, to locate a specific topic of interest, be sure to consult the A-Z Index Reference Guide, which starts on page 1 of this volume and which incorporates a glossary of terms to help you understand your body and your health.

THE EDITORS

The New Complete
MEDICAL
and HEALTH
ENCYCLOPEDIA

A-Z Index Reference Guide:

A Note on Using the Index

The pages that follow contain a reference tool that should be very useful for the layman. In using this glossary-index combination the reader will be able to find brief definitions for medical terminology and locate the pages where each major topic is discussed. Where appropriate, cross references to similar or related topics are given. Illustrations and photos are indicated by the page numbers which are in italics.

Reference Index

turn blue litmus paper red, and are capable of reacting with another compound (a base) to form a salt

acid burn, 162

acidosis: chemical imbalance in the blood marked by an excess of acid, sometimes affecting diabetics and leading possibly to diabetic coma, 1222, 1228, 1231

acidotic: having or marked by acidosis, 1228

acinous cell: cell in the pancreas that secretes digestive juice, as distinguished from the cells of the islets of Langerhans

acne: common eruptive skin disorder due to clogging or inflammation of the sebaceous glands, 299, 543-544, 800-801, *800*

acoustic nerve: auditory nerve

acromegaly: disorder of the pituitary gland characterized by enlarged head, hands, feet, and most body organs, 403, 1213

acrophobia: fear of heights, 486, 1325

ACTH/adrenocorticotrophic hormone, 403, *403*, 404

   in multiple sclerosis, 1100

   in rheumatic fever, 1148

ACTION, 683-684, *1045*

actinomycin D, 1293

activity vs. calorie expenditure, 225-227, 721-725, *725*

acupuncture: the Oriental art of traditional medicine in which needles are inserted at specific points through the skin to treat disease and induce anesthesia

acupuncturist: one skilled in acupuncture

acute: sudden and severe, as a disease. Compare *chronic.*

Adams-Stokes disease: temporary loss of consciousness caused by the heart's missing a beat, i.e., its failure to contract and pump blood on schedule, 273

addiction: the compulsive habitual use of a drug for other than medical reasons

   barbiturate, 556

   cigarettes and, 1198-1200

   heroin, 555-556, 1371-1373

   methadone, 1373

   morphine, 1370

Addison's anemia: anemia, pernicious, 116-117

Addison's disease: chronic hypofunction (underfunctioning) of the adrenal cortex, characterized by weakness, loss of body hair, and increased skin pigmentation, 1215

adenocarcinoma: carcinoma involving epithelial tissue of a gland

   endometrial, 1025-1026, *1025*

   of stomach, 943-944

adenoid(s): enlarged lymphoid growth behind the pharynx, 447, 952-954

adenoidectomy: surgical removal of the adenoids, 953-954

adenoma: benign tumor which can cause hyperfunction of the parathyroid glands, 1219

adenopathy: any glandular disease characterized by swelling of the lymph nodes

adenotonsillectomy: T and A operation

adhesions, 942-943, 992

adipose: of or pertaining to fat; fatty

adipose tissue: *see* fat, body

adolescents: age groups, teenagers, 444-445, 537-569

adoption, 447

adrenal cortex: the outer part of the adrenal gland, which produces several hormones that affect metabolism of foods, secondary sex characteristics, skin pigmentation and resistance to infection

adrenalectomy: surgical removal of an adrenal gland, 936-937

adrenal gland: either of two small ductless glands situated above each kidney, *401*, 404-405, *404*, 935-937, *936*, 1211, 1214-1215, *1214*

   disorders of, 935-937, 1214-1215

   nicotine and, 551-552

adrenaline/epinephrine: adrenal hormone which acts to stimulate the heart, dilate the blood vessels, and relax bronchial smooth muscles, 404, 1215

for insect stings, 502

adrenal medulla: inner part of the adrenal gland, 1214, 1215

adrenal steroids, in nephrosis, 1256

adrenocorticotrophic hormone/ACTH: hormone secreted by the anterior lobe of the pituitary gland which stimulates the growth and function of the adrenal cortex, 403, *403*, 404

See also ACTH.

Adriamycin, 1293

Aedes mosquito, 1303

aerobic: capable of living only in air or free oxygen, as certain bacteria. Compare *anaerobic.*

aerobics: exercises that involve a workout for the lungs and heart as well as the muscles, 237, 549

aerosol cans, 162-163

aerosol sprays, eye injury from, 162-163

affect: emotion, as distinguished from thought or perception

affective reaction: *see* manic-depressive reaction

afferent: applied to nerves, receiving sensations; sensory. Compare *efferent.*

afferent nerves: nerves, sensory, *363,* 362-364

aflatoxin: toxic substance produced by a fungus that develops typically in stored grains or legumes such as peanuts and that is associated with cancer of the liver

aflatoxins, liver cancer and, 1284

African trypanosomiasis: *see* sleeping sickness

afterbirth/the placenta: so called when expelled from the uterus after the birth of a baby, 599

age

biological vs. chronological, 619-620

65 and over (U.S. population), 655

aggression, 1323

aggressiveness, children and, 447-449, *448*

aging

and bone atrophy, 1069

care of

closed care, 334

nonorganized care, 334

open care, 334

cellular therapy for, 688-689

and central nervous system, 363

diabetes and, 621-622, 1232-1234

and diseases, 621-622

hormone therapy for, 688-689

and mental ability, 654, 656

mental attitude and, 656, 689, *689*

problems of, 629-636

senses and, 273, 654, 656, 1235

of skin, 355, 778-779

Aging, State Commission on, 685

Aging, U.S. Administration on, 663

agoraphobia: fear of open spaces

agranulocytosis: acute disease characterized by almost total disappearance of neutrophils from the blood, and often following the use of certain drugs, 1122-1123

Agricultural Extension Service, 744

AHF: antihemophilic factor, 1112, 1114

ailurophobia: fear of cats

air conditioning and dry skin, 780

air pollution, *754,* 756-762, *757, 759,* 1200-1202, *1201*

colds and, 830

eye irritation and, 758, 855

air travel and health, 273

airway: 1. passageway for air 2. plastic breathing tube for administering artificial respiration from rescuer's mouth to victim's mouth

American trypanosomiasis: *see* Chagas' disease

amino acid: any of a group of compounds that form an essential part of the protein molecule, 386, 389

amitriptyline, 196

ammonia, aromatic spirits of, 847

amnesia: loss or impairment of memory, sometimes temporary

amniocentesis/prenatal diagnosis: procedure for determining whether a fetus is afflicted with an inherited disorder by sampling the amniotic fluid of a pregnant woman, 583, *584*

amnion/amniotic sac: membranous sac enclosing the embryo in mammals, birds, and reptiles

amniotic fluid/bag of waters: the fluid within a membrane surrounding an embryo in the uterus of a pregnant woman, 592

amoebic dysentery: form of dysentery caused by an amoeba, 1162-1163

amphetamine/Benzedrine: any of a class of drugs that stimulate the central nervous system, used medically to treat depressive mental disorders and sometimes to retard appetite, and used illicitly to induce a state of abnormal alertness and excitement, 556, 730, 1362-1367

Amphotericin B: antibiotic substance used to treat histoplasmosis and other deep-seated fungus infections, 1192

ampicillin, 196

ampulla *(pl., ampullae):* any dilated part or sac, as the base of each of the semicircular canals of the inner ear, *416*

amputate: to remove surgically by cutting, as a gangrenous limb

amputation

    accidental, 986-987

    for gangrene, 1126

amyotrophic lateral sclerosis, 363

anabolism: the process by which nutrients are built up into the living organism; constructive metabolism. Compare *catabolism.*

anaerobic: capable of living without air or free oxygen, as certain bacteria. Compare *aerobic.*

anal fissure: crack, split, or ulceration in the area of the two anal sphincters that control the release of feces, 853

analgesia: incapacity to feel pain

analgesic: drug that lessens or eliminates the capacity to feel pain

anal pruritus, 794, 853

anal sphincter: the ring of muscle fibers surrounding the anus and controlling the passage of wastes from the body

anaphylactic shock: allergic shock, 144, *145*

anatomy, drawings of, *343, 372*

Ancylostoma, 1170

androgen: any of various hormones found in males which control the appearance and development of masculine characteristics, also present although in smaller amounts in females

androgen therapy, in testicular failure, 636

androsterone: an androgen secreted in the urine, 407

anemia: deficiency in the amount or quality of red blood corpuscles or of hemoglobin in the blood, 846, 1115-1118

    hemolytic: form of anemia caused by an abnormally high rate of breakdown of red blood cells, exceeding the capacity of the bone marrow to replace them with new cells, 1115-1116

    hemophilic: anemia caused by bleeding into joint cavities in advanced hemophilia, 1112-1114

    iron-deficiency: anemic condition caused by insufficient iron in the diet, *1116,* 1118

    pernicious/Addison's anemia: anemia characterized by the enlarged size and reduced number of red blood cells, caused by the body's inability to absorb vitamin B_{12}, 1116-1117

    sickle cell, 1117-1118

    and skin color, 778

anterior: toward the front

anterior lobe hypophysis: the anterior part of the pituitary gland that produces growth hormones and hormones that stimulate other glands

anterior urethra: the meatus, or external opening, of the urethra in the penis

anthrax: malignant, infectious disease of sheep, cattle, and other animals, caused by a bacillus and sometimes transmitted to humans

anti-: against; opposed to; opposite to

antibiotic(s): any of a large class of substances, such as penicillin and streptomycin, produced by various microorganisms and fungi that have the power to destroy or arrest the growth of other microorganisms, including many that cause infectious diseases, 748, 1185, *1185*

and acne, 801

in agranulocytosis, 1123

allergic reaction to, 865, *865*

in bronchitis, 854

in colitis, 1169

in ear infections, 856, 1244

gonococcus and, 1005

in influenza, 830

in jaundice, 1174

in meningitis, 1101

in moniliasis, 996

in pneumonia, 1185

in pyelonephritis, 1257

in rheumatic fever, 1149

antibody: substance produced by the body to counteract infection and in response to specific antigens, 274, 405, 861, *1173*

and rheumatic fever, 1146

and *Rh* factor, 582

in tuberculosis, 1189, *1189*

anti-clotting compounds: anticoagulant

anticoagulant: substance that retards clotting of the blood, 905, 1124, 1128

anticonvulsant: medicine used to control epileptic seizures

antidepressant: drug that stimulates physiological activity, thereby tending to alleviate depression, 1334-1335

antidiuretic hormone: vasopressin, 402, *403*, 1218

antidote: anything that neutralizes or counteracts the effects of a poison

antigen: any of several substances, including toxins, enzymes, and proteins, that cause the development of antibodies when introduced into an organism, 982-984, 1146, *1173*

antihelminthic: drug or remedy used to destroy intestinal worms, or helminths, 1169

antihemophilic factor/AHF: substance that causes clotting and stops bleeding in hemophiliacs, 1112, 1114

antihistamine: any of a number of drugs that counteract the nasal engorgement and vasoconstrictor action of histamine in the body, often used in the treatment of hay fever, 832, 871, 1194

antimetabolite: chemical that interferes with cell metabolism

antimony medications, 1306, 1313

antiperspirant: astringent preparation which acts to diminish or prevent perspiration, 295-296, 781

antiseptics, 1047-1048

in foot care, 674

antitoxin: antibody produced in response to the presence of a specific toxin, which it neutralizes

antivenin: antitoxin to venom or serum prepared to counteract the effects of venom

anuria: inability to urinate, 1249, 1255

anus: the opening at the lower extremity of the alimentary canal, *379*, 383, 391, *937*, *1156*

anvil/incus: the middle of the three ossicles of the middle ear, the bone between the hammer and the stirrup, 414, *417*, 955, *955*

anxiety, 365, 450-451, *450*, 830

and food, 514, 752

anxiety reaction: neurosis characterized chiefly by anxiety unrelated to any apparent cause, 1323-1324

aorta: the large artery originating from the left ventricle of the heart that forms the main arterial trunk from which blood is distributed to all of the body except the lungs, 366, *367*, 375, *965*

aneurysm of, 1001-1002

coarctation of, 964-965

aortic valve: the membranous valve between the left ventricle of the heart and the aorta, 1148

Apgar system: system of rating the health of newborn babies, 599-600

aphasia: partial or total loss of the power of articulate speech due to a disorder in the cerebrum of the brain, 1128

aplasia: arrested development or congenital absence of a part or organ of the body

aplastic: marked by aplasia; underdeveloped

apnea: cessation or interruption of breathing

apocrine glands, 295

apoplexy: stroke, 275

appendectomy: surgical removal of the vermiform appendix, 391, 938-939, 1169

appendicitis: inflammation of the vermiform appendix characterized by pain in the right lower abdomen, nausea, and vomiting, 391, 937-939, 1169

treatment for, 164-165

appendicular skeleton: skeleton

appendix vermiformis: vermiform appendix, *379*, *384*, 391, 937, *937*, 1169

appetite

of infant, 700, 703

in later years, 660

loss of, 718

regulation of, 361

apples, nutrients in, 705

appliances, prosthetic, for fractures, 970, *971*

apricots, nutrients in, 705

aptitudes of children, 446

aqueous humor: the clear, limpid alkaline fluid that fills the anterior chamber of the eye from the cornea to the lens, *410*, 413, *957*, 960

arachnoid: the middle of the three membranes that envelop the brain and spinal cord

arches, fallen, 841-842

arch supports, 629, 842

areola: the dark circular area around the nipple of a breast or around a pustule

arm(s), 344, *351*, 352, *352*

relief of tension in, 625

severed, reattachment of, 986-987

arrest: slow or stop the progress of, as a disease

arrhythmia: variation from the normal heartbeat, 1138

arsenic

skin cancer and, 765, 1274

in water pollution, 765

arterial: having to do with or carried by the arteries

arterial bleeding, control of, 141-142

arteriogram: X-ray picture of an artery

arteriography: technique of injecting an opaque substance into the coronary arteries and observing the material by X ray as it runs its course through the heart muscle, 1136

arteriole: small artery, especially the one that leads to a capillary, 366, *366*, 1144

arteriosclerosis: thickening and hardening of the walls of an artery, with impairment of blood circulation, 1133

cerebral, 1103, 1104

arteritis: inflammation of an artery, 1124

artery: any of a large number of muscular, tubular vessels conveying blood away from the heart to all parts of the body, 366, *367*

axillary, *367*

brachial, *142, 143, 367*

carotid, *367*

coronary, 375, 1132-1134, *1133*

femoral, *142, 143, 367*

hardening of: *see* atherosclerosis

iliac, *367*

peroneal, 367

pulmonary: artery that delivers oxygen-poor blood from the heart to the lungs, *374*, 374, 392, *393*

radial, *367*

renal, 367, *419*, 420, 421, *420, 1249, 1254*

subclavian, *367*

tibial, *367*

ulnar, *367*

artery-capillary-vein sequence, *366*

arthritis: inflammation of a joint, characterized by pain, swelling, and tenderness, 1051-1066

chronic gouty, 1061-1062

exercises for, 671, *1055, 1057*, 1058

and fever, 275

and foot problems, 673, 674

fungal, 1064

gonorrheal: complication of gonorrhea affecting the joints, 1005, 1062-1063

hemophilic: painful swelling and bleeding in joint cavities, 1113-1114

in later years, 671

and nail deformity, 791

new drugs for, 1057-1058

and overweight, 651

pyrogenic: form of arthritis characterized by fever, 1062

rubella, 1063

transient, of hip, 1054

treatment of, 275

tuberculous, 1063

voluntary agencies, 307-309, *309*

See also rheumatoid arthritis.

Arthritis Foundation, 307-309, *309*, 1057

arthropathy: any disease of the joints

articulate: form a joint, as one bone with another

artificial insemination, *573*

artificial respiration: artificial maintenance of respiration in someone who has ceased to breathe, especially mouth-to-mouth resuscitation, 140-141

asbestos, lung disease and, 755, 1207-1208, *1208*

ascaris: roundworms, 1171-1172

ascorbic acid/vitamin C: white, odorless, crystalline compound found in citrus and other fresh fruits and green leafy vegetables, and also made synthetically, that prevents scurvy, 212, 697, 863

and common cold, 739, 830

formula-fed baby and, 703

asepsis: prevention of infection by the maintenance of sterile conditions

aseptic: free from disease-causing microorganisms

aseptic meningitis: *see* meningitis, aseptic

asparagus, nutrients in, 702

asphyxiation: loss of consciousness caused by too little oxygen in the blood, generally as a result of suffocation by drowning or the breathing in of noxious gases, 183

aspirate: withdraw by suction

aspiration: act or process of aspirating

aspiration, vacuum: *see* vacuum aspiration

aspirin (acetylsalicylic acid): analgesic drug that has fever-reducing properties, widely used to treat symptoms of the common cold, rheumatoid arthritis and many other conditions, 197

allergic reaction to, 865

in arthritis, 275, 671, 1054, 1056-1057

and clotting, 275-276

side effects of, 275, 1056

in toothache, 275

assassin bugs, 1307, 1309-1310

assimilation: the process by which digested food is made an integral part of the solid or fluids of an organism

Association for Voluntary Sterilization, 324-325

asthenia: lack or loss of strength; weakness

asthma: chronic respiratory disorder characterized by recurrent paroxysmal coughing caused by spasms of the bronchi or diaphragm, and due in many cases to an allergic reaction, 451, 1192-1193, 1203

allergic, 274, 864, 865, 1194-1195

emergency treatment for, 165

smog and, 758

astigmatism: distorted vision caused by an uneven curvature of the cornea, 483, 1236-1237

asymptomatic: condition in which antibodies for a disease are present in the blood but no symptoms of the disease can be observed. Compare *symptomatic.*

ataxia: absence or failure of muscular coordination

atherosclerosis: hardening of the inner walls of the arteries, resulting in a loss of elasticity, and accompanied by the deposit of fat and degenerative tissue changes, 289, *1125,* 1126, 1133, *1133*

diet and, 736, 739

and intermittent claudication, 968

athetosis: derangement of the nervous system in which the hands and feet, especially the fingers and toes, keep moving or twitching, 1088

athlete's foot: ringworm of the foot, caused by a parasitic fungus, 674, 796-797, *796*

athletic supporter, 1216

atrioventricular block: disruption of normal transmission of signals between the upper and lower chambers of the heart, as from scar tissue, that may affect

blood flow to the brain and cause blackouts or convulsions, 1154

atrium (*pl., atria*)/auricle: one of the two upper chambers of the heart, which receive blood from the veins and transmit it to the ventricles, 374, *374, 965*

atrophy: the wasting or withering away of the body or any of its parts, as from disease or lack of use

bone, 1069

muscle tissue, 353

atropine (belladonna, hyoscyamine), 197, 1090

attention span, child's, *442,* 443

attenuated: weakened in strength, as a microorganism for use in a vaccine

audiologist: one who specializes in the treatment of those with hearing problems, 668, *1243*

audiometer: device that measures hearing, 896, 1244

auditory canal/auditory meatus: either of two passageways, the *external auditory canal* leading from the outer ear to the tympanic membrane or eardrum, and the *internal auditory canal* passing through the temporal bone to the brain, 414, *415, 955,* 1243, *1243*

infection of, 1244-1245

auditory nerve/acoustic nerve: nerve consisting of the cochlear nerve and the vestibular nerve and connecting the inner ear with the brain, conveying the sense of hearing and of equilibrium, *361,* 414, *415, 417, 955*

aura: subjective, momentary sensory perception of an unusual nature that occurs just before the onset of an epileptic convulsion, 1093, 1094-1096

Aureomycin: trade name for the antibiotic tetracycline

auricle: atrium, 374, *374, 965*

auscultation: diagnostic procedure of listening, as to sounds in the chest with a stethoscope, 879-880, *879*

authorization for therapy, 907-908

loss of hair on the crown of the head until only a fringe remains around the sides and in the back, often called *male pattern baldness*, 630-632, 786-787

from curling iron, 784

heredity and, 542

patchy/alopecia **areata:** sudden but usually temporary loss of hair in patches, 631

from sebaceous cysts, 799

ballet dancing, stress fractures and, 1075

bananas, nutrients in, 705

Banting, Frederick, 1220

barbell exercises, 234, *265-266*

barber's itch: sycosis, 798

barbiturates: any of a class of drugs derived from barbituric acid that depress the central nervous system, used medically as sedatives and sleeping pills and in the treatment of epilepsy and high blood pressure, and illicitly to counteract the effects of stimulant drugs, **556, 841, 1367-1368**

alcohol and, 1347

in anesthesia, 914

overdose of, 177

barium: metallic element used in compounds, especially barium sulfate, in radiography of the gastrointestinal tract because it is radiopaque—impervious to X rays

barium enema: enema in which a barium mixture is used to visualize the inner walls of the large intestine by X ray, used to detect cancer and other diseases, **892-893, 1177**

barium meal: liquid containing barium taken orally for the visualization of the upper gastrointestinal tract by X ray, **890, 892**

barium sulfate: an insoluble barium compound used to facilitate X-ray pictures of the stomach and intestines, **890, 892, 1177**

barium swallow: X-ray examination of the esophagus as the patient swallows a liquid containing barium, **890**

Barnard, Christiaan, 985

baroreceptors/barostats: sensitive nerve cells that respond to changes in blood pressure and may help to regulate it, 1145

Basal Body Temperature/BBT: accurate measure of body temperature taken under uniform conditions, used to determine a woman's day of ovulation, 572, 573

basal caloric state, 727, 729

basal cell cancer, 666

basal ganglia: group of nerve cells embedded in the cerebral hemisphere, the largest part of the human brain

basal metabolism: the minimum energy, measured in calories, that the body needs to maintain essential vital activities when it is at rest

basal thermometer: thermometer scaled in tenths of degrees instead of fifths, used by women to determine the time of ovulation

Basic Food Groups, 658-659, 704, 705

bathing, 778-779, 794

of bedridden patient, 1042-1043

skin care and, 627, 779-780

battered child syndrome, 453-454

See also child abuse.

BBT: *see* Basal Body Temperature

BCG (basille Calmette Guerin) vaccine, 1036

beaches, polluted, 763, 765

beans, nutrients in, 701-702

beard, growth of, 787, *788*

Becker type muscular dystrophy, 1107

bed, accessories for, in home nursing, 1041, 1046

bed linen, changing, in home nursing, 1043

bedpan, 1043, 1048

bed rest

in congestive heart failure, 1154

hazards of, 1078, 1129-1130

in rheumatic fever, 1148

bedridden patient, home care of, 1041-1048

bedtime, child's, 454

atrophy: decalcification

brittle: osteogenesis imperfecta

broken: fractures

bruises to, 167-168

cancer of, 1073

development of, 346, 347, 542, 1049

disorders of, 347-348, 1067-1073

functions of, 339

inflammation of: osteomyelitis

injury to, 1074-1083

softening and thickening: Paget's disease

tumors of, 1072-1073, *1073*

bone marrow, 347, 1115

   disorders of, 890, 892, 1119, 1121-1123, 1290

   transplant of, 322, 985-986

booster shots, 500, 532

boredom, in child, 454-456, *455*

boric acid, 1048

bottle feeding, 431-432, *432*, 600-601

botulism: poisoning caused by eating spoiled or improperly prepared or canned food and characterized by acute gastrointestinal and nervous disorders, *168*, 168-169, *739*, 1172, *1172*

bouillon cubes, nutrients in, 716

bowed legs, 487

bowel, large: *see* intestine, large

bowel habits, change in, 364, 672, 1272-1273

bowling, 662

Bowman's capsule: dilated structure surrounding a glomerulus as part of the nephron of a kidney, *420*, 421, *1254*

boy *(slang):* heroin

brain, 358, 359-361, *360*

   cranial nerves of, *361*

   degenerative diseases of, 1103-1104

   diagnostic procedures for, 888-890, *889*

   in later years, 685

   "lesser brains": cerebellum and nervous system, 360-365

brain cage: cranium

brain damage: tissue destruction of the brain caused by an injury before, at, or after birth, 456, 1322

   alcohol and, 1346

   mechanical injury and, 974-976, 1080

   minimal: *see* minimal brain dysfunction

   in stroke, 1127

   in tertiary syphilis, 1263

brain death: biological death

brain scan: procedure of injecting a radioactive substance into the brain tissue or fluid and recording its movement by X rays, 888-890, *889*, 974, *975*, *1086*, *1285*, *1286*

brain scanning: *CAT scanning* of the brain

brain stem: all of the brain except the cerebellum, cerebrum, and cerebral cortex; the midbrain, 360, *360*

brain surgeon: neurosurgeon

brain surgery, 972, 974-976

brain tumor, 364, 973-974, 1284-1285, *1285*

brain waves, 888

   recording of: electroencephalography

brandy, 1341

bran flakes, nutrients in, 711

breads, nutrients in, 711

breakfast, 640, 729

   modified menus for, 728, 734, 735, 740, 743, 746, 750

breastbone: *see* sternum

breast(s)

   abscess of, 1016

   cancer of, 1027-1036, *1032*, *1034*, *1036*

   cosmetic surgery of, 979-980

   cysts of, 1015-1016

   enlargement of: mammoplasty

   inflammation of, 601

   reduction of: mastoplasty

   self-examination of, *313*, 1028, *1029*

breast feeding, 429-431, *430*, 600-601, *600*

breath

   bad: halitosis, 849, 1158

immunosuppressive chemicals and, *313*, 983, *1274*

and immunotherapy, 1035-1036

of kidney, 1258-1259, 1282-1283

of larynx, 1285-1287

in later years, 635, 666, 671-672

leukemic, 1121-1122, 1290-1292

of lip, 951

liver, 1283-1284

lung, 277, 962-963, 1268

of lymphatic system, 1269, 1288-1290, 1292, 1293

in middle years, 635, 1121

oral, 950-952, 1275

ovarian, 1026-1027

of pancreas, 1283

of prostate, 674-675, 1260

skin, 298, 666, 755, 765, 779, 1273-1275

stomach, 943-944, 1267, 1275-1278, *1276*

thyroid, 1287-1288

of tongue, 951-952

of uterus, 689, 1023-1026

voluntary agencies, 309-313, 325

warning signals of, 671-672, 1277

cancer-producing agents: carcinogens

candidiasis: *see* moniliasis

candy, nutrients in, 716

canine teeth: the sharp, pointed teeth, two in the upper jaw (called *eye teeth*), and two in the lower jaw, located between the incisors and the molars, 380, **806, 807**

canker sore: small ulcerous lesion in the mouth near the molar teeth, inside the lips or in the lining of the mouth, **849,** 1158

cannabidiol, 1377

cannabinol, 1377

cannabis: hashish or marihuana, 1376-1378

Cannabis sativa: the Indian hemp plant, from whose flowering tops are derived marihuana and hashish, 1376, *1376*, 1377

cannula: narrow tube inserted into a body cavity or vessel, as to extract a substance or introduce a medication

canoeing, 624

cantaloupes, nutrients in, 705

capillary(ies): minute blood vessel, 366, *366*, 372

in kidney, *420*, 421

in lungs, 392-393, *393*

of lymphatic system, 373

in skin, *354*

capillary bed, 366, *366*

caput succedaneum: swelling under a newborn baby's scalp soon after birth, that usually dissolves in a few days, **427**

carbohydrate(s): any of a group of compounds, including sugars, starches, and cellulose, that contains carbon combined with hydrogen and oxygen, essential in the metabolism of plants and animals

in diet, 696-697, *708*, 730

metabolism of, 380, 386, 389-390, 394

in diabetes, 1220-1222

smoking and, 587

carbolic acid/phenol: powerful caustic poison distilled from coal tar oil and used as a disinfectant, 162, 674, 1048

carbonated beverages, nutrients in, 716

carbon dioxide

role of, in respiration, 392, 393, 394-395

surgical uses of, 630, 1135-1136

carbon monoxide: colorless, odorless gas that is highly poisonous when inhaled since it combines with the hemoglobin in the blood and thus excludes oxygen, **539, 758, 759, 1202**

poisoning, treatment for, 183

in tobacco smoke, 552-553, 1197

carbon tetrachloride: colorless liquid that can be poisonous if inhaled over a long period, and often used as a fire extinguisher or cleaning fluid

carbuncle: painful, extensive inflammation of the skin, marked by hardness and the discharge of pus, 172, 299, 797-798

carcinogen: cancer-producing agent, 754-756, 758-759, 768, 1269

carcinogenic: causing cancer or increasing the incidence of cancer in a population

carcinoma: malignant tumor that arises in the tissue that lines body cavities and ducts (epithelial tissue), 1268

cardia: the opening between the esophagus and the stomach, 383

cardiac: of or relating to the heart

cardiac arrest: a stopping of the heartbeat

  treatment for, 145-147, 1140-1142

cardiac catheterization: the advancing of a catheter, or thin tube, through the veins to the heart chamber, in order to detect abnormalities and obtain blood samples, 890-891, 1152

cardiac insufficiency, 1152

cardiac massage/cardiovascular pulmonary resuscitation/CPR: emergency procedure consisting of the application of rhythmic pressure on the chest in order to compress the heart and start it beating again, 145-147, 1140-1141

cardiac monitor, 1138

cardiac muscle: the striated but involuntary muscle of which the heart is composed, 350, 374-376, 392

cardiac output, exercise and, 623

cardiac shock, 144-145

cardiac sphincter: ring of muscle at the entrance of the stomach, or cardia, that opens to allow food to enter from the esophagus

cardiac X-ray series: chest X rays taken after the patient has swallowed an opaque liquid such as barium sulfate, 890

cardiogram:

  1. record produced by a cardiograph

  2. electrocardiogram

cardiograph:

  1. instrument for recording the force of the movements of the heart

  2. electrocardiograph

cardiologist: physician specializing in the diagnosis and treatment of heart disease, 873, 890

cardiology: the branch of medical science dealing with the heart, its physiology and pathology, 873

cardiopulmonary development, exercise and, 549, 550

cardiovascular: pertaining to the heart and blood vessels

cardiovascular disease/heart disease: disorders affecting the heart and blood vessels

  cholesterol and, 739

  life style and, 219-220

  noise pollution and, 773

cardiovascular pulmonary resuscitation: *see* cardiac massage

cardiovascular specialist: physician specializing in the diagnosis and treatment of diseases of the heart and blood vessels, 873

career guidance, teenagers and, *561*

caries: decay of a bone or tooth *(dental caries)*; *see* tooth decay

cariogenic: causing caries, or tooth decay

carisoprodol, 198

carotene: orange or red crystalline pigment converted to vitamin A in animal metabolism, 778

carotid artery: either of two major arteries of the neck supplying blood to the head

carpal(s): pertaining to the bones of the carpus, or wrist, *344*

carpus: the wrist

carrier: person who is immune from infection of specific disease-causing bacteria that his body carries and that can be transmitted to others who are not immune

  dysentery, 1163

  in muscular dystrophy, 1106

  of sickle-cell trait, 1118

  typhoid, 1164

carrots, nutrients in, 702

cartilage: tough, elastic supporting tissue, 344, 347

torn, 970, 972

cartilage plate/epiphysis: extremity of a long bone, originally separated from it by cartilage but later consolidated with it by ossification

carnuncle, urethral, 1009

castile shampoo, 785

cast(s): bit of tissue, often microscopic, having taken the shape of a vessel or cavity in which it was formed, that is found in excretions and may indicate the presence of disease

urinary, 885-886

casts, plaster, 1077

catabolism: the destructive aspect of metabolism, in which living matter breaks down nutrients into simpler substances. Compare *anabolism.*

catalepsy: abnormal condition characterized by lack of response to stimuli and by muscular rigidity, often associated with a psychological disorder

catalyst: substance or agent that causes a chemical reaction while remaining stable, such as an enzyme or hormone in the human body

cataract: the gradual clouding and opacity of the lens of the eye, leading to impaired passage of light and loss of vision, 672, 958, *958,* 1238-1239

congenital, 581

senile: cataract affecting elderly people due to degenerative changes in the lens, 316

voluntary agency, 315-316

catatonic schizophrenia: *see* schizophrenia, catatonic

cathartic: medicine for purging the bowels, 673

hemorrhoids and, 853

catheter: slender tube for drawing off fluid from a body cavity, especially urine from the bladder

catheterization: the introduction of a catheter into the body

cat, pet, 514-515, 1194

and toxoplasmosis, 303

CAT scanner/body scanner: computerized X-ray machine used in *CAT scanning,* 889, 891, *1086,* 1087

CAT (computerized axial tomography) scanning/body scanning: procedure for producing a cross-sectional, computer-generated, composite X-ray picture of the body or an organ, as the brain, by rotating about a site and taking a series of radiographs directed to it, 888-889, *889,* 891, *893,* 974, *1086,* 1087, 1152

cost of, 898

cat scratch fever, 172-173

caudal: situated at the tail end or bottom; posterior

caudal anesthesia/caudal/caudal block: form of anesthesia in which the patient is injected in the region of the lower spinal cord (sacral canal) to block pain in the pelvic area, 595

caul: membrane *(amnion)* surrounding the fetus if it is unruptured and intact about the baby's head at delivery, 592

cauliflower, nutrients in, 702

cautery, chemical: chemosurgery

cavities: dental caries; *see* tooth decay

CBC: complete blood count; *see* blood count

cc: cubic centimeter

cecum: blind pouch or cavity open at one end, esp. the cavity below the ileocecal valve that forms the first section of the large intestine, *384,* 387, 391

celery, nutrients in, 702

celiac: pertaining to the abdomen

celiac disease: *see* malabsorption syndrome

cells

cancerous, *1020, 1024, 1025,* 1267-1269, *1267, 1279*

nerve, 362-363, *363*

respiration in, 394

sense receptor, 408

taste: *see* taste bud

cellular death, 694

cellular therapy: treatment for the process of aging in which a person is injected with cells from healthy embryonic animal organs with the idea that the animal cells from the particular organ injected will then migrate to the same organ in the aging body and reactivate it, **688-689**

cementum: the layer of body tissue developed over the roots of the teeth, **339,** *339, 807,* **808**

central nervous system: the portion of the nervous system that contains the brain and spinal cord and controls voluntary action and movement, **350, 358-359, 361-362**

aging and, **620**

alcohol and, **1343**

amphetamines and, **1362-1367**

anesthetics and, **914**

caffeine and, **638**

cocaine and, **1366**

and food intake, control of, **722-724**

marihuana and, **554-555**

narcotics and, **1369, 1371**

centrifuge:

1. *(n.)* rotary machine employing centrifugal force to separate substances having different densities, as the constituents of blood
2. *(v.)* subject to a whirling motion to separate component parts, as of blood, that have different densities

cephalhematoma: swelling under a newborn baby's scalp, that usu. dissolves within a few weeks, **427**

cereal foods, requirements of, **658-659,** *708*

cerebellum: large section of the brain located below and behind the cerebrum, consisting of a central lobe and two lateral lobes, and which coordinates voluntary muscle movements, posture, and equilibrium, *360,* **360-361**

cerebral arteriogram: an X-ray picture of the brain used to investigate brain damage, esp. after a hemorrhage or stroke, and made by injecting opaque dye into the blood vessels serving the brain and X-raying them, **889-890,** *889*

cerebral arteriosclerosis: degenerative changes in the arteries of the brain

cerebral cortex: the cells and fibers that look like a convoluted layer of gray matter and that cover the cerebral hemisphere of the brain, **359-360,** *360*

cerebral hemisphere: one of the two halves into which the brain is divided, **359-360**

cerebral hemorrhage: hemorrhage into the cerebrum of the brain or within the cranium, **1128**

cerebral palsy: inability to control movement caused by nonprogressive brain damage resulting from a prenatal defect or birth injury, *459,* **459-460, 1087-1089,** *1088*

voluntary agencies, **313**

cerebrospinal fluid/CSF: the clear, colorless fluid that surrounds the brain and spinal cord, **359**

diagnostic use of, **279, 1085, 1101**

cerebrospinal meningitis: inflammation of the membranes that cover the brain and spinal cord, **359, 1101**

cerebrovascular: of or relating to the vessels supplying blood to the brain

accident, **1084**

cerebrum: the upper anterior part of the brain, consisting of two hemispherical masses which constitute the chief bulk of the brain in man and is assumed to be the seat of thought and will, **359-360**

cervical:

1. pertaining to the cervix of the uterus
2. pertaining to the neck or any neck-like part

cervical cap: contraceptive device made usu. of soft plastic which fits over the cervix, *607,* **608**

cervical mucus, in fertility test, **574**

cervical polyp, **1016**

cervical spine: cervical vertebrae

cervical vertebrae/cervical spine: the top seven vertebrae of the backbone, which are located in the neck and support the head, **339-340,** *341,* **342**

esophagal varices and, 1158

clams, nutrients in, 701

clap: *see* gonorrhea

claudication, intermittent, 968

claustrophobia: fear of being in an enclosed place, 486, 1325

clavicle: the bone connecting the shoulder blade and breastbone; the collarbone, 339, 342,

cleansing cream, 780, 781-782

cleft lip/harelip: genetic defect in which the upper lip is not completely joined, 463, 977, 1050

cleft palate: genetic defect in which the hard palate is not completely joined, 463, 977, 1050

climacteric, female: *see* menopause

climacteric, male: in men, the psychological equivalent of the menopause, characterized by forgetfulness, depression, and declining sexual interest, 635-636

climate

choice of, in later years, 693

effect of

on allergies, 275

in multiple sclerosis, 1100

on rheumatoid arthritis, 1054

on sinusitis, 275

clinical: pertaining to or based on the actual process or symptoms of a disease as observed, as distinguished from those described as typical from a statistical or theoretical point of view

clinical death: cessation of respiration and heartbeat. Compare *biological death.*

Clinoril: sulindac, 1057

clitoris: small, erectile organ of the female in the front part of the vulva

clonic: of or characteristic of clonus

clonic phase: the period during a grand mal epileptic convulsion when spasms of rigidity and relaxation (or jerking) occur in rapid succession, 1093

clonus: muscular spasm characterized by rapid alternation of contraction and relaxation. Compare *tonus.*

closed bite: form of malocclusion, a severe overbite in which upper teeth extend far over lower teeth when the jaws are together

closed-chest massage: *see* external cardio-pulmonary resuscitation

closed fracture/simple fracture/complete fracture: fracture in which bone is completely broken, but without accompanying break in the skin

Clostridium botulinum, *739*

clothing, children's, 463-464, *464*

clotting, 370, 1111, 1112-1114

effect of aspirin on, 275-276

clotting concentrates, 318, *318*

clotting-deficiency diseases: hemorrhagic diseases

clubfoot, 464-465

clumsiness, 473-474

as symptom, 1108

coagulation: clotting, as of blood

coal derivatives and skin cancer, 1274

coal dust, inhalation of, 1207-1209, *1209*

coal, low-sulfur, 758

coal soot, cancer and, 754

coarctation: stricture or contraction, as of a cavity or blood vessel

of aorta, 964-965

coated tongue: condition in which the tongue is coated with a whitish substance, consisting of food particles and bacteria, which can indicate fever, illness, or a temporary lack of saliva

cobalt, 698, 765

cocaine: white, bitter, crystalline alkaloid used as a local anesthetic and a narcotic, 1366-1367, *1366*

co-carcinogen: substance which is not cancer-producing but reacts with other substances to produce cancers, 552, 1269

coccidioides fungus: fungus, the spores of which can cause coccidioidomycosis

coccidioidomycosis/desert rheumatism/valley fever: infectious disease caused by fungus spores and characterized by symptoms resembling pneumonia and tuberculosis and the formation of reddened bumps, 1192

coccyx: the tail end of the spinal cord, 344

cochlea: spiral-shaped structure of the inner ear containing the essential organs of hearing, including the organ of Corti, 414, *414*, *417*, 955, *1247*

cochlear nerve: the part of the auditory nerve leading from the cochlea of the inner ear to the brain, conveying the sense of hearing

codeine: white, crystalline alkaloid, derived from morphine and used in medicine as an analgesic and to suppress coughing, 199, *1371*, 1373

coffee, caffeine in, 638

coitus: sexual intercourse

coitus interruptus: contraceptive method whereby the male withdraws before he ejaculates, 609-610

cola, caffeine in, 638

cold

allergic reaction to, 868

sensation of, 354, 409

cold application, in home care, 1045-1046

cold, common: viral infection of the respiratory tract, 278, *829*, 829-831, 1179, 1181-1183

ascorbic acid and, 739

children and, 466

diet and, 736

fatigue and, 626

cold cream, 667, 781

cold sores: herpes simplex, 174, 798-799

colic, 465

colitis: inflammation of the colon, 1168-1169

collagen: fibrous protein that forms the chief constituent of the connective tissues of the body, such as cartilage, skin, bone, and hair, 654

collapsed lung: pneumothorax, 1210

collarbone: clavicle, 339, 342

collards, nutrients in, 702

collecting, as hobby, 496

college, teenagers' plans and, 558, 559

colon: the part of the large intestine extending from the cecum to the rectum and divided into the ascending colon, transverse colon, descending colon, and the sigmoid, *384*, 391, 937, 938, 1157

ascending: the section of the colon extending up from the cecum along the right side of the abdomen, *379*, *1156*

cancer of, 944-946, 1272-1273

descending: the section of the colon leading from the transverse colon and extending down the left side of the abdomen, *379*, *1156*

disorders of, 1160, 1161, 1168-1172

colon and rectal surgeon, 874, 892

colonoscope: speculum used to examine the colon, 893

color

eye, 413

skin, *356*, 777, 778

color blindness: inherited vision defect consisting of the total or partial inability to discriminate between certain colors, usu. red, green, and blue, 465-466, 1238'

color vision, 410-411

colostomy: the formation of an artificial opening in the colon through which solid wastes can pass, 1273

colostrum: the creamy, yellowish, milklike substance rich in proteins, that is produced by a mother's breasts the first few days after having given birth, 430-431, 601

colposcopy: microscopic technique for visual examination of the cervix and vagina, 1022-1023, *1022*

coma: prolonged loss of consciousness, 194

diabetic, 175-176, 1226

comminuted fracture: fracture in which bone is splintered or crushed

common bile duct: duct formed by the juncture of the hepatic and cystic ducts,

contraception: the prevention of conception, 605-610

contraceptive: device or substance designed to prevent conception, 605-610

oral/the pill: the birth control pill, which is composed of synthetic hormones that suppress ovulation and thus prevent pregnancy, 605-607

contraindication: symptom or sign that makes a particular course of treatment inadvisable

contusions, 169-170

conversion hysteria: see conversion reaction

conversion reaction/conversion hysteria: neurosis characterized by manifestation of physical symptoms, such as blindness or deafness, without organic cause, as an expression of psychic conflict, 1324

convulsion/seizure: spontaneous violent and abnormal muscular contraction or spasm of the body

in barbiturate withdrawal, 1368

in encephalitis, 1101

in epilepsy: see epileptic seizure

in infant, 175, 486

in pregnancy, 579

treatment for, 174-175

See also focal convulsion, grand mal.

cookies, nutrients in, 713

cooking, for one or two, 660-661

Cooley, Donald G., 243

Cooley's anemia: see thalassemia

cooperative: housing owned jointly by stockholders who are residents

coordination

in children, 440

loss of, 364

copper, 697-698

copperhead snake, bite of, 189-190

coral snake, bite of, 189-190

cordials, 1341

corium: dermis

corn(s): horny thickening of the cuticle common on the feet, 286, 796, 843-844

corn bread, nutrients in, 713

cornea: the transparent lens surface of the eye, 410, 411-412, 413

lesions of, in Bell's palsy, 1089

transplant of, 286, 959-960, 959, 984-985

cornflakes, nutrients in, 713

corn grits, nutrients in, 713

corn, nutrients in, 713

cornstarch, as skin dressing, 521

coronary: encircling or crowning, such as the two arteries branching from the aorta and encircling the heart

coronary arteries and veins: the network of arteries and veins that nourishes the muscle and tissue of the heart

coronary artery disease: fatty obstructions in the coronary vessels that nourish the heart, thus impairing adequate delivery of oxygen to heart, 1132-1134

surgery in, 917, 1134-1137

coronary attacks: heart attacks

coronary care unit (CCU), 1138-1139

coronary insufficiency: insufficient blood circulation through the coronary arteries

coronary occulusion: closure of the coronary artery, due to buildup of fatty deposits or coronary thrombosis, 1137

coronary thrombosis: interference with the blood supply to the heart muscle because of a blood clot in the coronary artery, 1137. See also heart attack.

corporal punishment, 519

corpus callosum: fibrous tissue connecting the two hemispheres of the cerebrum of the brain

corpuscle: one of the cells that make up blood, either a red corpuscle (erythrocyte) or a white corpuscle (leukocyte)

corpus luteum: mass in the ovary formed by the rupture of a Graafian follicle that releases an ovum during each menstrual cycle, 404

corpus luteum cyst, 1015

cortex: the outer layer or covering of an organ or part, as of the cerebrum or cerebellum of the brain (called gray *matter*), of the adrenal glands, or of the kidneys

corticoids: any of the hormones manufactured in the adrenal cortex, 405

corticosteroid:

1. any of the steroids secreted by the cortex of the adrenal gland

2. any steroid hormone resembling in its effects the steroids secreted by the adrenal gland, 871, 1293

corticosterone: steroid hormone of the adrenal cortex associated with blood sugar levels and other metabolic functions

Corti, organ of: *see* organ of Corti

cortisol, 202

cortisone: powerful hormone extracted from the adrenal cortex and also made synthetically, 405

anesthesia and, 905

in Bell's palsy, 1089

in multiple sclerosis, 1100

in polymyositis, 1109

in rheumatic fever, 1148

in rheumatoid arthritis, 1058

cortisone cream, in anal pruritis, 794

coryza: inflamed mucous membranes in the nose, with discharge of mucus characteristic of a head cold

cosmetics, 781-782, *782*

acne and, 544, 801

advertising claims for, 781, 785

as allergens, 868

cosmetic surgeon: physician specializing in cosmetic surgery, 629-630, 976-977

cosmetic surgery: plastic surgery concerned with improving the appearance of parts of the body, 629-630, 976-982

costal: pertaining to or near a rib or ribs

costs, hospital diagnostic tests, 897-898

cottage cheese, nutrients in, 698

cotton dust, lung disease and, 755, 1207

cough: to expel air or phlegm from the lungs in a noisy or spasmodic manner

coughing, 854

importance of, after surgery, 919

in lung cancer, 1272

in obstructive airway disease, 1203-1204

cough medicines, 854

cough plate, 301

cowpeas, nutrients in, 702

cowpox: live calf lymph virus, used in smallpox vaccinations

coxa: the hip or hip joint

coxa vara: deformity of the hip joint caused by curvature of the femur toward the joint, thus shortening the affected leg and causing a limp, 1070

Coxsackie virus: any of a group of viruses causing various diseases in humans, including a form of meningitis

crab lice, 1007-1008

crabmeat, nutrients in, 701

crackers, nutrients in, 713

cradle cap: disease of the scalp, esp. in babies, marked by yellowish crusts, 466

crafts, in later years, 682-683

cramps, muscular, 188, 364, 673, 845

cranberry sauce, nutrients in, 706

cranial nerves: the twelve pairs of nerves that originate within the brain, 361-362, *361*

cranial sutures, in microcephaly, 1050

cranioplasty: surgical correction of the skull, as to repair a congenital defect

craniotomy: any surgery involving an opening in the skull, 974

cranium: the part of the human skull that encloses and protects the brain, 341

crash *(slang):* amphetamine

crash dieting, 640-641, 726

crawling, 434

cream cheese, nutrients in, 698

creams, skin, 781-782

medicated, 782, 801

creativity, need for, 682

in pregnancy, 811-812

prepaid, 675

in teen years, 809-810, *810*

See also tooth decay.

dental caries/cavities: ulceration and decay of teeth; *see* tooth decay

dental clinics, 473, 675

dental floss: strong, silky filament for cleaning between the teeth, 813-814, *814*

dental surgeon: *see* oral surgeon

dentin: the hard calcified substance that forms the body of a tooth, 807-808, *807*

dentist: one who specializes in the diagnosis, prevention, and treatment of disease affecting the teeth and their associated structures

dentistry: the branch of medical science that concerns the study, diagnosis, prevention, and treatment of diseases of the teeth, gums, and associated structures

specialties in, 887

dentition: the kind, number, and arrangement of the teeth in the mouth

denture(s): frame of plastic or other material adapted to fit the mouth and containing one, several, or a complete set of artificial teeth to replace natural teeth that have been lost, 658, 821-823, *823*

ill-fitting, 848

deodorants, 295-296, 780-781

Department of Health, Education, and Welfare, Public Health Service, National Institutes of Health, 1098

depilatory: chemical product capable of removing or loosening hair, 542-543, 790

depressant: drug or other substance that reduces or calms the physiological processes of body or mind, 1367-1369. Compare *stimulant.*

depression:

1. mental state marked by melancholy, pessimism, or dejection

2. psychotic condition characterized by stuporous withdrawal from reality and intense guilt feelings, 717, 830, 994, 1323, *1325*

depressive reaction:

1. neurosis characterized by persistent feelings of depression and pessimism unrelated to any apparent cause

2. (involutional melancholia) psychosis usu. occurring in women around the time of menopause, and in men during their 50s, characterized by hopeless melancholy, anxiety, weeping, and often delusions, 1324-1325, 1330

dermabrasion: the removal of layers of skin by planing with an abrasive tool to dispose of wrinkles or skin blemishes, 299, 629-630, 667

Dermacentor variabilis (dog tick), 502

dermal: of or relating to the skin

dermal layer, 777

dermatitis: inflammation of the skin, 792

contact: dermatitis caused by a hypersensitive reaction to external contact with a substance or material, 520, 792, *792*, 862, 866

dermatologist: physician specializing in the diagnosis and treatment of disorders of the skin, 874, 888

dermatology: the branch of medical science dealing with disorders of the skin, 874

dermis/corium/true skin: the inner layer of the skin, which contains blood vessels, nerves, connective tissue, sweat glands, and sebaceous glands, *354*, 355, 777, *777*

DES: *see* diethylstilbestrol

desert rheumatism: coccidioidomycosis, 1192

Desoxyn: methamphetamine, 1362

dessert, in child's meal, 709

destructiveness, 449-450, 473-474

detached retina/separated retina: eye disorder in which the membrane at the back of the eye (retina) is separated from its bed, as by being torn, thus impairing vision

detergents, water pollution and, 762, 763

developmental disability: any condition which interferes with a child's development, esp. one which will constitute a handicap throughout the individual's life, such as mental retardation or cerebral palsy

"devil's pinches," 279

dexamethasone, 199

Dexedrine: dextroamphetamine, 199, 1362

dextroamphetamine (d-amphetamine)/ Dexedrine: isomer of the amphetamine compound, considered to have a more stimulating effect on the central nervous system than amphetamine, 199, 1362

dextrose: form of glucose (a sugar) found normally in animals, used in intravenous feeding because it is readily assimilated by the blood

diabetes, chemical/prediabetic condition: condition indicating predisposition to development of diabetes, when blood sugar level remains abnormally high for too long after taking a glucose tolerance test, 1233

Diabetes Detection Drive, 314

diabetes insipidus: production of excessive amount of urine due to deficiency of antidiuretic hormone, 1219, 1220

diabetes mellitus: disease associated with inadequate production of insulin and characterized by excessive urinary secretion containing abnormal amounts of sugar, accompanied by emaciation, excessive hunger, and thirst, 406, 1220-1234

control of, 1229-1231

diagnosis of, 301, 302, 1223

diet and, 315, 731, 733-734, 1222-1224

early detection of, 474, 1233-1234

foot and leg problems with, 673, 843, 858, 859, 1126

and heredity, 1234

and impotence, 688

insulin pump, 1227

in later years, 672, 1232-1233

and overweight, 640, 724

and pregnancy, 1232

symptoms of, 672

treatment for, 1223-1228

voluntary agency, 314-315

diabetic: one who has diabetes

diabetic acidosis: advanced stage of diabetes treated with insufficient insulin, characterized by increasing buildup of ketone bodies, drowsiness, and, if untreated, coma, 1222, 1228. Compare *diabetic ketosis.*

diabetic coma: state of unconsciousness in a diabetic resulting from insufficient insulin, characterized by deep, labored breathing and a fruity odor to the breath, 175-176, 1226

diabetic gangrene, 1126

diabetic ketosis: early stage of diabetes treated with insufficient insulin, characterized by excessive urination, thirst, and hot, dry skin, 1227, 1228. Compare *diabetic acidosis.*

diabetic retinopathy: disease of the eye associated with diabetes in which new, abnormal blood vessels form on the surface of the retina, sometimes marked by bleeding, 286, 961, *1232*

diabetics

caloric needs of, 731, 733-734

children's camps for, 457, *458*

foot care for, 674, 843, 858-859

diacetylmorphine: heroin, 555-556, 1370-1373, *1371*

diagnosis: identification of a disease or disorder by its characteristic symptoms, or the conclusions reached in a particular instance

diagnostic procedures

general, 877-887

of specialists, 887-896

diagnostic tests, 279, 897-898

admission labs, 898

batteries, 897-898

dialysis: the separating of mixed substances by means of wet membranes, as the action of the kidneys, esp. applied to an artificial process to remove waste products and excess fluid from the bloodstream of a patient with defective kidneys, 319, 1251-1252, *1251, 1252*

Medicare coverage of, 1252-1253

diaper rash: rash caused by the ammonia produced by the urine in diapers, 520

diaphragm:

1. dome-shaped layer of muscle between the chest and abdomen whose contraction enlarges the rib cage for inflation of the lungs in breathing

2. contraceptive device of molded rubber or soft plastic material used to cover the cervix and prevent entry of spermatozoa

cervical, 608

contractions of: *see* hiccups

respiratory, 395-396, *962, 1179*

diaphragmatic hernia: hernia, hiatus, 496, 941-942

diarrhea: frequent and fluid evacuation of feces, 474-475, 736, 851-852, *852,* 1161-1162, 1168

emergency treatment of, 176

diastole: the instant when the heart is relaxed as the ventricles fill with blood prior to contraction and pumping (systole), 377

diastolic pressure: measure of blood pressure taken when the heart is resting, the lower of the two figures in a reading, 881, 1145

diathermy: treatment by means of heat generated within the body by high-frequency radiation

diazepam (Valium), 199, 1369

dicetylmorphine: heroin

dicyclomine, 199

diet(s)

and acne, 544, 801

and aging, 620

bland: diet that is not irritating or abrasive, as the diet recommended for peptic ulcer patients

bland soft, 732, 735, 921

and constipation, 852-853

and dental health, 812, 815

diabetic, 731, 733-734, 1223-1224

juvenile, 1224, 1231

and diarrhea, 852

and disease prevention, 739, 742

and gastritis, 849-850

and gastroenteritis, 851

and gout, 1062

and heart attack, 1143

individual differences in, 736

infants, 700, 703

in later years, 658-661, 717-718

low calorie, 728

low fat, 736, 745-746

low sodium, 737-740, 922, 944, 1153

in middle age, 620, 639-641

minimal residue, 736, 749-750, 922

modified fat, 736, 741-743, 922

in nephrosis, 1256

post-operative, 921-923

in pregnancy, 577-578, 717

salt-free, 734-736

soft, 732-734

teenagers, 544-547, 712

ulcers and, 1165

diet drugs, 1366

diethylcarbazine, 1311

diethylstilbestrol/DES/stilbestrol: synthetic hormone resembling estrogen implicated in the formation of vaginal and cervical cancers in the daughters of women who had taken the hormone during pregnancy, *989,* 1025

differential blood count: blood count

digestion: process of dissolving and chemically changing food in the alimentary tract so that it can be assimilated by the blood and its nutrients can be absorbed by the body, 1155, 1157

duration of, 378, *384*

products of, 386

digestive system, 377-392, *379,* 1155-1157, *1156*

diagnostic procedures in, 892-894

diseases of, 1157-1177, *1161, 1162, 1163, 1166, 1167, 1170, 1175*

digestive tract: *see* gastrointestinal tract

digitalis: the dried leaves of foxglove, containing several glycosides, often used as a heart tonic, 1153

digitalis drugs, 905, 1153

digitoxin, 200

digoxin, 200

Dilantin, 1096

dilate: to become larger, as the pupil of the eye in diminished light

dilation and curettage/D and C: enlarging the opening into the uterus and the scraping of the uterus with a curette, 587, 992, 995

Dilaudid, 1373

dimethyltryptamine: *see* DMT

dinner, modified menus for, 728, 734, 735, 740, 743, 746, 750

diphenhydramine, 200

diphenylhydantoin: phenytoin, 208, 1096

diphtheria: respiratory, bacterial disease marked by the formation of a false membrane that obstructs breathing, 475

immunization, 433, 500, 581

diplopia: *see* double vision

disability

chronic disease and, 620, 621

developmental, 474

learning, 478

disagreement, expression of, 1319

discharges, unusual, 672

discipline, *475*, 475-476, 519, 618

disclosing tablets: tablets which, after being chewed, leave a temporary stain on plaque remaining on teeth after brushing, 814

dishonesty, parental models and, 476

disinfectants: germicides, 1047-1048

disk, intervertebral, 340

slipped/herniating disk: painful displacement (herniation) of one of the fibrous disks of the spinal column between two vertebrae, such that it presses against nerves and may cause sciatica, 968-969, 1068-1069

dislocation(s): the partial or completed displacement of one or more of the bones at a joint, 1074

congenital, of hip, 1050-1051

elbow joint, 1074

finger, 181

jaw, 186

disobedience, 477

displacement: transference of intense anxiety unconsciously felt about a particular conflict to a substitute, which is regarded consciously with the same intensity of anxiety, a manifestation of the phobic reaction, 1325

dissociative reaction: neurosis characterized by escape from a part of the personality by means of dream states, amnesia, forgetfulness, etc., 1325

distal: relatively remote from the center of the body, or from a point considered as central. Compare *proximal*.

distal muscles: the muscles of the extremities (the hands and the feet)

distillation: separation of the more volatile parts of a substance from the less volatile by boiling and condensing the vapors into separate liquids, 1338

diuresis: excessive excretion of urine, 1250

diuretic(s): substance stimulating the secretion of urine

in congestive heart failure, 1153

in gout, 1061

in hypertension, 1146

in nephrosis, 1256

diverticula (*sing., diverticulum*): pouches or sacs opening off the large intestine, 1166-1167, *1166*

diverticulitis: inflammation of diverticula in the digestive tract, esp. in the colon, 736, 1166

diverticulosis: the presence of diverticula in the digestive tract, 1166-1167

diverticulum (*pl. diverticula*): abnormal pouch or bulge protruding from an organ or part, as from the colon of the intestines, 1166-1167, *1166*

diverticulum (urethral), *1009*, 1010

divorce, 602, 649-653

dizziness, 176, 364, 1142, 1246

DMSO (dimethylsulfoxide), 1057-1058

DMT/dimethyltryptamine: synthetic hallucinogen, 1375-1376

doctor-patient relationship, 279-285, *388*, 897-899

dog, as pet, 515

dog tick, 502, 1298-1299, *1298*

Dolly *(slang)*: methadone

Dolophine (methadone), 203, 1373

DOM/STP: synthetic hallucinogen, 1376

dopamine: chemical compound found in the brain, needed in the synthesis of norepinephrine and epinephrine, 1090

Doriden: glutethimide, 1368

dorsal: toward, near, or in the back. Compare *ventral.*

double vision/diplopia: condition in which a single object is perceived as two images due to inability to coordinate focusing of the eyes, 1110

douche, vaginal, 609-610, 997

douching: flushing of a body part or cavity, esp. the vagina, with water as a means of cleansing, 609-610, 997

doughnuts, nutrients in, 715

downers, 556. *See also* barbiturates.

Down's syndrome/Mongolism: congenital mental and physical retardation due to a chromosomal anomaly, accompanied by variable signs including a flat face and pronounced epicanthic folds, *508*, 509, 583, 1322, *1322*

downs/downers/goof balls *(slang):* barbiturates or other drugs that depress the central nervous system

Doxorubicin, 1292

doxylamine, 200

DPT injection: injection to provide immunity against diphtheria, pertussis (whooping cough), and tetanus, *433*, 436, 500, 536, 581

Dramamine: proprietary drug used to counteract motion sickness

dreamer *(slang)*: morphine

dreams
bad, 477-478

Freudian view of, 1319, 1332-1333

drinking, 1338-1339, *1339*

driving and, 1347-1348, *1348*, *1349*

driving
alcohol and, 649, 1347-1348, *1348*, *1349*

defensive, 307

epileptics and, 1097

voluntary agency, 307

drooling, 1088, 1089

dropsy: former term for edema, esp. when caused by cardiac insufficiency, 1155

drowning, emergency treatment of, 176-177

drug(s):

1. any substance other than food that changes or has an effect on the body or mind

2. narcotic drug, 285, 1359-1378

allergies and, 831-832, 865-866, 1362

childbirth and, 593-596

and children's growth, 300

consumption of, 1359, 1364, *1364*, 1369

dependence on: physical or psychological accommodation to the periodic or continuous presence of a drug in the body's system, 555-556. *See also* physical dependence, psychological dependence.

generic (table), 195-212

overdose of, 177

over-the-counter, 1360, *1363*

pregnancy and, 576-577

prescription, 1360-1362, *1361*

psychomimetic, 555

and secondary gout, 1061

side effects of, 1361-1362

standards on, 1360

teenagers and, 553-556

voluntary agencies, 315, 323-324

drug resistance, malaria and, 1302

dry socket: painful complication of a tooth extraction in which underlying tissue of the alveolar bone is exposed to infection, 817-818

DTs: delirium tremens, 278-279, 1354

Duchenne's muscular dystrophy: pseudo-hypertrophic muscular dystrophy, 1106-1107

duct/hepatic: either of two ducts of the liver that join to form the common hepatic duct and that carry bile

ductless glands: *see* endocrine glands

Duke University study on sexuality, 685

dumbbells, exercises with, 235-236, 267-269

dumdum fever: *see* kala-azar

duodenal ulcer: ulcer of the duodenum of the small intestine, 939-941, 1164-1166 *See also* peptic ulcer.

duodenum: the first section of the small intestine, leading from the stomach to the jejunum, 379, 384, 385-386, 937-938, *1156*, 1157

dura mater: the tough, fibrous, outermost membrane of the three membranes covering the brain and spinal cord

dust, 758, 863, 865

dwarfism: disorder characterized by stunted growth, 403, 1213

dyes
  aniline, 755, 1280
  hair, 784

dye stripping, 785

dying, attitude toward, 693-694

dysentery: severe inflammation of the mucous membrane of the large intestine, characterized by bloody stools, pain, cramps, and fever, 1162-1163

dysfunction: impairment or abnormal functioning, as of an organ

dyslexia:
  1. impairment or loss of the ability to read, as from a stroke
  2. in children, impairment of ability to acquire language skills due to motor or perceptual disabilities, 478

dysmenorrhea: painful menstruation, 993, 1018

dyspareunia: painful sexual intercourse, 1009, 1010, 1018-1019

dyspepsia: indigestion, characterized by heartburn, nausea, pain in the upper abdomen, and belching, 736, 1160

dysphagia: difficulty in swallowing, 1108, 1160

dysphasia: disorder of the cerebral centers characterized by difficulty in understanding or using speech

dyspnea: labored, difficult breathing

dystrophy:
  1. defective or faulty nutrition
  2. any of various neurological or muscular disorders, as muscular dystrophy

dysuria: difficult, painful, or incomplete urination, 1009, 1249

ear, 414-417, *415, 416, 417,* 954-956, 1243, *1243*

  blockage of, 285, 856

  cosmetic surgery on/otoplasty, 981-982

  diagnostic procedures for, 883, 895-896

  disorders of, 957, 1243-1247

  foreign body in, 178, 479

  infection of, 478-479, *668,* 856, 1181-1183, *1244*

  injury to, 771-772, 1245

  ringing in: tinnitus, 667, 856-857, 1245-1246

  surgery on, 954-956

earache, *479,* 478-479, *668,* 856, 1182, *1244*

emergency treatment for, *177,* 178

ear canal, 955

eardrum/tympanic membrane/tympanum: drumhead membrane separating the middle ear from the external ear, 414, *415, 417,* 954, *955,* 1243, *1243*

noise and, 771

perforation of, 480, 954

ear lobes, 666

earphones, hearing loss and, 775

electrocardiograph: machine used to record the electric current produced by the heart muscle

electrocardiography: technique of producing electrocardiograms and interpreting them

electrocoagulation, 790

electrocution, accidental, 178-179

electroencephalogram/EEG: graph recording the pattern of electric impulses produced by the brain, used in the diagnosis of neurological disorders, 888, *889, 1084,* 1085

in epilepsy, *179,* 1091-1092

electroencephalograph: machine used to record the electric current produced by the brain

electroencephalography: technique of producing electroencephalograms and interpreting them

electrolysis: technique for removing unwanted hair by destroying the hair root with an electric current, 543, 790

electromyogram/EMG: graph recording the electrical activity of a muscle

electromyography: technique of producing electromyograms and interpreting them, 888, 969, 1106, *1106*

electronic amplification, ear damage and, 774

electronic equipment in intensive care unit, 918, *918*

electron radiograph, *1277*

electroshock: describing a form of treatment for psychological disorders in which a controlled electric current is passed through the patient's head, producing convulsions and unconsciousness, usu. given in series, 1335

electrosurgery/surgical diathermy: surgical procedure utilizing electricity to destroy tissue, 667

elephantiasis: lymphatic edema, esp. of the legs and scrotum, a symptom of filariasis, 1310-1311, *1310*

embolism: the stopping up of a vein or artery, as by a blood clot, that has been brought to the point of obstruction by the bloodstream

phlebitis and, 967

prolonged bed rest and, 1130

pulmonary: embolism in the pulmonary artery or one of its branches, 1129-1130, 1209-1210

stroke and, 1127, 1128

embolus: object moving within the bloodstream, as a blood clot or air bubble, that is capable of causing an obstruction (embolism) in a smaller vessel

in phlebitis, 967-968, 1124

embryo: the rudimentary form of an organism in its development before birth, usu. considered in the human species to be the first two months in utero, 577

movement of, 221

emergencies

everyday, 222-223

medical, alphabetical guide to, 161-194

emergency cardiac care (ECC), 1139

emergency room (ER), *901,* 902-903

emergency services

ambulance, 158

hospital, 158

physician, 158

poisoning, 150-156, 158

emergency surgery, 901-902

emetic: medicine or substance used to induce vomiting

EMG (electromyograph), 1106

emotional disorders, 1318-1336

emotional maturity, 1319

emotional needs of infant, 436-437

emotional pressures, in middle age, 642-643

emotional problems

physical symptoms and, 642-643

posture and, 517-518

psychiatric help for, 1330-1332

treatment for, 1332-1335

emotions and nervous system, 365

emphysema: puffed condition of the alveoli or air sacs of the lungs (or other tissues or organs) due to infiltration of air and consequent loss of tissue elasticity, 1202-1207, *1203, 1205, 1207*

smog and, 758

smoking and, 552, 637, 1197

enamel: the layer of hard, glossy material forming the exposed outer covering of the teeth, 339, *339*, 806-807, *807*

encephalitis: inflammation of the brain, 364, 539, 1101

encephalogram: X-ray picture of the brain made by encephalography

encephalography: X-ray visualization of the brain following the removal of cerebrospinal fluid and its replacement with air or other gases

encounter groups, 297

encyclopedia, child's, 469

endarterectomy: surgical procedure in which carbon dioxide is forced through hardened arteries to ream out fatty blockages, 1135-1136

endemic: confined to or characteristic of a given locality, as a disease

endocarditis: inflammation of the membrane (endocardium) lining the chambers of the heart, sometimes caused by bacteria, 375, 1150

bacterial: bacterial infection of the membrane (endocardium) lining the chambers of the heart

subacute bacterial: bacterial endocarditis resulting as a complication of rheumatic fever, usu. fatal

tooth decay and, 816

endocardium: the delicate membrane that lines the chambers of the heart, 375

endocrine gland: one of several ductless glands that release secretions (hormones) directly into the blood or lymph and that exert powerful influences on growth, sexual development, metabolism, and other vital body processes, 400-408, *401, 403, 404, 405,* 1212

disorders of, 894, 1211-1234

endocrinologist: physician specializing in endocrinology

endocrinology: the branch of medical science dealing with the structure and function of the endocrine glands and their hormones, 402, 873

endoderm: innermost layer of tissue

endodontics: branch of dentistry dealing with root canal work and the dental pulp, 818

endodontist: dentist specializing in root canal work

endogenous insulin: self-produced insulin

endolymph: fluid within the semicircular canals of the inner ear, 416

endometrial: of or pertaining to the endometrium

endometrial polyp, 1016-1017

endometrioma: mass of tumorlike endometrial cells as a result of endometriosis, 1018

endometriosis: condition in which tissue that lines the uterus (endometrium) grows outside the uterus in the pelvic cavity, 1018-1019

endometrium: the lining of the uterus, 567

cancer of, 1023-1025, *1024*

hormonal control of, 404

endoscope: instrument for examining a hollow organ or an internal cavity, as the urinary bladder or the urethra

endoscopy: examination with an endoscope

enema: liquid injected into the rectum as a purgative or for diagnostic purposes, 853, 907, 1161

administration of, in home nursing, 1044

barium, 1177

energy

bodily, 377, 394

of light, in vision, 409-411

of sound waves, 771

ENT: otolaryngology (ear, nose and throat) doctor, 874-875

enteric: pertaining to the intestines

enteric fever: *see* typhoid

slipped: the slipping or dislocation of the end of a bone (epiphysis), as of the femur at the hip joint, 1070

episiotomy: incision made during labor to enlarge the vaginal area enough to permit passage of the baby, 596

epistaxis: nosebleed

epithelial: pertaining to the epithelium

epithelium: membranous tissue that lines the canals, cavities, and ducts of the body, as well as all free surfaces exposed to the air

Equanil (meprobamate), 203, 1369

equipment, sickroom, 1047-1048

erection: enlarged and firm state of the penis when sexually stimulated, 565

erector pili muscle, 354, 777

ergotamine, 200

eruption:

1. emergence of a tooth through the gums

2. a breaking out of a rash on the skin

erysipelas: acute bacterial skin infection characterized by bright red patches, 798

erythema: redness of the skin, a symptom occurring in various forms in different conditions having various causes, as from infection or a burn

erythremia: polycythemia vera, 1119

erythrityl tetranitrate, 201

erythrocyte/red blood cell/red corpuscle: cell found in the bloodstream, often lacking a nucleus, the carrier of hemoglobin, 1114-1115

See also red blood cell.

erythromycin, 201

erythrophobia: fear of blushing

eschar: dry crust or scab left by a burn caused by heat or corrosive chemical action

Escherichia coli: see E. coli

esophagoscope: device inserted into the esophagus to permit its inspection, 893

esophagus (gullet): the tube through which food passes from the mouth to the stomach, 378, 379, 381, 384, 397, 937, 962, 1155, 1156, 1159

disorders of, 1158-1160

essential: of unknown cause, as a disease or condition

essential hypertension: see hypertension, essential

estrin, 584

estrogen: any of several hormones found in the ovarian fluids of the female which promote growth of secondary sex characteristics and influence cyclical changes in the female reproductive system, 201, 403, 407-408, 540, 1217

cancer and, 1025, 1034, 1036

breast, 1027-1028

prostate, 1281

uterine, 689

conjugated estrogens, 201

esterified estrogens, 201

estrogenic substances, 201

estrone and equilin, 201

ethanol: ethyl alcohol

ethchlorvynol (Placidyl), 1368

ether: colorless, volatile, flammable chemical compound used as an anesthetic, 595, 914

ethinamate (Valmid), 1368

ethmoid bone: sievelike bone at the base of the skull behind the nose, 418

ethnic groups

and alcoholism, 1352, 1352

and hirsutism, 789

and tuberculosis, 1186

ethyl alcohol/grain alcohol/ethanol: product of the distillation of fermented grains, fruit juices, and starches, used in beverages and having intoxicating properties, 1337

etiologist: physician specializing in studying the causes of disease

etiology:
1. the cause or causes of a disease
2. the branch of medical science dealing with the causes of disease

eunuch: in males, the failure at puberty to develop secondary sex characteristics due to disorder or removal of testicles, 1216

Eustachian tube: passage connecting the middle ear to the upper throat which equalizes air pressure on both sides of the eardrum, 285, 414, *415*, *417*, 955, *955*

blockage of, 856, 1182, 1245

Ewing's sarcoma: malignant tumor of the shafts of the long bones in children, 1073

examination
gynecological, 988-990
neurological, 1085-1087
physical, 876-899
pre-operative, 905-906

excise: cut out or remove by surgery

excision: act or procedure of cutting out or removing surgically

excrete: to eliminate, as waste matter, by normal discharge from the body

excretion:
1. the act of excreting
2. the body's waste matter, as sweat, urine, and feces

through skin, 354

exercise
in adolescence, *545*, 548-550
after illness or surgery, 243-245, 1142
childbirth, 245-246
mastectomy, 245, *1035*
for arthritis, 671, *1055*, *1057*, 1058
calorie equivalents of, 721, 722
children and, *227*, *481*, 481-482, 518
constipation and, 672-673, 853
and heart attack risk, 236, 1143
and hernia prevention, 353

jogging, 221, 623-624, 859-860
in later years, 246-247, 253-263, *661*, 661-665, 670
in middle years, 622-626, *624*
muscle strengthening, 247-248
muscles (table), 248
and weight control, 225, 303, 665, 724-725, *725*, 729, 731

exercise programs, 227-234, *229*, *549*, 548-550, 662-665
equipment for, 230-231
isometric, 236-237, 626
maximum performance plateau, 232-234
progressive indoor, 252-263
tension-relieving, 625-626
warm-up, 230-231, 249-251
weight-lifting, 234-236, *235*, *265-269*
for women, 241-243, *270-272*

exhibitionists, 688

exocrine gland: any of various glands, such as mammary or sebaceous glands, having ducts that carry their secretions to specific locations, 400, 1211. Compare *endocrine gland.*

exophthalmic goiter: hyperthyroidism

expectorant: medicine that promotes the discharge of mucus from the respiratory tract

expectorate: discharge from the mouth, as saliva or phlegm

exploratory: performed for the purpose of making a diagnosis: said of a surgical operation

exploratory activity, toddler and, 501

extension: state of being extended or straightened, 352

extensor: muscle whose function is to extend or straighten a part of the body, *352*

external cardiac massage: cardiac massage

external cardiopulmonary resuscitation (ECPR), 145-147, 1140-1141

external oblique abdominals, 248

extraction: surgical removal of a tooth from the mouth

extrinsic: originating or situated outside an organ or part

exudate: substance filtered through the walls of living cellular tissue, sometimes as a result of disease or injury, as in the case of inflammation

eye(s), 378, 409-414, *410*, *412*

　chambers of, *410*, 413

　control of, 360-362

　diseases of, 286, 1004, 1235-1242

　　examination of, 882-883, 895-896

　　　for children, 316, 467

　　voluntary agency, 315

　injury to, 1240-1241

　　aerosol spray and, 162-163

　　blow and, 165-166

　　chemical burn and, 174

　　foreign body and, 180, 1240-1241

　in later years, 672

　muscles of, 350, 412-413, *412*, 957-958, *957*

　See also vision; blindness.

eyeball, 361, 413

eye bank, 959

eyebrows, plucking of, 790

eye color, 413, 542, 778

eyeglasses, 482-483, 668, 1236

eyeground: the inner side of the back of the eyeball

eyegrounds, in diabetes, 1233

eyelids, 413

　cosmetic surgery of, 630, 981

　drooping, 1110

　inflammation of: *see* sty

eye makeup, 782

eye socket, creation of, 328

eyestrain: disorder caused by excessive or improper use of the eyes and characterized by fatigue, tearing, redness, and a scratchy feeling in the eyelids, 856

eye surgery, 957-961

eye teeth: the upper canine teeth; *see* cuspids

face

　birth defects of, 1050

　injury to, 1080-1081

　paralysis of, 1090

face lift: rhytidoplasty, 630, 904, 980

facial canal: Fallopian canal

facial nerve, 362

　inflammation of, 1089

　paralysis of: Bell's palsy

facial neuralgia: *see* trigeminal neuralgia

facial plasty: rhytidoplasty

fainting: brief loss of consciousness, 144, 847-848

fallen arches, 841-842

Fallopian canal/facial canal: bony canal in the skull

Fallopian tubes: the pair of tubes connecting the ovaries and the uterus, through which the egg must pass at the time of ovulation, *566*, 566, *567*, 996

falls, 273

family doctor, 282, 872-873

family health records, 494, 500, 1047

family life education, voluntary agency, 324

family planning, voluntary agency, 316-317

　See also birth control.

Family Service Association, 678

family therapy: form of group therapy in which the patient group are members of the same family, 1334

fantasies, children's, 483-484, *483*

farina, nutrients in, 715

farsightedness/hypermetropia/hyperopia: inability to see nearby objects clearly, 483, 1236-1237

fascia: fibrous tissue in the form of sheets that connect, surround, and support muscles and organs of the body

fascitis: inflammation of the fascia

fat: chemical compound forming an important food reserve and a source of

fovea: shallow rounded depression in the retina, directly in the line of vision at a point where vision is most acute, 410, *410*, 957

fracture: break in a bone; *see* closed fracture, complete fracture, incomplete fracture

in children, 1071

and diet, 922

of facial bones, 1080-1081

first aid for, 181-182

healing of, 347, 1075-1080

internal appliances for, 970, *971*, 1076, *1077*, *1078*, 1079

jaw, 1080-1081

long bones, 970

nose, 1080

pelvis, 1077-1079

pubic, 1079

rib, 1081-1082

skull, 1080

spine, 970, 1082-1083

spontaneous, 1073

types of, 1074-1075

Framingham Study, 219-220, 225, 662

frankfurter, nutrients in, 701

fraternal twins: twins who are not identical, derived from separately fertilized ova

frauds in health aids, 679

freckle: small, brownish or dark-colored spot on the skin, 803

free association: psychoanalytic technique in which the patient talks freely about anything that comes to mind, 1333

freezing of skin: cryosurgery

Freud, Sigmund: Austrian neurologist (1856-1939) who founded psychoanalysis and shaped the course of modern psychiatry, 1319, 1321, *1321*, 1332, *1332*

friends, child's, *469*, 487-488, *488*

frigidity: sexual unresponsiveness in women, 605, 644

Froehlich's syndrome: failure of secondary sex characteristics to develop in males due to anterior pituitary disease, 1216

frontal bone, 343

frontal lobe: the front portion of each cerebral hemisphere of the brain, whose functions are uncertain, 360

frontal lobotomy: rarely performed surgical operation of cutting into the frontal lobes of the brain to alter behavior

frontal thighs, 248

frostbite: partial freezing of a part of the body, esp. of the extremities or ears, 794-795, 840

frozen section, 301

fructose/levulose: very sweet crystalline sugar, 639

fruit

daily requirement of, 658

nutrients in, 705-708, 711

frustration, 365, 488-489

FSH: follicle-stimulating hormone, 403-404

fulguration: destruction of tissue, esp. malignant growths, by electric cautery, 1279

functional:

1. able to function, esp. in spite of structural defect

2. affecting performance, as in illness, but lacking any verifiable physical basis

functional hypertension: hypertension, essential

fundus: the rounded base or bottom of any hollow organ

fungal diseases

arthritis, 1064

respiratory, 1191-1192

of skin, 796-805

thrush, 1158

fungus (*pl., fungi*): any of a group of plants including the mushrooms, molds, yeasts, and various microorganisms, some of which cause diseases in human beings

funnel chest/pectus excavatum: congenital deformity in which the sternum is depressed, 286-287

furuncle: *see* boil

fusion of spinal joints: *see* spondylitis, rheumatoid

gait, as diagnostic clue, 881

galactosemia: hereditary condition affecting infants who lack an enzyme that converts galactose (a sugar) into glucose in the blood

diet and, 736

gall bladder/cholecyst: small pear-shaped pouch situated beneath the liver that serves as a reservoir for bile, *379*, *384*, 385, 387, 389, 390, *405*, *937*, *1156*, 1157, *1175*, 1175-1176

removal of (cholecystectomy), 390, 922, *946*, 948

gallstone(s): solid substance formed in the gall bladder that can obstruct the flow of bile and prevent the digestion of fats, 287, 390, 946-948, 1174, *1175*, 1175-1176

diet and, 736

emergency treatment for, 182-183

nonsurgical treatment for, 287, 948

See also gall bladder, removal of.

Gambian sleeping sickness, 1307-1309, *1307*, *1308*

games, as exercise, 623-625

gamete: either of two mature reproductive cells, an ovum or sperm cell

gamma globulin: component of blood serum which contains various antibodies, 582

gamma ray source, 1122

ganglion *(pl., ganglia):*

1. cluster of nerve cells outside of the central nervous system

2. cyst of a tendon, as on the wrist, 364

gangrene: death of tissues in a part of the body, caused by lack of adequate blood supply, 859, 1074, 1126

garbage disposal, 763

gardening, 680-681

gases, noxious, in air pollution, 1202

gas exchange in lungs, 393

gas poisoning, first aid for, 183

gastrectomy: surgical removal of all or part of the stomach, 940-941

gastric analysis: extraction and study of gastric juices, 892

gastric juice: the acid fluid secreted by the glands lining the stomach, containing several enzymes, 1166

gastric ulcer: ulcer of the mucous membrane of the stomach, 302-303, 385, 939-941, 1164-1166

diet and, 731, 732-735, 922, 1165, 1166

See also peptic ulcer.

gastritis: inflammation of the stomach, 849-851, 1168

acute: sudden, sharp attack of gastritis, 849-850, 1168

chronic: recurrent and persisting attacks of gastritis, 850-851

toxic: gastritis caused by the swallowing of a poisonous substance, 850

gastrocnemius: the large muscle at the back of the calf of the leg

gastroduodenal fiberscope, 893

gastroenteritis: inflammation of the mucous membrane that lines the stomach and intestines, 851

gastroenterologist: physician specializing in the diagnosis and treatment of gastrointestinal disorders, 892

gastroenterology: the branch of medical science dealing with the study of the stomach and intestines and the disorders affecting them, 873, 892

gastrointestinal disorders, 736, 752, 1176-1177

gastrointestinal (GI) series, 892, 1177

gastrointestinal tract (alimentary canal; digestive tract), 352, 377, 382, *384*, 890, 1155

gastroscope: device that allows inspection of the interior of the stomach, 893

gastroscopy: examination of the stomach with a gastroscope

GC: *see* gonorrhea

gelatin dessert, nutrients in, 716

gene: hereditary unit contained within a chromosome and associated with specific physical characteristics transmitted from parents to offspring

general paresis, 1002

general practitioner/GP: physician whose training is not specialized and includes some preparation in pediatrics, surgery, and obstetrics and gynecology, thus enabling him to care for an entire family, 282

generation gap, 568-569

genetic counseling, 470, 516, 582-583

genetic counselor: specialist, usu. a physician, who counsels couples on the probability of genetic disorders occurring in their offspring, 470, 516, 582-583

genitalia: genitals

genitals/genitalia: the reproductive organs, 424-425, *424*, *996*

size of, 541

genitourinary tract: urinogenital tract, 423

genus: class or category of plants and animals ranking next above the species, as the genus *Homo* in *Homo sapiens*

gerbils, 515

geriatrics: branch of medicine dealing with diseases and physiological changes associated with aging and old people

German measles: *see* rubella

germicidal soaps, 780

germicide: disinfectant or other agent capable of killing disease germs

gerontologist, 656

gerontology: scientific study of the processes and phenomena of aging

gestation: the total period of pregnancy, from conception to birth

GI: gastrointestinal

giant, 1213

giardia lamblia, *852*

gifted: having ability or intelligence above the normal range

gigantism/giantism: disorder due to oversecretion of somatotrophin by the pituitary gland and resulting in excessive growth, 402-403

gin, 1342

gingiva: mucous membrane and soft tissue of the gums surrounding the teeth

gingival: pertaining to the gums, 820

gingivitis: inflammation of the gum tissues, 808, 819, *819*

gingivitis, necrotizing ulcerative: *see* trench mouth

girdle, maternity, 579

GI series/gastrointestinal series: X rays of the esophagus, stomach, and intestines utilizing an opaque substance swallowed by the patient, 892, 1177

glabrous: without hair

gland(s): any of various organs that secrete substances essential to the body or for the elimination of waste products, 400. *See also* endocrine system.

ductless: *see* endocrine gland

prostate, inflammation of: *see* prostatitis

submandibular: *see* submaxillary gland

glandular fever: mononucleosis, infectious, 1123

glaucoma: disease of the eye characterized by increased pressure on the eyeball and leading to the loss of vision if untreated, 414, 672, 1238

tests for, 895, 1238, *1238*

treatment for, 960-961, 1378

voluntary agency, 316

glomeruli (*sing.*, *glomerulus*): tiny tufts of capillaries in the kidneys through which the blood passes in the filtering of wastes, *420*, 421, 1254, *1254*

glomerulonephritis: inflammation of the glomeruli, 1254-1255

glossitis: inflammation of the tongue, characterized by a bright red or glazed appearance, 849

glossopharyngeal nerve: the nerve that supplies sensation to the throat and rear of the tongue, *361*, 418

glottis: the passage between the vocal cords at the upper opening of the larynx

gloves, disposable rubber, 1048

glucagon: hormone produced by the islets of Langerhans in the pancreas, 406

glucose/blood sugar: sugar found normally in blood and abnormally in urine, as in the case of diabetes mellitus, 389-390, 394

metabolism of, 406

in diabetes, 1222, 1223

in urine, 1220, 1222, 1223

glucose-glycogen balance, in diabetes, 1222

glucose tolerance test/GTT: test that determines the rate at which glucose in the blood is reduced, or metabolized, used as an indicator of chemical diabetes or a prediabetic condition, 1233

glucosuria: condition, as diabetes mellitus, in which the urine contains glucose

See also renal glucosuria.

gluten: protein component of wheat and rye, 459, 863

glutethimide (Doriden), 1368

gluteus: any of the three muscles that form each buttock

glycerol/glycerin: sweet, oily alcohol, one of the components of natural fat, 386, 390, 697

glycogen: animal starch usu. stored in the liver for conversion to glucose when the body needs energy, 389-390

in diabetes, 1222

glycosuria: glucosuria

renal, 1223

goiter: enlargement of the thyroid gland, often due to lack of iodine in the diet, 407, 954, 1214

exophthalmic: hyperthyroidism, 1214

golf, 623, 662, 725

gonad(s): male or female sex gland; ovary or testicle, 407-408, 1211, *1212*

See also ovaries, testicles.

gonadotrophic hormone/gonadotrophin/gonadotropin: any of three hormones that stimulate the gonads and are secreted by the anterior pituitary gland, 404, 407-408, 540

gonioscope: specialized ophthalmoscope for examining the angle between the cornea and the iris, 895

gonococcal (gonorrheal) arthritis, 1004, 1062-1063

gonococcus: parasitic bacterium that can cause gonorrhea, 1003, 1005, 1264

gonorrhea (clap; GC): contagious venereal disease transmitted by sexual contact, 568, 1003-1005, 1062-1063, 1264

goof balls (*slang*): barbiturates

gooseflesh, *354*, 777

gout: metabolic disease characterized by painful inflammation of a joint, as of the big toe, and an excess of uric acid in the blood, 287, 841, *841*, 1060-1062, *1062*

alcohol and, 1346

gouty arthritis, chronic: form of gout characterized by urate deposits and consequent joint stiffness

Government Printing Office, 681

GP: general practitioner

Graafian follicles: small sacs in the ovaries that contain the developing ova, 403-404

cyst in, 1014

grades, school, 489

graft: piece of tissue removed from one organism and inserted in a new site in the same organism or in a different organism

grafts, types of, 983

graham crackers, nutrients in, 713

Graham, Dr. James, 243

grain alcohol: ethyl alcohol, 1337

grain products, nutrients in, 711, 713

grand mal: major epileptic seizure, characterized by falling, loss of consciousness, and spasmodic jerking of the arms and legs, **481, 1093**. Compare *petit mal*.

grandparents, 489-490, *490*

granulation: process of forming new tissue in the healing of wounds

granulation tissue/proud flesh: new, temporary, vascular tissue formed in a wound as a stage in the healing process, usu. soft and moist

granulocyte: *see* neutrophil

granulocytic leukemia: *see* leukemia, granulocytic

granuloma: small tumor composed mainly of granulation tissue

granuloma inguinale/granuloma venereum: chronic venereal disease that produces lesions in the genital or anal regions, **1006**

grapefruit juice, nutrients in, 706-707

grapefruit, nutrients in, 706

grape juice, nutrients in, 707

grapes, nutrients in, 707

grass (*slang*): marihuana

gravid: pregnant

Grawitz's tumor/hypernephroma: malignant tumor of the kidney, found chiefly among men, 1282-1283

gray matter: cortex, 359

green soap, tincture of, 785

greenstick fracture: incomplete fracture, with the bone bending on the unbroken side, more common in children than adults, 1075

grippe: influenza

griseofulvin, 201

groin: the fold or depressed area where the thigh joins the abdomen

group therapy/group psychotherapy: psychotherapy in which interactions within a group under the direction of a therapist are intended to provoke therapeutic insights and lead to improved social adjustment, 296-297, 1334

growing pains, 523

growth hormone/growth-stimulating hormone/somatotrophin: hormone secreted by the posterior lobe of the pituitary gland that stimulates growth, 287, 402-403, 538, 1213

growth rates, birth to 36 months

  boys, *492*

  girls, *493*

growth, stunted, 287

GTT: glucose tolerance test

"guard hairs": vibrissae, nasal, 399

guilt, feeling of, 365, 1319

  in children, 448, 490

  sudden infant death and, 530

  in working mothers, 612

guinea pigs, pet, 515

gullet: *see* esophagus

gum disease: *see* periodontal disease

gumma: rubbery tumor that develops within organs in the late stages of syphilis

  syphilitic, 1001

gums: *see* gingiva

  inflammation of: *see* gingivitis

gurney: stretcher mounted on wheels, commonly used to move nonambulatory patients in hospitals

Guthrie test, 301

gym equipment, 230-231

gynecologist: physician specializing in gynecology, often an obstetrician as well, *575*, 874

gynecology: the branch of medical science that deals with the care and treatment of women and their diseases, esp. of the reproductive system, **874, 988**

H (*slang*): heroin, 1370

haddock, nutrients in, 701

hair(s), 353, 355, 356-357, 783-790

  color of, 542, 784-785

  curling of, *783*, 784

  ingrown, 788

  loss of, 631, *1289*. *See also* baldness.

  removal of, 787-790

  straightening of, 784

hebephrenic schizophrenia: *see* schizophrenia, hebephrenic

heels, height of, 627, 629

heights, average, birth to 36 months, *492, 493*

Heimlich maneuver: emergency treatment for obstruction of the windpipe in which sharp pressure is applied just below the rib cage so that the air in the lungs ejects the obstruction, 148-150, *148*

Heine-Medin disease: *see* poliomyelitis

helminth: parasitic worm that invades the intestines, most often via food or water, 1169

hemal: of or relating to blood

hemangioma: reddish, usu. raised birthmark consisting of a cluster of small blood vessels near the surface of the skin, 804

hematocrit:

1. instrument for measuring the relative amount of plasma and red corpuscles of the blood by centrifuging it (whirling it around to separate parts having different densities)

2. measurement of relative amount of plasma and red corpuscles by a hematocrit, 886

hematological tests, 891-892

hematologist: physician specializing in the study of the blood and in the diagnosis and treatment of blood diseases, 873, 890

hematology: the branch of medical science dealing with the blood, including its formation, functions, and diseases, 873

hematoma: blood tumor, 167

subdural: mass of blood clots or partially clotted blood in the space beneath the outermost (dura mater) and middle (arachnoid) membranes covering the brain, 1080

hematuria: blood in the urine, 1249

hemiplegia: paralysis of one side of the body, involving both the arm and leg

hemiplegic: one affected by hemiplegia

hemispheres of the brain, 277, 360

hemodialysis: *see* dialysis

hemoglobin: pigment of red blood corpuscles serving as the carrier of oxygen and carbon dioxide, 369-370, *369*, 392, 393, 778, 1114-1115

and anemia, 846

and carbon monoxide, 553

and iron, 546, 698

in sickle-cell anemia, 1117

hemophilia: inherited disorder characterized by an incapacity of the blood to clot normally, thus resulting in profuse bleeding even from slight cuts, typically affecting males only, 1111, 1112-1114

voluntary agency, *317, 318*, 318-319

hemophiliac/bleeder: one afflicted with hemophilia, 1112-1114

hemorrhage: discharge of blood from a ruptured blood vessel, 372

See also bleeding.

hemorrhagic disease, 1112-1114

hemorrhoidal:

1. of or pertaining to the blood vessels in the rectal area

2. of or pertaining to hemorrhoids

hemorrhoidectomy: surgical removal of hemorrhoids

hemorrhoids/piles: swollen varicose veins in the rectal mucous membrane, 794, 853, 949-950, 1167

prolapsed: hemorrhoids that protrude from the anus

hemotoxic: (of certain poisonous snakes) transmitting venom that is carried by the bloodstream of the toxified animal. Compare *neurotoxic*.

Henle's loop: U-shaped part of a tubule of the kidney, *420*, 421, 1254

heparin: chemical compound that prevents coagulation of the blood, 1112

hepatic: of or relating to the liver

hepatic duct, 389

hepaticologist: physician specializing in the diagnosis and treatment of liver diseases

hepaticology: branch of medical science concerned with the study, diagnosis, and treatment of diseases of the liver

hepatitis: inflammation of the liver, 1173, 1174-1175

infectious: inflammation of the liver caused by a viral infection usu. transmitted by food and water contaminated by feces from an infected person, *1173*, 1174

serum: form of infectious hepatitis usu. spread by blood transfusions or by infected hypodermic needles, *1173*, 1174

hereditary: acquired through one's genetic makeup by inheritance, as physical characteristics, disease, etc. **Compare** *congenital.*

heredity

aging and, 620-621, 666

allergies and, 1193

baldness and, 542

chronic kidney failure and, 1250

diabetes and, 1233-1234

genetic counseling for characteristics of, 582-583

mental retardation and, 509

migraine and, 833

muscular dystrophy and, 1106

obesity and, 722

peptic ulcer and, 1164

physical traits and, *542*, 542

sickle-cell anemia and, 1115, 1117-1118

hernia/rupture: protrusion of an organ or part, as the intestine, through the wall or body cavity that normally contains it, 353, *948*, 1167

in children, 496

in digestive tract, 948-950

femoral, 949

hiatus/diaphragmatic hernia: hernia in which the lower end of the esophagus or stomach protrudes through the diaphragm, 290-291, 496, 941-942, 1159, 1167

inguinal: protuberance of part of the intestine into the inguinal region (near the groin), 496, 900, 948-949, *948*, 1167, *1167*

strangulated: hernia that has become tightly constricted, thus cutting off blood supply, 949, 1167

umbilical: hernia in which an abdominal part protrudes through the abdominal wall at the navel, 496

of vaginal wall, 1011-1012, *1012*

ventral: projection of part of the intestine into the abdominal wall, 1167

herniate: slip away from its proper position as an organ or part to form a hernia, 1167

herniating disk: slipped disk, 968-969, 1068-1069

herniation: forming of a hernia

heroic: extraordinary or extreme, as measures undertaken when life is in immediate danger

heroin/diacetylmorphine: addictive narcotic drug derived from morphine, illegal in the U.S., 555-556, 1370-1373, *1371*

addicts, 1371-1373

herpes: any of various acute viral diseases characterized by the eruption of small blisters on the skin and mucous membranes

herpes simplex: virus that causes cold sores and other skin conditions in humans, 291. *See also* cold sores.

Type 1/HSV-1: variety of herpes simplex that causes cold sores, 799, 997

Type 2/HSV-2: variety of herpes simplex that often affects the genital region and can result in congenital damage to the baby of an infected mother, 799, 997-998, *998*

herpes zoster (shingles), 364, 799

heterograft/xenograft: tissue graft taken for transplanting from a donor of a different species from that of the patient receiving it, 983

hexachlorophene: antibacterial agent used in some soaps

hiatus hernia: *see* hernia

hiccup/hiccough: involuntary, spasmodic grunt caused by spasms of the diaphragm and the abrupt closure of the glottis, 185, 855

high *(slang):* amphetamine

high blood pressure: *see* hypertension

hiking, 224, *224,* 646, *664*

hip bone: ilium

hip joint: acetabulum, 344

artificial, 1054, 1079

congenital dislocation of, 1050-1051

disorders of, 1069-1070

fractures of, 1078-1079

osteoarthritis of, *1053,* 1054

replacement of, 1054, 1079

hips, exercises for, 242-243, *271*

Hirschprung's disease, 291

hirsutism: abnormal or excessive hairiness, especially in women, 789

histamine: substance found in animal tissues that can cause allergic symptoms when allergens stimulate the body to produce it in large amounts, 274, 831, 861, 868, 1194

histoincompatibility: incompatibility between tissues, as between the tissues of a patient and the tissues of a transplanted organ or part, 982-983

histoplasma: fungus that can cause histoplasmosis

histoplasmosis: chronic fungus disease of the lungs, 1191-1192

hives/urticaria: skin condition marked by large, irregularly shaped swellings that burn and itch, 793, 864, 866, 868

hoarseness, 854

hobbies

children's, 496-497

in later years, 681-682

in middle years, 646-647

Hodgkins's disease: disease of the lymph system, characterized by chronic, progressive enlargement of the lymph nodes, lymphoid tissue, and spleen, 458, 1061, 1266, 1288-1290

Holter monitor, 1142-1143

home care, 1037-1048

home care programs of voluntary agencies

arthritis, 308

cancer, 311

Home Delivered Meals, 675

home dental service, 675

home health services, 329, 333, 334-335

Homemaker-Home Health Aide service, 675

homeopathy: system of medicine in which disease is treated by administering minute doses of medicines that would in a healthy person produce the symptoms of the disease treated

homeostasis: maintenance of uniform physiological stability within an organism and between its parts

Home Safety Inventory, 307

homework, 526

homograft/allograft: tissue graft taken for transplanting from a donor of the same species as the patient receiving it, 983

honeymoon, 604

honeymoon cystitis, 1009

hookworm: parastic intestinal worm whose larvae usu. enter the body by penetrating the skin of the feet of people who go barefooted, 1170-1171, *1170*

hormone: internal secretion released in minute amounts into the bloodstream by one of the endocrine glands or other tissue and stimulating a specific physiological activity, 400-402, 1211

ACTH (adrenocorticotrophic hormone), 403, *403,* 404, 1100, 1148

adrenal cortex, 405

and aging, 621, 688-689

androgen, 538

anterior pituitary, 403-404

antidiuretic, 1218, 1219

in breast cancer, 1027-1028

in breast feeding, 1028

chorionic gonadotropic, 584

corticoids, 405

deficiency in, and osteoporosis, 1070

in digestive process, 386

in endometrial cancer, 1023

estrin, 584

follicle-stimulating (FSH), 403, 540

growth, excess production of, 1213

and hair growth, 789

and heartbeat, 376

lactogenic, 403, 404

luteinizing (LH), 403-404

and menopause symptoms, 633

in miscarriage, 584

in oral contraceptives, 605-606

in pregnancy, 579

pressor, 422

prolactin, 601

in prostatic cancer, 674, 1260

and puberty, 538-540

sex, 407-408, 540

thyroid-stimulating (TSH), 403-404

thyrotropic, 403-404

thyroxin, 403, 406-407, 1213-1214

transported by blood, 368

and undescended testicles, 541

horn cells, anterior, in poliomyelitis, 1101-1102

hornets, 185-186, 866

horny layer of epidermis: stratum corneum, 356

horse *(slang):* heroin, 1370

hosiery and foot care, 628

See also elastic stockings.

hospices, 330-331, *331*

hospital insurance, Medicare, 676-677

hospitalization, children and, 497-499, *497, 498*

hospitals

coronary care unit (CCU) in, 1138-1139

emergency services of, 158, 902-903

hospice program in, 331

intensive care unit (ICU) in, 1139

and social services, 334

hotels, retirement, 692

hot flashes, 1218

hot water bags, 674, 1045-1046

hot weather

exercise in, *838,* 839

salt tablets and, 837

housemaid's knee: chronic inflammation of the bursa in front of the knee due to pressure from constant kneeling or injury, 844, 1051

housewife, average, 604

housework, working mothers and, 612

Housing and Urban Development Agency/ HUD

retirement housing and, 692

housing, in later years, 689-693

HSV-1: *see* herpes simplex, Type 1

HSV-2: *see* herpes simplex, Type 2

Hubbard tank: large, specially designed tub in which a patient may be immersed in water for exercises as a means of physical therapy

Human Sexual Inadequacy, 643

Human Sexual Response, 643, 687

humerus: the long bone of the arm from elbow to shoulder, 343, 345, *351*

humors, body, *1329*

humpback, hunchback: kyphosis, 1066, 1067

hunger, in diabetes, 672

hyaline membrane disease/respiratory distress syndrome: disease of newborn babies characterized by severe respiratory distress caused by the presence of a membrane lining the alveoli of the lungs, 499

hydatidiform mole: benign tumor formed from a placenta that has degenerated into a mass of grapelike cysts, 586-587

hydralazine, 201

malignant: form of essential hypertension with an acute onset and rapid rise in pressure, 1146

oral contraceptives and, 607

overweight and, 640

pregnancy and, 579

secondary: hypertension arising as a consequence of another known disorder

sexual activity and, 687

stroke and, 1127

hypertensive heart disease: *see* heart disease, hypertensive

hyperthyroidism: abnormal and excess activity of the thyroid gland, resulting in oversecretion of thyroxin and an abnormally high metabolism, characterized by fatigue, weight loss, rapid pulse, intolerance to heat, and sometimes by protruding eyes (in which case the disorder is called *exophthalmic goiter*), 406-407, 1214

hypertonic: characterized by an abnormally high degree of tension, as muscle

baby, 449

hypertrophic: characterized by hypertrophy

hypertrophic arthritis: *see* osteoarthritis

hypertrophy: excessive development of an organ or tissue due to enlargement of the size of its constituent cells

hyperventilation: abnormally fast or deep breathing, resulting in loss of carbon dioxide from the blood and sometimes causing dizziness and muscle spasms

hypnosis, in childbirth, 597-598

hypnotic: tending to produce sleep

hypoallergenic: less likely to produce an allergic reaction

makeup, 782

hypochondria: extreme anxiety about one's health, usu. associated with a particular part of the body and accompanied by imagined symptoms of illness

hypochondriac:

1. *(n.)* one suffering from hypochondria

2. *(adj.)* pertaining to the upper right or left parts of the abdomen

hypodermic: pertaining to the tissue just under the skin or to an injection made under the skin

hypofunction: disorder of an endocrine gland, characterized by too little secretion of a hormone

hypogastric: pertaining to the lower middle part of the abdomen

hypogastrium: the lower middle (hypogastric) part of the abdomen

hypoglossal nerve, *361*

hypoglycemia/low blood sugar: abnormally small amount of glucose in the blood, which can lead to insulin shock, 752, 1225, 1228

hypoglycemic drug: drug intended to reduce the amount of glucose in the blood by stimulating the release of insulin from the pancreas, 1227-1228

hypophysis: *see* pituitary gland

hypophysis cerebri: pituitary gland

hyposensitization: program for desensitizing allergy patients by injecting them with progressively larger doses of pollen or other allergens to build tolerance levels, 1195

hypotension: excessively low blood pressure, 422

hypothalamus: region of the brain below the thalamus, important in regulating the internal organs and associated with the functioning of the pituitary gland, 402, 540, 1213

hypothermia: artificially low body temperature produced by gradually cooling blood, used to slow metabolism and reduce tissue oxygen need so that heart and brain can withstand short periods of interrupted blood flow during surgery, 1152, *1153*

hypothyroidism: deficient functioning of the thyroid gland, resulting in undersecretion of thyroxin and an abnormally low metabolism, characterized by lack of energy, thick skin, and intolerance to cold, 406, 1213-1214

hypotonic: characterized by an abnormally low degree of tension, as muscle

hysterectomy: surgical procedure in which the uterus is completely removed, 633, 1024

ovarian hyperfunction and, 1218

radical: surgical removal of the uterus, cervix, ovaries, and Fallopian tubes

total: surgical removal of the uterus and cervix

hysteria: neurotic condition characterized by impulsive, demonstrative, and attention-getting behavior and sometimes by symptoms of organic disorders

hysteria, conversion: *see* conversion reaction

hysterogram: X-ray examination of the uterus and surrounding areas, 574

ice bag, 1045-1046

ice cream, nutrients in, 546, 658, 690

ice milk, nutrients in, 658, 690

ice-skating, 519, 860

id: the concealed, inaccessible part of the mind, the seat of impulses that tend to fulfill instinctual needs, 1321

identical twins: twins having the same genetic makeup, derived from a single fertilized egg

identification: mental process, often unconscious, by which a person associates with himself the attributes of another with whom he has formed an emotional tie

identification, medical warning

for allergies, 145, 871

for diabetes, 1226, *1226*

for epilepsy, *1098*

identity, search for, 560

idiopathic: (of diseases) originating spontaneously or of unknown cause

ileitis: inflammation of the ileum of the small intestine

ileocecal valve: the valve between the ileum of the small intestine and the cecum, the first section of the large intestine, *384*, 387

ileum: the last section of the small intestine, following the jejunum and leading to the large intestine, 385, 387

iliac: pertaining to or near the ilium

ilium: the large upper portion of the hip bone, 342, 1069

illusions, in epilepsy, 1095-1096

immune: protected from a communicable or allergic disease by the presence of antibodies in the blood

immune defenses

deficiency in, 291-292

and thymus, 408

immune reaction

infertility and, 572

rheumatic heart disease and, 1146-1147

Rh factor and, 1120-1121

in transplants, 982-984

immunity: resistance to infection or lack of susceptibility of an organism to a disease or poison to which its species is usu. subject, either by means of antibodies produced by the organism itself *(active immunity)* or by another and subsequently introduced into its body *(passive immunity)*, as by injection

immunization: act or process of making immune, esp. by inoculation

of children, 291, 433, 436, 499-501

and pregnancy, 581-582

and Rh disease, 1121

immunize: make immune, as by inoculation

immunoglobulin: any of various proteins of the body that are active as antigens or otherwise contribute to the formation of antibodies

immunoglobulin E and skin allergies, 866-867

immunologist: physician or specialist in the study of immunity

immunology: the branch of medical science concerned with the phenomena and techniques of immunity from disease, 291

immunosuppressive: acting to suppress natural immune responses, as to foreign tissue in an organ transplant

immunosuppressive drugs, 983, 1100

immunotherapy: therapy to relieve allergic response consisting of a series of injections of a dilute allergen, gradually increased in strength, 871

and cancer, 1035-1036, 1100

impacted tooth: tooth wedged between the jawbone and another tooth so as to prevent its eruption

impaction: state of being firmly packed or tightly wedged, as feces in the rectum or a tooth in the jaw; *see* impacted tooth

imperforate: lacking a normal opening

impetigo: contagious bacterial skin infection characterized by blisters that break and form yellow encrusted areas, 798

impotence: in men, the inability to have sexual intercouse, 605, 636, 642-644, 687

impression (dental), 810

incision:

1. cut or gash, as of a wound

2. cut or slit made in a surgical operation

incisor: one of the four upper and four lower cutting teeth near the front of the mouth, 380, 806, *807*

incompetence: inadequate performance, as of the heart valves

incomplete fracture: partial fracture of a bone in which continuity of the bone is not destroyed, 1074

incontinence: inability to control the flow of urine or the evacuation of the bowels

incoordination, in cerebral palsy, 1088

incubation period: the period between the entry of a disease-causing organism in the body and the onset of the symptoms of that disease

incubator baby, *589*

incus: anvil, 414, 416, *417*, 955, *955*

independence, children's need for, 501-502, 558-559, 1318

Indian hemp, 1376

indigestion (dyspepsia), 292, 736, 1160

indomethacin: analgesic and anti-inflammatory drug used for arthritic disorders, often as a substitute for aspirin, 1057

infant

behavioral development of, 436-438, *436*

care of, 294, 428-429, 433-436, *530*

instruction in, 572

diet of, 434, 435, 700, 703

feeding of, 429-432, *430*, 600-601, 748-750

"infant Hercules": myotonia congenita

See also newborn.

infantile paralysis: *see* poliomyelitis

infantile sexuality: the sexual interest and pleasure that infants and young children take in their genitals and other body parts

infarct: tissue rendered necrotic (dead) by an obstructed blood supply, as because of a thrombus (clot) or an embolus

infarction: death of tissue due to deprivation of blood caused by an obstruction, as in a coronary thrombosis (heart attack)

infection(s): communication of disease by entrance into the body of disease-causing organisms

and alcohol, 1346

ear, 856, 1244-1245, *1244*

of female reproductive tract, 995-1006

lung, 1179

of nervous system, 1101-1103

personal hygiene and, 626-627

of skin, 796-799

spinal, 1068

of upper respiratory tract, 829-831

infectious: (of a disease) transmitted by organisms, as bacteria, 292

infectious hepatitis, 1174-1175

infectious mononucleosis/glandular fever/ kissing disease: acute communicable disease marked by fever, malaise, and swollen lymph nodes, esp. in the throat, 1123

inferior vena cava: the large vein that brings blood from the lower part of the body to the heart

infertility: inability to conceive or to produce offspring, 570-576

inflammation: localized reaction to infection, injury, etc., characterized by heat, redness, swelling, and pain

of arterial walls: arteritis

of bladder: cystitis

of bone: osteomyelitis

of brain: encephalitis

of brain coverings: meningitis

of bursa: bursitis

of Fallopian canal, 1089

of femoral head: Legg-Perthes' disease

of glomeruli: nephritis

of gums: gingivitis

of joints: arthritis

in kneecap, 972

of larynx: laryngitis

of liver: hepatitis

of mucous membrane: laryngitis

of prostate: prostatitis

of skin: dermatitis

of spinal joints: spondylitis, rheumatoid

of stomach lining: gastritis

of tendons: tendinitis

of tendon sheath: tenosynovitis

of tongue: glossitis

of veins: phlebitis

of vertebrae: osteomyelitis, spinal

influenza/flu/grippe: acute, contagious, sometimes epidemic disease caused by a virus and characterized by inflammation of the upper respiratory tract, fever, chills, muscle ache, and fatigue, 830, *1181*, 1183

in pregnancy, 581, 830

shots, 830-831, 1183

Information and Referral Service, local, 676

informed consent, 897

ingrown toenail: toenail that has grown into the surrounding flesh, 628

prevention of, 292, 674

inguinal: pertaining to or near the groin

inguinal canal, *948*, *1167*

inguinal hernia: *see* hernia

inhalants, as allergens, 832

INH (isoniazid), 1190

injection sites, insulin, 1225, *1225*

inner ear: the innermost part of the ear, containing the essential organs of hearing within the cochlea, the auditory nerve, and the semicircular canals that govern equilibrium

innervation: distribution or supply of nerves to a part

inoculate:

1. immunize by administering a serum or vaccine to

2. introduce microorganisms into (a culture medium)

inoculation: act or process of inoculating

inoperable: characterized by a condition that excludes surgery as a course of treatment

inpatient, 902

insecticide, 1304

Anopheles mosquito and, 1302

insect stings, 502, 866, *866*

treatment for, 185-186

venom in, allergic reaction to, 866

insecurity, social, of teenagers, 562

in situ: in its original site or position

insomnia: chronic inability to sleep, 642, 840-841

depression and, 1325

inspiration, position of diaphragm in, *1179*

insufficiency: inability to function adequately, as the heart (cardiac insufficiency)

insufflation: tubal insufflation

insulin: protein hormone secreted by the islets of Langerhans in the pancreas that checks the accumulation of glucose in the blood and promotes the utilization of sugar in the treatment of diabetes, 202, 390-391, *405*, 406, 1224-1225

discovery of, 1220-1221, *1221*

dosages of, 1224-1225, *1225*

injection of, 1224, 1225, *1225, 1226, 1227, 1230*

rapid-acting, 1224, 1228

surgery and, 905

types of, 1224, 1228

insulin pump, 1227

insulin shock: condition caused by too low a level of blood sugar, and characterized by sweating, dizziness, palpitation, shallow breathing, confusion, and ultimately loss of consciousness, 1225-1226

emergency treatment for, 176

insulin shock therapy: former method of treating psychotic patients involving large injections of insulin, inducing coma, 1334

insult: injury to tissue caused by stress or trauma

insurance, medical, 293

integument: skin, 354

intellectual stimulation, need for, 647

intelligence, child's, 503, 508-509

in cerebral palsy, 1088

in epilepsy, 1091

intelligence quotient/IQ: a score obtained from standardized tests indicating the level of a person's intelligence

intensive care unit (ICU): section of a hospital specially equipped and staffed to monitor the vital systems of patients and provide close, round-the-clock care for a relatively brief period, as for patients just removed from surgery or for those in an unstable or critical condition, 890, *891*, 918, 1139

intercostal muscles: the muscles between each of the ribs that contract when air is exhaled, 248, 396

intercourse: sexual intercourse

interferon, *1274*

intermittent claudication: vascular disease associated with aging and marked by muscle fatigue and pain, esp. in the legs, due to atherosclerosis, 968

intermittent positive pressure breathing (IPPB), 1205-1206

intern: advanced medical student or graduate (M.D.) undergoing resident training in a hospital, 873

internal medicine: the branch of medical science that deals with the study, diagnosis, and nonsurgical treatment of diseases of the internal organs, 282-283, 873, 874

International Association of Laryngectomees, 311

internist: physician specializing in internal medicine, 282-283, 872, 873, 894

interstitial calcinosis: condition characterized by deposits of calcium salts in the skin and subcutaneous tissue, 1065

intestinal obstruction, 1161, *1161*, 1171

intestinal tract, 377

intestine(s): tubular part of the alimentary canal, linking the stomach to the anus, 352, *379, 384, 386, 937, 1156*

cancer of, 944-946

diseases of, 937-938, 939-940, 1160-1172

large: the lower part of the intestine, of greater diameter than the small intestine and divided into the cecum, colon, and rectum, 391-392

small: the convoluted upper and narrower part of the intestines, where most nutrients are absorbed by the bloodstream, between the pylorus and the cecum, divided into three parts, the duodenum, jejunum, and ileum, 385-387, *405*

intoxicated: in legal use, having more than 0.10% alcohol in the bloodstream

intoxication, 1343

intracutaneous: within the dermis

intramuscular: situated within or injected into a muscle or muscular tissue

intrauterine device/IUD: contraceptive device consisting usu. of a plastic coil, spiral, or loop that is inserted and left within the uterus for as long as contraception is desired, **607-608**

intravenous: into or within a vein, as an injection

intravenous feeding, post-operative, 919-920

intrinsic: originating or situated within an organ or part, as a disease

introitus: entrance into a body cavity, esp. into the vagina

intussusception: the turning inward or inversion of a portion of the intestine into an adjacent part, thus obstructing it, found esp. in male infants, **1161**

in utero: in the uterus, prior to birth

invasive: invading or spreading to tissues other than at the place of origin: said of malignant growths

inversion, temperature, 756-757, *756*

involuntary (smooth) muscle, 350

involutional melancholia: *see* depressive reaction

iodine

antiseptic use of, 674

dietary, 546, 1213-1214

radioactive, hyperthyroidism and, 1214

in thyroxin, 406, 407, 1213-1214

IQ: intelligence quotient

IQ tests, 503

and mental retardation, 508-509

iris: colored, circular, contractile membrane between the cornea and the lens of the eye, whose central perforation is occupied by the pupil, *410, 412,* 412-413, 957

pigment in, 413

iron

in bile, 389

deficiency of, in anemia, 540, 846, 1118

loss of, in menstruation, 540

requirements, 540, 546, 698

sources of, 546, 659, 846

storage of, in liver, 372

ironing

hair, straightening by, 784

iron tonics, 659

irradiation: process of exposing a part of the body to radiant energy, as X rays

irrigate: wash out or cleanse, as a body cavity or a wound, with a flow of water or other liquid

irrigation: act or process of irrigating a body cavity, wound, etc.

ischemia: localized deficiency of blood, as from a contracted blood vessel, 1126

ischium: the part of the hip bone on which the body rests when sitting, *341, 342*

islands of Langerhans: islets of Langerhans

islets of Langerhans/islands of Langerhans: small, cellular masses in the pancreas which produce and secrete insulin, *391, 401, 405,* 406, *1212, 1220*

isomer: compound with the same molecular weight and formula as another, but with a different arrangement of its atoms, resulting in different properties

isometrics: means of strengthening muscles by forcefully contracting them against immovable resistance, **236-237, 242,** 626

in rheumatoid arthritis, 1058

isoniazid/INH: isonicotinic acid hydrazide, a chemical compound used in the treatment of tuberculosis, 202, 1190

isoprenaline/isoproterenol, 202

isopropamide, 202

isopropyl: chemical in the family of methyl alcohol, used as a rubbing alcohol, 1048, 1338

isoproterenol/isoprenaline, 202

isosorbide dinitrate, 202

isotopes, radioactive, diagnostic tests with, 892

itching (pruritus), 794, 1146

diabetes and, 672, 1223

in later years, 666

pubic lice and, 1008

itch, the: scabies, 797

IUD: intrauterine device, 607-608

jackhammer, 770

Jacksonian epilepsy: form of epilepsy characterized by recurrent focal seizures, spasmodic movements or tingling or burning sensations, as of an arm, leg, or facial area, caused by a condition affecting a motor area of the brain, 1094

Jacksonian seizure: form of focal seizure that characterizes Jacksonian epilepsy, 1094

jams, nutrients in, 716

jaundice: yellowish tint to the skin and tissues, as the whites of the eyes, caused by excessive bile in the blood, a symptom of certain disorders, 1173-1174

jaw

dislocation of, 186, 1080

fracture of, 1080, 1081

malformations of, 1050

jawbones, 338, *341*

jejunum: the middle section of the small intestine, between the duodenum and the ileum, 385, 386-387

jellies, nutrients in, 717

jellyfish sting, 186

jerking, nocturnal, 299-300

jet lag, 292

jet planes, pollution and, *754*

jewelry, allergies and, 868

"jogger's ankle," 859

jogging, *218*, 221, *237*, *241*, 623-624

and foot care, 238-239, 859-860

jogging shoes, proper choice of, 239-241, 859

Johnson, Virginia E., 643, 644, 687

joint(s): place where two or more bones or separate parts of the skeleton meet, 344-345

aging and, 671, 1052-1053

artificial, 1054

bleeding in, 1113-1114

diagnostic procedures, 887

diseases of, 1051-1066

inflammation: arthritis

Jones criteria for rheumatic fever, 1147

Jones, Ernest, *1332*

judgment, impairment of, 1103

jumping, spinal injury from, 1082

junction nevus, 299

Jung, Carl G., *1332*

junk *(slang)*: heroin, 1370

juvenile insulin dependent diabetes (JIDD), 1231

diet for, 1231

juvenile rheumatoid arthritis: *see* rheumatoid arthritis, juvenile

kala-azar/black fever/dumdum fever/visceral leishmaniasis: form of leishmaniasis that is usually fatal if not treated, 1304

kaolin-pectin compound, 852

keratin: horny substance that is the main constituent of nails and hair, and in nonhuman animals of claws and horns, 356, 783, 790, 866

keratosis: disease of the skin characterized by an outer layer of horny tissue

ketamine, 914

keto-acidosis: *see* ketosis

ketone bodies: organic compounds that are a by-product of fat metabolism, 1222, 1228

ketosis (keto-acidosis)

diabetic, 1227-1228, 1231

kidney: one of a pair of organs located at the rear of the abdomen near the base of the spine, whose function is to filter the fluid portion of the blood in regulating the composition and volume of body fluids, and to dispose of waste in the form of urine, *367*, *404*, 418-422, *419*, *938*, 1248, *1249*

artificial, 1251, *1251*, *1252*. *See also* dialysis.

cysts of, 935

diagnostic procedures for, 896

infection of, 1257-1258

removal of, 932, 934

organs within the abdominal cavity, 575

lapidary, as hobby, 683

lapse attack or seizure: *see* petit mal

lard, nutrients in, 716

laryngeal cartilage, *381*

laryngectomy: surgical removal of all or part of the larynx, 1286-1287

voluntary agency, 311

laryngitis: inflammation of the mucous membranes of the larynx, causing the voice to become hoarse or disappear altogether, 18̄7, 854

chronic: permanently hoarse voice resulting from thickened, toughened mucous membrane in the larynx, due to too many attacks of laryngitis, **854-855**

laryngologist: physician specializing in the diagnosis and treatment of disorders of the throat, 217

laryngology: the branch of medical science concerned with the study and treatment of the throat and related areas, 216

laryngoscope: instrument for inspecting the larynx

larynx/voice box: the organ of voice in humans and most other vertebrates, consisting of a cartilaginous box in the upper part of the trachea across which are stretched vocal cords whose vibrations produce sound, 382, 396, *397, 962*

cancer of, 1285-1287

smoking and, 1197

laser beam, 755

in retinal surgery, *672, 960,* 961

latent: not visible or apparent, as symptoms of a disease at an early stage

lateral:

1. relating to or directed toward the side

2. more distant from the midline of the body, as compared to a nearer (medial) position

later years, 654-694, *656, 663, 681, 682, 683, 684*

daily food requirements in, 705

diet in, *659,* 717

progressive exercises for, 246-247, 253-263

surgery in, 923-924

latissimus dorsi, 348

lavage: cleansing or washing out of an organ, as the stomach

Law of Use, 221, 622

laxative: substance that has the power to loosen the bowels, as milk of magnesia, 292, 852, 853, 1160, 1176

L-dopa/levodopa: medicine used in treating the symptoms of Parkinson's disease, 1090

lead poisoning, 503, 758, 759-760, *760, 761*

mental retardation and, 503, 509

lead pollution

atmospheric, 758

sources of, 759-760

water, 765

leaflet: flap of a heart valve, 1147-1148

learning disability: condition in which a child cannot acquire certain skills or assimilate certain kinds of knowledge at or near the normal rate, 478, 504

learning, in later years, 656, 685

leeches, to remove, 187

left-handedness, 277, 288, 435

leg biceps, 348

Legg-Perthes' disease: inflammation of the bone and cartilage in the head of the femur (thigh bone), 1070

legs

bowed, in Paget's disease, 1071

cramps in, 845

pregnancy and, 580-581

exercises for, 276, 625

shaving of, 787, 789

vascular disorders in, 276, 966-968, *967*

leiomyoma: benign tumor consisting of smooth muscle tissue, 1259

leishmaniasis: tropical disease resembling malaria in which an animal parasite is transmitted by the sandfly, 1304-1306, *1305* leishmaniasis protozoa, life cycle of, 1306

leishmaniasis, visceral: *see* kala-azar

leisure activities

in later years, 680-689

in middle years, 646-649

lemonade, nutrients in, 707

lens: biconvex transparent body behind the iris of the eye that focuses entering light rays on the retina, 410, *410*, 411-412, *412*, 957

lepromatous: characterized by nodular skin lesions, as a form of leprosy, 1316, *1317*

leprosy/Hansen's disease: chronic bacterial disease characterized by skin lesions, nerve paralysis, and physical deformity, 288, 1315-1317, *1315*, *1316*, *1317*

lesion: any abnormal change in an organ or tissue caused by disease or injury

lettuce, nutrients in, 702

leukemia: form of cancer involving the blood and blood-making tissues, characterized by a marked and persistent excess of leukocytes, 1121-1122, *1122*, 1269, 1290-1292

and secondary gout, 1061

granulocytic: form of leukemia characterized by predominance of granulocytes (or neutrophils), 1290
acute, 1290

lymphocytic: form of leukemia characterized by uncontrolled over-activity of the lymphoid tissue, 1290

new drugs for, 1291-1292

voluntary agency, 325-326

Leukemia Society of America, 325-326

leukemic: of or characteristic of leukemia

leukocyte/white blood cell/white corpuscle: white or colorless cell found in the bloodstream important in providing protection against infection, *368*, 370

bone marrow transplants and, 985-986

diseases of, 1121-1123

leukopenia: abnormal reduction in the number of leukocytes in the blood, 1123

leukorrhea: whitish, viscid discharge from the vagina, 995

levodopa: medicine used in treating the symptoms of Parkinson's disease, 203, 1090

levulose: fructose, 639

LGV: *see* lymphogranuloma venereum

LH: luteinizing hormone, *403*, 404

libido: the instinctual craving or drive behind all human activities, esp. sexual, the repression of which leads to neurosis

testicular hypofunction and, 1216

library services, 681

Librium: chlordiazepoxide, 639, 1369

lice

head, 786, 1007, *1007*

pubic, 1007-1008, *1007*

and typhus, 298

lidocaine: chemical used as a local anesthetic, 1140

life expectancy

alcohol and, 1346

obesity and, 640, 724

Life Extension Institute, 221

lifetime care facilities, 692

lifting, *264*, *351*, 673

ligament(s): band of tough, fibrous connective tissue that binds together bones and provides support for organs, 351, *351*

ligate: tie or close off with a ligature

ligation: the act of tying or binding up, as an artery

of Fallopian tubes, 610

of varicose veins, 967

See also tubal ligation.

ligature: thread, wire, etc., used to close off or tie a vessel

lightening: during the last few weeks of pregnancy, a shift in fetal pressure from the upper abdomen to the pelvic region as the head of the fetus moves toward the birth canal, 590

lighting, eyestrain and, 856

lightning shock, 187-188

light waves, sight and, 409

lumbar: pertaining to or situated near the loins

lumbar puncture: *see* spinal tap

lumbar vertebrae, 340-342, *341*

lumen: space enclosed by the walls of a blood vessel, duct, etc.

lumpectomy, 1035

luncheon, modified menus for, 728, 734, 735, 740, 743, 746, 750·

lung: either of two porous organs of respiration in the chest cavity of humans, having the function of absorbing oxygen and discharging carbon dioxide

lung cancer, 962-963, 1269-1272, *1270, 1272*

　air pollution and, 1202

　in asbestos workers, 755

　obstructive airway disease and, 1203-1204

　smoking and, 277, 1197, 1266, 1270-1272

lung diseases, 1179, 1183-1185, 1186-1190, 1196-1210

　air pollution and, 1200-1202

　occupational exposure and, 755, 1207-1209

　smoking and, 1196-1200

lungs, 368, 396-400, *397*, 1178

　capacity of, 398, *399, 1199*

　circulation to, 374-375, 392-393

　collapsed, 397-398

　injury to, by fractured ribs, 1081

　surgery of, 398, 961-963

lung tissue, *1198, 1203*

　of coal miner, *1209*

　in emphysema, *1203, 1205, 1207*

　of heavy smoker, *1198*

　in tuberculosis, *1188*

lung transplant, experimental, 986

lunula: the living part of the nail, the pale, half-moon shape at the nail base, 357

luteinizing hormone/LH: a hormone secreted by the anterior lobe of the pituitary gland that stimulates a Graafian follicle to release an ovum

during each menstrual cycle and converts the follicle into corpus luteum, *403*, 404

luteotrophic hormone: lactogenic hormone, *403*, 404

luteotrophin: lactogenic hormone, *403*, 404

lye (alkali) burns, 163, 173-174

lying, 476-477

lymph: transparent fluid resembling blood plasma that is conveyed through vessels (lymphatic vessels) and lubricates the tissues, 373-374

lymphangiogram: the visualization by X ray of lymph nodes after injection of an opaque fluid, 892

lymphatic: pertaining to or conveying lymph

lymphatic system, 373-374

　invasion of, in filariasis, 1310

lymph gland: *see* lymph node

lymph node/lymph gland: one of the rounded bodies about the size of a pea, found in the course of the lymphatic vessels, that produce lymphocytes, 373, 400

　biopsy of, 892

　swollen, 373, *855*

　　in bubonic plague, 1295

　　in Hodgkin's disease, 1289

lymphoblast: young cell that matures into a lymphocyte

lymphocyte: variety of leukocyte formed in the lymphoid tissue, 373, *1117*, 1121

　in infectious mononucleosis, 1123

lymphocytic leukemia

　acute, 458, 1266

　chronic, 1290

lymphogranuloma inguinale: *see* lymphogranuloma venereum

lymphogranuloma venereum/LGV/lymphogranuloma inguinale: venereal disease affecting the lymph nodes, 1005

lymphoid: pertaining to lymph or to the tissue of lymph nodes

lymphoma: abnormal (neoplastic) growth of lymphoid tissue, symptomatic of various diseases, as lymphocytic leukemia or Hodgkin's disease,1269, 1288, 1292

new drugs for, 1293

lymphosarcoma: malignant growth of the lymphatic system,1292

lysergic acid diethylamide: LSD, 555, 1373-1375

lysol, 674, 1047

lysozyme: enzyme present in tears that is destructive to bacteria,414

lyssophobia: fear of becoming insane, 1325

M *(slang):* morphine,1370, *1371*

macaroni, nutrients in, 715

mackerel, nutrients in, 701

macrobiotic: of or pertaining to macrobiotics

macrobiotics: the idea, Oriental in origin, that an equilibrium should be maintained between foods that make one active (Yang) and foods that make one relax (Yin),504, 748

macrocephalic: individual with macrocephaly

macrocephaly: excessive head size,1050

macula: spot or discoloration. *See also* macula lutea, senile macula degeneration.

macula lutea: yellowish area in the retina related to color perception and marked by most acute vision,410

magnesium, in teenage diet, 547

magnesium trisilicate, 1165

mainlining: injection of heroin directly into a vein

malabsorption syndrome/celiac disease: syndrome characterized by bulky, foul-smelling stools and other symptoms due to the inability of the body to absorb certain nutrients from the intestinal tract,459

malaise: feeling of being run-down, listless, uncomfortable, weary, and generally unwell

in influenza, 1183

malaria: disease caused by certain animal parasites transmitted by the bite of the infected Anopheles mosquito, causing intermittent chills and fever, *1300*, 1300-1303, *1301*

pregnancy and, 581

male pattern baldness, 630-631, 786-787

malignancy:
1. malignant tumor
2. state of being malignant

malignant: so aggravated as to threaten life, usu. resistant to treatment, and often having the property of uncontrolled growth, as a cancer

malignant hypertension, 1146

malleus: hammer,414, *417*, 955, *955*

malnutrition: nutritional deficiency, as of essential proteins, vitamins, or minerals, causing impairment of health and certain specific diseases,717-718

in children, 504

maternal, 509

teenagers and, 544

malocclusion: faulty closure of the upper and lower teeth,824-826, *824*, *825*, *826*

chewing and, 848-849

periodontal disease and, 821

Malta fever: *see* brucellosis

mammary glands (milk glands), 400, 1015, 1028

mammogram: X-ray picture of the breast by the technique of mammography,*1031*

mammography: specialized X-ray examination of the breasts,1030-1031, *1032*

mammoplasty: surgical procedure to augment the size of the breasts,979-980

mandible: the lower jawbone,343

manganese, 698

mania: psychotic condition characterized by excessive activity, elation, extreme talkativeness, and agitation,1328

manic-depressive reaction/affective reaction: psychosis characterized by mania or depression or by the alternation of both,1328-1330

manners, 504

margarine, nutrients in, 716

marihuana: the dried leaves and flowers of the hemp plant *(Cannabis sativa)*, which if smoked in cigarettes or otherwise ingested can produce distorted perception and other hallucinogenic effects, 554-555, *554*, 1376-1378, *1376*, *1377*

marriage, *603*

    early, 602

    sexual compatibility in, 604-605

marriage counseling, 602-604

marriage license, syphilis test and, 1003

marrow: either of two types of soft, vascular tissue found in the central cavities of bones—*red marrow* which produces red blood cells, and yellow marrow, composed mainly of fat cells; *see* bone marrow

marshmallow, nutrients in, 716

mascara, 782

Massachusetts General Hospital alcoholism study, 1355

massage

    of feet, 628

    for osteoarthritis, 671

    rheumatoid arthritis and, 1058

mastectomy: surgical removal of the breast, 1033-1035, *1033*

    exercise following, 244-245, *1035*

    and immunotherapy, 1035-1036

    modified radical, 1034, 1035

    pre-surgical staging, 1033

    radical: surgical removal of the breast, underlying chest muscles, and lymph glands in the armpit, 1034, 1035

    rehabilitation after, 244-245, 311

    simple: surgical removal of the breast only, 1035

    voluntary agency, 311, *1035*

    wedge excision, 1035

master gland: pituitary gland

Masters, William H., 643, 644, 687

mastitis: inflammation of the breast, 601

mastoiditis: inflammation of the air cells in the mastoid process

mastoid process: process of the temporal bone behind the ear

mastoplasty: surgical procedure to reduce the size of the breasts, 979

masturbation: the touching or rubbing of the genitals for sexual pleasure and usu. orgasm, 512, 564, 688, 1321

materia alba: white, viscous mixture of mucus, molds, tissue cells, and bacteria adhering to teeth or to the spaces between teeth and gums, a potential source of disease, 815

maxilla: the upper jawbone, 343

maxillary sinus: *see* paranasal sinus

MBD: *see* minimal brain dysfunction

MD: *see* muscular dystrophy

M.D.: Doctor of Medicine

mead, 1341

meals

    atmosphere at, 660, 709, 751

    for bedridden patient, 1044-1045

    preschool child and, 748-751

    schedule of, 641, 659

measles/rubeola: contagious viral disease, esp. of children, marked by rash, fever, and conjunctivitis, sometimes having severe complications, 504-505

    German: *see* rubella

    immunization, 499-500, *500*, 504, 505

meat group of foods, 658, 705, *706*

meatus: passage or canal in the human body, esp. one with an external opening, such as the anterior urethra of the penis

    of male urethra, 425, *565*

meatwrappers' asthma, 865

meclizine, 203

medial:

    1. middle, or relatively near the middle

    2. nearer to the midline of the body, as compared to a more distant (lateral) position

Medicaid program, 679

medical:
1. of or relating to medicine
2. of or relating to the treatment of disease by nonsurgical means

Medical Assistance for the Aged, 679

medical care, financing, 675-679

medical checkups

children, 460-461, *460*

later years, 657

middle age, 620-622

and nutrition, 718

oral contraceptives and, 607

prenatal, 426, 577

teenage, 547

Medic Alert Foundation, 145, *1098*, 1226, *1226*

medical history: the questions asked by a doctor of a patient that are designed to give an outline of the patient's state of health, 877-878, *877*, 904-905

medical records

automated, 622

family, 494, 500

in home care, 1047

transferral of, 283

Medicare, 675, *676*, 676-677, 679, 1252-1253, 1254

Medicare Coverage of Kidney Dialysis and Kidney Transplant Services, 1252-1253, 1254

Your Medicare Handbook, 677

medicated creams, 782

medicated soaps, 780

medications

and anesthesia, 905

appetite loss and, 718

children's, 505-506

outdated, 506

in pregnancy, 576-577

medicine:
1. the profession dealing with the maintenance of health and the treatment of physical and psychological disorders
2. the treatment of disease by nonsurgical means

medulla:
1. medulla oblongata: the lower part of the brain continuous with the spinal cord that controls certain involuntary processes such as breathing, swallowing, and blood circulation, 360, *360*, 395
2. the inner portion of an organ or part, as of the kidneys or the adrenal glands

adrenal, 404, *404*

of bone, *345*

of kidney, *419*, 1249

melancholia, involutional: *see* depressive reaction

melancholic disposition, 1329

melanin: dark brown or black pigment of the skin, 356, 778, 784

melanin cell clusters: *see* moles

melanoma/black cancer: malignant tumor formed of cells that produce melanin, 1274-1275

membrane(s)

amniotic, 592

intact: caul, 592

hyaloid: the delicate membrane that envelops the vitreous humor of the eye

periodontal: the membrane covering the bony tissue (cementum) around the roots of teeth

tympanic: eardrum

memory loss, 1099, 1103

menarche: the first menstrual period of a girl, 297, 537-540, 990, 991

Ménière's disease/Ménière's syndrome: symptoms including vertigo, ringing or buzzing sensations (tinnitus), nausea, and vomiting, associated with disease of the inner ear and often leading to progressive deafness of one ear, 1246

Ménière's syndrome: *see* Ménière's disease

meninges: the membranes that cover the brain and spinal cord, 359, 1101

meningioma: uncontrolled new cell growth in one of the membranes (arachnoid) covering the brain and spinal cord, 1068

meningitis: inflammation of the membranes that cover the brain and spinal cord, 359, 364, 506, 1101

   aseptic/viral meningitis: meningitis thought to be caused by a virus instead of a bacterium, 1101

   viral: aseptic

meningococcal: pertaining to meningococcus, a bacterium

meningococcus: bacterium that causes a form of meningitis, 1214

meningoencephalitis

   mumps, 510

menopausal: of or occurring during the menopause

menopause/change of life/climacteric: the cessation of menstruation and the end of a woman's capacity to bear children, normally occurring between 40-50 years of age and often marked by hot flashes, dizzy spells, and other physical and emotional symptoms, 632-635

   bleeding after, 995

   loss of hair at, 630

   male counterpart of, 635-636

   premature, 1218

   surgical: abrupt onset of menopause in women due to surgical removal of the uterus and ovaries, 633

menorrhagia, 992

menses: menstruation

menstrual: of or relating to menstruation

menstrual cycle, 539, 566-567

   fertile period of, 571-572, 609

   hormonal control of, 408, 1217

   oral contraceptives and, 606, *606*

   ovarian cysts and, 1015

   regularity of, 990, 991

menstrual discharge

   blood clots in, 994

   composition of, 567, 990, 991

   odor and, 994

menstrual disorders, 990-995, 1218

menstruation/the menses: periodic bloody discharge of the unfertilized ovum and tissue from the uterus of a female of child-bearing age

   activities during, 540, 993-994

   anovulatory, 539

   onset of: *see* menarche

mental abilities, aging and, 654, 656

mental health, physical fitness and, 229

mental illness, 1318-1330

   in children, 506-508

   genetic factors in, 507, *507*

   noise and, 772

   organic, 1321-1322

   treatment of, 1330-1336

   voluntary agencies, 319-320

mental retardation: failure in mental development that is severe enough to prevent normal participation in everyday life, 508-509

   PKU and, 516

   protein deprivation and, 718

   Rh factor and, 582

   voluntary agencies, 327-328, 329

mentoplasty: plastic surgery of the chin, esp. a procedure to build up an underdeveloped chin, 978-979, *980*

menus

   bland soft diet, 735

   low calorie diet, 728

   low fat diet, 746

   low sodium diet, 740

   minimal residue diet, 750

   modified fat diet, 740

   salt free diet, 734-736

   soft diet, 734

meperidine/pethidine/Demerol: medicine used as an analgesic and sedative, 203

meprobamate/Equanil/Miltown: tranquilizer used as a sedative and muscle relaxant, 203, 1369

mepyramine/pyrilamine, 210

mercaptan, 1317

mercury poisoning/"hatter's disease," 508, 754, 765-766

mercury, water pollution by, 765-767

mescaline: chemical extracted from the peyote cactus that induces hallucinations in its users, 555, 1375, *1375*

mesentery: the fan-shaped fold of the membrane (peritoneum) that enfolds the small intestine and connects it with the abdominal wall, 387

mesoderm: middle layer of tissue

metabolic: of or relating to metabolism

metabolic abnormality

    hereditary gout and, 1060-1061

    kidney stones and, 1258

    malnutrition and, 504

    overweight and, 729

metabolic rate, 361

    corticoids and, 405

    exercise and, 623

    thyroxin and, 406

metabolism: aggregate of all physical and chemical processes continuously taking place in living organisms, including those which build up and break down assimilated materials, 695-696

metacarpal: any of the five bones of the metacarpus, *344*

metacarpus: the five bones of the hand connecting the wrist to the fingers (phalanges), 337

metachromatic leukodystrophy, 293

metal plate, in skull fracture, 976

metals, heavy, and water pollution, 765

metastasis: the transfer of a disease or its manifestations, as a malignant tumor, from one part of the body to another, 1268

metatarsalgia: painful inflammation of the nerves in the region of the metatarsus of the foot, 628-629

metatarsals: the bones of the metatarsus, *344*

metatarsus: the five bones of the foot connecting the ankle to the toes (phalanges)

methacycline, 203

methadone/Dolophine: synthetic opiate used as an analgesic and experimentally as a substitute for heroin in the treatment of addicts, 203, 1373

methamphetamine/Methedrine/Desoxyn: chemical compound that allays hunger and has a more stimulating effect on the central nervous system than does amphetamine or dextroamphetamine, 1365

methanol: methyl alcohol

Methadrine: methamphetamine "methhead," 556, 1362, 1365

methaqualone, 204

methotrexate: drug used in the treatment of psoriasis and leukemia, 1064, 1291

methyl alcohol/wood alcohol/methanol: flammable liquid obtained through the distillation of wood or made synthetically, poisonous if taken internally, 1338

methyclothiazide, 204

methylphenidate (Ritalin), 204, 300, 1364, 1366

methyprylon (Noludar), 1368

metiamide, 1166

metric system, conversion tables for

    body temperatures, 1040

    food measures, 698

metrorrhagia: erratic or unpredictable menstrual bleeding, 993

Mg.%, 300

microcephalic: individual with microcephaly

microcephaly: abnormal smallness of the head, with imperfect development of the cranium, 1050

micrograph, *1181*

molluscum contagiosum: contagious viral disease marked by raised lesions containing waxy material, 1006-1007

molybdenum, 698

money, children and, 456, 509-510

Mongolism: congenital disorder characterized by mental retardation, *508,* 509, 583, 1322

moniliasis/candidiasis: fungus infection involving the skin or mucous membranes of various parts of the body, such as the mouth, esp. in babies (when it is called thrush), or the vagina, 996

monitoring equipment

cardiac, *1138,* 1139

premature baby, *589*

monocyte: relatively large leukocyte, 370

mononucleosis: infectious mononucleosis, 1123

monovalent: pertaining to a form of the Sabin polio vaccine in which each dose gives protection against a different strain of polio, 517. Compare *trivalent.*

morning sickness: nausea and vomiting experienced by some pregnant women in the morning hours, esp. in early pregnancy, 578

morphine: addictive narcotic drug derived from opium, used medically to relieve pain, 555-556, 1370, *1371*

as anesthetic, 594, 914

morphinism: abnormal condition of the body system caused by an excessive dose or habitual use of morphine, 1370

Morton's toe: painful inflammation of the nerves in the region of the metatarsus of the foot (metatarsalgia) between the third and fourth toes, 628-629

mosquito(s)

control of, 502, *1304,* 1312

disease and, 950, 1300-1301, 1302-1303, *1303,* 1303-1304, 1310

mother

new, advice to, 428-429

single, 653

working, 611-617

and child care, 484-485

motion sickness: nausea and sometimes vomiting caused by the effect of certain complex movements on the organ of balance in the inner ear, typically experienced in a moving vehicle, ship, or airplane, 188, 511

motor area in cerebral cortex, 360

motor nerve/efferent nerve: nerve that conveys information from the central nervous system to a muscle with a directive for action, 358

motor (efferent) neurons, *363*

polio and, 1101-1102

mouth, 378-383, *379, 381*

cancer of, 950, 951, 1197, 1275

disorders of, 848-849, 1157-1158

examination of, 883

mouth breathing, 399, 447

mouth-to-mouth respiration/mouth-to-mouth resuscitation: form of artificial respiration in which the rescuer places his mouth over the victim's mouth and breathes rhythmically and forcefully to inflate the victim's lungs and start respiration

mouth-to-mouth and mouth-to-nose artificial respiration, 139-141, *141*

mouthwashes, and bad breath, 849

MS: multiple sclerosis

mu: micron

mucocutaneous lymph node syndrome, 293

mucosa: mucous membrane

mucosal: of or pertaining to the mucous membrane

muscosal test for allergens, 870-871

mucous: pertaining to, producing, or resembling mucus

mucous glands, 400

mucous membrane/mucosa: membrane that lines many of the body's inner surfaces, kept moist by glandular secretions

mucus: viscous substance secreted by the mucous membranes

stomach, 384

National Society for the Prevention of Blindness, 315-316

Natulan: procarbazine, 1293

natural childbirth, 596-597

natural foods: foods processed minimally, although not necessarily organically grown, 748

nausea: feeling of sickness or dizziness usu. accompanied by the impulse to vomit

navel/umbilicus: the depression at the middle of the abdomen where the umbilical cord of the fetus was attached, 427

navy beans, nutrients in, 701

nearsightedness/myopia: inability to see distant objects clearly, 482-483, 1235-1236, *1236*

nebulizer, 1205-1206

Necator, 1170

neck

blood vessels of, *366*

injury to, 1082-1083

neck ribs, extra, 1050

neck stiffness, 1101, 1102

neck vertebra: vertebra, cervical

necrosis: death of a group of cells, tissue, or a part of the body

necrotizing ulcerative gingivitis: *see* trench mouth

needle biopsy: the excising of a tissue sample for biopsy by means of a long needle, 892, 896

negativism, in child, 440

nematode: any of a class of roundworms, many of which, such as the hookworm or pinworm, are intestinal parasites in man and other animals, 1171

neonate: newborn baby

neoplasm: any abnormal growth of new tissue, as a tumor, which may be benign or malignant

neoplasms, benign, in female reproductive system, 1013-1019

neoplastic: of or characteristic of neoplasms

neoplastic diseases, tests for, 892

nephrectomy: surgical removal of a kidney, 932, 934-935

nephric: renal, 214

nephritis/Bright's disease: inflammation of the kidneys, 1254-1255

nephroblastoma: *see* Wilm's tumor

nephrologist: physician specializing in the diagnosis and treatment of diseases of the kidney, 215

nephrology: branch of medical science dealing with the structure, function, and diseases of the kidney, 214

nephron: one of the basic filtration units of the kidney, consisting of Bowman's capsule, a glomerulus, and tubules, *419, 420,* 421, *1249, 1254*

nephrosis/nephrotic syndrome: disease of the kidneys characterized by degenerative lesions of the renal tubules and loss of protein (albumin) through the urine, 1255-1256

nerve block/plexus block: form of local anesthesia in which the anesthetic is injected into nerve trunks leading to the area in which surgery is to be performed, 915, 916

nerve bundle, master: *see* spinal cord

nerve cell:

1. one of the cells of the nervous system

2. the cell body of a neuron

See also neuron.

nerve deafness, 667, 957

nerve endings, in skin, 354, 777

nerve fibers, 359, 362-364

nerve impulse, 358, 360, 362-364

nerves

cranial, 361-362, *361*

lingual: nerve beneath the floor of the mouth that conveys taste sensations to the brain motor, 358, 418

olfactory: the special nerve of smell, *361,* 418

optic: the special nerve of vision connecting the retina with the occipital lobe of the brain, *361* sensory/afferent nerve: nerve that conveys information and stimuli from the outside world to the central nervous system, 358

spinal: the thirty-one pairs of nerves that originate in the spinal cord, 362

nervous breakdown: popular, nontechnical term for any debilitating or incapacitating emotional disorder

nervous habits, 511-512

nervous system, 359, 361-362, 1084

aging and, 363, 620

diagnostic procedures for, 888-890, *890*, 1085-1087, *1086*

disorders of, 363, 364-365, 1084-1104

infections of, 1101-1104

neural: of or relating to a nerve, 216

neuralgia: acute pain along the course of a nerve

facial: *see* trigeminal neuralgia

trigeminal/facial neuralgia/tic douloureux: acutely painful neuralgia of a region of the face, with paroxysmal muscular twitchings, associated with branches of the trigeminal (cranial) nerve in the affected area, 302, 972-973

neuritis: inflammation of a nerve

neuroblastoma: malignant tumor of the nerve tissue of the adrenal glands, found esp. in children, 458

neurofibroma: tumor on a nerve fiber, 1068

neurogenic shock: shock resulting from impairment of the regulatory capacity of the nervous system due to pain, fright, or other stimulus, 144

neurological surgery, 874

neurologist: physician specializing in the care and treatment of the nervous system, 217, 888, 1085

neurology: the branch of medical science that deals with the nervous system, 216, 888

neuromuscular ailments, free diagnosis of, 326-327

neuron: nerve cell with all its processes and extensions, such as the axon and dendrites, 359, 362-364, *363*

motor: horn cells, anterior

neuropathologist: physician specializing in neuropathology, 217

neuropathology: the branch of medical science that deals with the study, diagnosis, and treatment of diseases of the nervous system, 216

neuropharmacology, 294

neurosis/psychoneurosis (*pl.*, *neuroses*): mental disorder having no organic cause and less severe than psychosis, 1323-1325

neurosurgeon: physician specializing in surgery of the nervous system, 217, 874, 888

neurosurgery: the branch of medical science that deals with the treatment of disease of the nervous system by means of surgery, 972-976, *973*, *975*

neurosyphilis: syphilis of the brain and spinal cord, 1263

neurotic:

1. one who has a neurosis

2. of or relating to neurosis, 1323

neurotoxic:

1. (of certain poisonous snakes) transmitting venom that directly affects the nervous system and brain of the toxified animal, 189. Compare *hemotoxic.*

2. causing destruction or damage to nerve tissue

neutrophil/granulocyte/polymorphonuclear leukocyte: granular leukocyte that can be stained with dyes that are neither acid nor alkaline (i.e., neutral), 370, 1121, 1122

nevus: birthmark or congenital mole junction, 299

newborn, 426-432, *595*

blood pressure of, *1151*

contact with mother, *599*

eye care of, 316

gonorrhea and, 1003

health rating of, 599-600

Rh disease in, 1120-1121

siblings of, 512

nystatin, 205

oat cereal, nutrients in, 715

obesity: excessive accumulation of body fat, 640-641, 713, 718-725, *726, 836,* 836-837

aging and, 620

back problems and, 673

children and, 457, 547, 720-721, 722, 723, 724

diabetes and, 724, 1233

exercise and, 303, 623

heart disease and, 219, 669, 724, 1143

hiatus hernia and, 1159

life expectancy and, 640, 718, 724

metabolic abnormality and, 723-724

physical fitness and, 225-227

pinch test for, 640, 719

pregnancy and, 577

psychological factors in, 722, 724, 837

ob-gyn specialist: physician trained as an obstetrician and gynecologist, 217

objective: (of symptoms) of a kind that can be observed or measured by the examining physician through diagnostic techniques. Compare *subjective.*

obsession: persistent, unwanted idea or feeling, a symptom of certain neuroses, 1324

obsessive-compulsive reaction: neurosis characterized by obsessions that are relieved temporarily by the compulsive performance of certain acts, 1324

obstetrician: physician specializing in obstetrics, often a gynecologist as well, 217, 874

obstetrics: the branch of medical science dealing with pregnancy and childbirth, 216, 874

obstructive-airway disease: condition characterized by the presence of chronic bronchitis and pulmonary emphysema, and involving damage to lung tissue and the bronchi, 1203-1204

obturator: special device inserted into a cleft palate to close it against the flow of air, 463

occipital: of or relating to the lower back part of the skull (occiput)

occipital bone, *341*

occipital lobe: the rear portion of each cerebral hemisphere which receives messages from the optic nerve,360, 411

occlusion:
1. the act of closing or shutting off so as to block a passage, as a blood vessel
2. the manner of being shut, as the teeth of the upper and lower jaws

occupational disease: disease resulting from exposure in one's occupation to toxic substances or other hazards to health, 754-755, 1207

occupational therapist, *459*

oceans, pollution of, 762-767

ocular: of or relating to the eye

ocular muscle, *410, 957*

ocular muscular dystrophy, 1108

oculist: ophthalmologist, 215

oculomotor nerve, 361

oculopharyngeal muscular dystrophy, 1107

odor, perspiration, 295, 358, 780-781

Oedipal complex: repressed sexual attachment of son to mother, analogous to the Electra complex involving the daughter and father, **443-444**

oil glands: glands, sebaceous

oils, nutrients in, 716

oil spills, 763-765

okra, nutrients in, 702

Older Volunteers in the Peace Corps, 684

olfaction: the act, sense, or process of smelling

olfactory: pertaining to the sense of smell or the capacity to smell

olfactory bulb, 417-418

olfactory lobe: the portion of each cerebral hemisphere of the brain on the underside of the frontal lobes, the centers for smelling, 360

olfactory nerve: *see* nerve, olfactory

oliguria: decreased production of urine, 1249, 1250

Olympic competitors, *233, 264*

onchocerciasis: form of filariasis transmitted by a blackfly and sometimes leading to blindness, 1311, *1311*

oncologist: physician specializing in the diagnosis and treatment of tumors, 217

oncology: the branch of medical science concerned with the study of tumors, 216

Oncovin: vincristine, 1292, 1293

onions, nutrients in, 702

oophorectomy: *see* ovariectomy

open bite: form of malocclusion in which incisors of the upper and lower jaws do not meet when the jaws are together

open fracture: compound fracture, 1075

open-heart surgery, *1136*

  in infants, 1152, *1153*

open surgery: surgery involving an incision and opening of the skin

operating room

  equipment, 911-912, *913*

  personnel, 908-911, *909*

ophthalmic: of or pertaining to the eye, 214

Ophthalmological Foundation, 316

ophthalmologist/oculist: physician specializing in the care and treatment of the eyes, 215, 874, 876

ophthalmology: the branch of medical science dealing with the structure, function, and diseases of the eye, 214, 874

ophthalmoscope: optical instrument for examining the interior of the eye, 882, 895

opiate: drug derived from opium, as morphine, 555-556

  synthetic, 1373

opium: narcotic drug obtained from the opium poppy from which morphine, codeine, heroin, and other drugs are derived, 1369-1370, *1370, 1371*

optic/optical: pertaining to the eye or to vision

optician: one who makes or sells eyeglasses and other optical equipment

optic nerve: special nerve of vision, conveying sensations from the retina to the brain, *361, 410,* 411, *957*

optometrist: one who practices optometry

optometry: profession of measuring the power of vision and prescribing corrective lenses

oral: pertaining to or situated near the mouth

oral cancer: *see* mouth

oral contraceptives, 605-607, *606,* 991, 994, 1217

  embolism and, 1209, 1210

  syphilis and, 999

oral hygiene, 629, 657-658, 812-814, *814*

oral irrigating devices, 814

oral surgeon/dental surgeon: dentist who specializes in oral surgery, 217, 887

oral surgery: the diagnosis and surgical treatment of diseases, injuries, and defects of the mouth and jaw, 216

orange juice, 707

  allergy to, 863

  oranges, nutrients in, 707

orbit: either of the bony sockets of the eyes

orchidopexy/orchiopexy: surgical correction of an undescended testicle, 929-930

orchiectomy: surgical removal of one or both testicles, 980

orchiopexy: *see* orchidopexy

orchitis: inflammation of the testicles

  mumps and, 510

organic:

  1. of or pertaining to an organ of the body

  2. having a physical basis, as a disorder

  3. of or pertaining to animals or plants

  4. pertaining to foods grown only with natural fertilizers of animal or plant origin

organic foods: foods grown with the use of organic fertilizers only, such as compost or animal (not human) manure, and without the use of pesticides or herbicides, 747-748

organ of Corti: the true center of hearing within the cochlea of the inner ear, a complex spiral structure of hair cells, 415

organ transplants, 670-674

orgasm: the climax of the sexual act, normally marked by the male's ejaculation of semen and by relaxation of tension of both male and female

female, 605

orifice: opening into a body cavity

orthodontia: orthodontics, 216

orthodontics/orthodontia: the care and treatment of irregularities and faulty positions of the teeth, including the fitting of braces, 216, 513-514, 550-551, 551, 824-827, 824, 825, 826, 827

orthodontist: dentist specializing in orthodontics, 217, 887

orthopedics: the branch of surgery dealing with the treatment and correction of deformities, injuries, and diseases of the skeletal system and its associated structures, as muscles and joints, 215

orthopedic surgeon: orthopedist, 215

orthopedic surgery, 874, 888, 968-972

orthopedist/orthopedic surgeon/orthopod: surgeon specializing in orthopedics, 215, 874, 887, 1076

orthopod: orthopedist, 215

orthoptist: medical technician trained to diagnose defects of the eye muscles and to provide corrective exercises, 467

orthotic device, 491

oscilloscope: instrument for visibly representing electrical activity on a fluorescent screen, 1106

Osgood-Schlatter disease, 295

osseous: osteal, 214

ossicle: one of the three small connecting bones of the middle ear, the hammer (or malleus), the anvil (or incus), and the stirrup (or stapes), that transmit sound from the eardrum to the cochlea, 339, 414, 415, 416, 417, 955, 1247

surgical procedures on, 955-956

ossification: conversion into bone

ossify: to convert or be converted into bone

osteal/osseous: of or relating to bone, 214

osteitis: inflammation of a bone

osteitis deformans: see Paget's disease 1

osteoarthritis/degenerative joint disease/ hypertrophic arthritis: chronic degenerative disease that affects the joints, 671, 1051-1054, 1052, 1053

osteogenesis: formation and growth of bones

imperfecta: condition in which bones are abnormally brittle and liable to fracture due to a deficiency of calcium, 1071, 1071

osteogenic: pertaining to osteogenesis

osteogenic sarcoma, 1073

osteomyelitis: inflammation of the bone tissue or marrow, 348, 1068, 1072

tooth decay and, 816

osteopath: physician trained in osteopathy, 217, 283

osteopathy: system of healing based on a theory that most diseases are caused by structural abnormalities that may best be corrected by manipulation, 216

osteophyte(s): abnormal bony outgrowth, 1052, 1054

osteoporosis: reduction in bone mass and increase in interior space, porosity, and fragility of bone, 1070

otitis media: inflammation of the middle ear, 955, 1245

nonsuppurative: inflammation of the middle ear resulting from a blocked Eustachian tube and fluid collection in the middle ear, causing hearing damage, 955

otolaryngologist: physician specializing in the diagnosis and treatment of the ear, nose, and throat, 214, 874, 895

otolaryngology: the branch of medicine dealing with the study and diseases of the ear, nose, and throat, 214, 874-875

otologist: one who specializes in the ear and its diseases, 215, 667

otology: the branch of medical science dealing with the functions and diseases of the ear, 214

2. cancerous disease of the breast marked by the inflammation of the areola and nipple

pain, 354, *363*, 409

back, 346, 673, 1069

chest: *see* chest pain

epigastric, 1168

in feet, 673-674

in lungs, absence of, 496

in muscles, 353

ovarian, 1218

post-operative, 918

in skeletal system, 348

in terminal illness, 694

from unknown cause, 364

pain threshold, for sound, 771

palate: the roof of the mouth

hard: the bony part of the roof of the mouth, 381, *381*

soft/velum: the soft, muscular tissue at the rear of the roof of the mouth, *379*, 381, *381, 397, 962, 1156*

palpation: diagnostic procedure of feeling, pressing, or manipulating the body

palpitation: rapid or fluttering heartbeat

palsy/paralysis: Bell's palsy, cerebral palsy

PAN: peroxyacl nitrate, 758

pancreas: large gland situated behind the stomach and containing the islets of Langerhans that produce insulin and glucagon, and secreting pancreatic juice via small ducts to the duodenum, *379, 384,* 387-389, 390-391, *401, 405,* 406, *937, 1156, 1212*

cancer of, 1283

duodenal ulcer and, 939

tissue transplant of, 986

pancreatic duct, *379, 384,* 389, *405, 937, 1156*

pancreatic enzymes, 385-386

pancreatic juice: secretion of the pancreas containing digestive enzymes

pancreatitis: inflammation of the pancreas

pandemic: epidemic occurring over a very large area or worldwide

influenza, 1183

Pantopon, 1373

Papanicolaou, Dr. George N.: developer of a test, called the *Pap smear* or *Pap test*, for detecting cancer of the cervix, 1020

Papanicolaou smear: Pap smear

papaverine, 205

Paperver somniferum, 1369

papillae *(sing., papilla):* tiny, nipple-shaped projections that cover the inner layer (dermis) of the skin and the surface of the tongue

renal, *419, 1249*

skin, *354,* 355-356, *355,* 777

of tongue, 380-381

papillary tumor:

1. papilloma: benign tumor of the papillae of the skin, as a wart or corn

2. malignant tumor of the bladder, so called because it is nipplelike in shape (Latin *papilla* means nipple), 1259, 1279

Pap smear/Papanicolaou smear/Pap test: method of early detection of cervical cancer consisting of painless removal of cervical cell samples, which are stained and examined, *312, 635,* 635, 998, 1020-1022, *1021,* 1266

Pap test: Pap smear

papule: pimple

para-aminosalicyclic acid (PAS), 206

paraffin baths, in rheumatoid arthritis, 1058-1059

paraldehyde, 639

paralysis

of face, in Bell's palsy, 1089

and muscle atrophy, 353

in poliomyelitis, 1101-1102

spinal injury and, 1082-1083

stroke and, 1127-1128, *1129*

paralysis agitans: Parkinson's disease

paralysis, infantile: *see* poliomyelitis

paranasal sinus: air cavity in one of the cranial bones communicating with the nostrils, **399-400**

paranoia, 1328

paranoid: describing a personality disorder in which the individual is extraordinarily sensitive to praise or criticism and subject to suspicions and feelings of persecution, 1327

paranoid reaction/paranoia: psychosis characterized by invariable delusion, usu. of persecution, sometimes of grandeur, 1328

paranoid schizophrenia: *see* schizophrenia, paranoid

paraplegia: paralysis of the lower half of the body

paraplegic: one who is paralyzed in the lower half of the body, including both legs

parasite(s): animal or plant that lives in or on another organism (called the host), at whose expense it obtains nourishment

intestinal, 1169-1172

parasiticide: medication designed to destroy parasites such as body lice

parasympathetic nervous system: the part of the autonomic nervous system that controls such involuntary actions as the constriction of pupils, dilation of blood vessels and salivary glands, and slowing of heartbeat, 362. Compare *sympathetic nervous system.*

parathormone/parathyroid hormone: hormone secreted by the parathyroid glands, important in regulating the amount of calcium in the body, 407

parathyroid glands: four small endocrine glands near or embedded within the thyroid gland, usu. two per side, that regulate blood calcium and phosphorus levels, *401*, 407, 1211, *1212*, 1219

parathyroid hormone: *see* parathormone

paregoric (camphorated tincture of opium), 206

parent(s)

abusive, 453-454

adoptive, 447

death of, 471-472, 652

estranged, 485, 651-652

single, 651, 652-653

parent-child relationship, 439, 443-444, 559-560, 646, 648, 1319

Parents Anonymous, 453-454

Parents Without Partners, Inc., 653

paresis:

1. partial paralysis

2. general paralysis *(general paresis)* caused by degeneration of the brain as a result of syphilis

parietal bone, *341*

parkinsonism: Parkinson's disease

Parkinson's disease/paralysis agitans/ parkinsonism: chronic, progressive nervous disease characterized by muscle tremor when at rest, stiffness, and a rigid facial expression, 364, 1090

parotid gland: either of two large salivary glands located below and in front of the ear, 378

mumps and, 510, 1157

paroxysm: sudden onset of acute symptoms, as an attack or convulsions

paroxysmal tachycardia, 847

parrot fever: psittacosis

particulate matter: fine particles in smoke that are dispersed by the wind and fall back to earth

in air pollution, 1202

parturition: act or process of giving birth

passive-dependent: describing a personality disorder in which the individual needs excessive emotional support from an authority figure, 1327

passivity, in children, 449

pasteurization, *1182*

patch test: skin test for determining hypersensitivity by applying small pads of possibly allergy-producing substances to the skin's surface

patchy baldness: alopecia areata

patella: the kneecap, *341*

pathogen: disease-causing bacterium or microorganism

pathogenic: disease-causing

pathologic: caused by or relating to disease, 214

pathologic fracture: fracture that occurs spontaneously, as because of pre-existing disease, without external cause

pathologist: physician or expert specializing in pathology, **215, 875**

pathology: the branch of medical science dealing with the causes, nature, and effects of diseases, esp. disease-induced changes in organs, tissues, and body chemistry, **214, 875**

patient-doctor relationship, 279-285, 897-899

PCBs/polychlorinated biphenyls: chemicals related to DDT and having many industrial uses, posing a potential threat to health as a water pollutant from industrial wastes, **767**

Peace Corps, 683-684

peaches, nutrients in, 708

peanuts, nutrients in, 702

pears, nutrients in, 708

peas, nutrients in, 702

pectorals, 348

pectus carinatum: *see* pigeon breast

pectus excavatum: *see* funnel chest

pedal: of or relating to the foot

pediatric dentist: dentist specializing in the care and treatment of the teeth of children, **217, 887**

pediatrician: physician specializing in the care and treatment of children, **215, 875, 875**

pediatrics: the branch of medicine dealing with the care and treatment of children and their diseases, **214, 875**

pedodontics: branch of dentistry specializing in the care of children

pedodontist: dentist specializing in pedodontics, **513**

pellagra: disease caused by a vitamin deficiency and characterized by gastric

disturbance, skin eruptions, and nervous symptoms

pelvic girdle: the part of the human skeleton to which the lower limbs are attached, **338, 342**

pelvis:
1. the part of the skeleton that forms a bony girdle or basin joining the lower limbs to the body, and consisting of the two hip bones and the sacrum

2. the central area of the kidney from which urine drains into the ureter

fracture of, 1077-1078

penicillamine, 1058

penicillin: powerful antibacterial substance found in a mold fungus and prepared in several forms for the treatment of a wide variety of infections, *1184*

allergy to, 865

in dental surgery, 1150

nephritis and, 1255

pneumonia and, 1184

scarlet fever and, 525

syphilis and, 1002-1003, 1264

penicillin G, 206

penicillin V, 206

penis: tubular male organ of sexual intercourse and excretion of urine, located at the front of the pelvis, **565, 565**

tumors of, 929

pentaerythritol tetranitrate, 206

pentamidine, 1308

pentobarbital, 206

Pentothal/sodium Pentothal/thiopental: trademark for an ultra-short-acting barbiturate used as an anesthetic, as in dentistry, **914, 1367**

peppers, nutrients in, 703

pep pills: *see* amphetamines

pepsin: enzyme secreted by the gastric juices of the stomach, 384-385

peptic ulcer: ulcer of the mucous membrane of the stomach (gastric ulcer) or small intestine (duodenal ulcer) caused by the action of acid juices, 302-303, 385, 1164-1165

diet and, 731, 732-735, 922, 1165

surgery for, 940-941, *940*

perception, through skin, 354

percussion: diagnostic procedure of striking or tapping the body with instruments or with the fingers

method of, 879-880

perfectionism, 450-451, 1323

perfumes, allergies to, 274

perianal: situated around the anus

pericarditis: inflammation of the pericardium

pericardium: the membrane that surrounds and protects the heart, 375

peridental: periodontal

perimeter: device for determining peripheral vision, 895-896

perinatologist, 294

perineal: of or pertaining to the perineum

perineum: region of the body at the lower end of the trunk, between the genital organs and the anus

periodontal/peridental: situated around a tooth, 216

periodontal disease, 657-658, 808, 810, 816, 819-821, *819*

periodontal membrane: membrane, periodontal, *339*, *807*, 808, *820*

periodontia: periodontics, 216

periodontics/periodontia: the branch of dentistry dealing with the diagnosis and treatment of periodontal (gum) diseases, 216

periodontist: dentist who specializes in periodontics, 217, 887

periodontitis: inflammation of the tissues around a tooth, leading to destruction of the alveolar bone, 820

periodontium: the supporting structures of the teeth, comprising the gingiva, alveolar bone, and periodontal ligaments, 808

periosteum: the tough, fibrous membrane that surrounds and nourishes bones, *345*, 346, *351*

peripheral nervous system: the nerves and ganglia outside the brain and spinal cord, 362

peripheral smear, 891-892

peripheral vision, 410-411

peristalsis: wavelike muscular contractions of the alimentary canal that move the contents along in the processes of digestion and excretion, 382, 392, 1157

peristaltic wave: the alternate contraction and relaxation of muscles in the alimentary canal in peristalsis

peritoneoscopy: technique for examining the female reproductive organs within the abdominal cavity, 575

peritoneoscope/laparoscope: instrument used for examining the organs within the abdominal cavity, esp. the female reproductive organs

peritoneum: the serous membrane that lines the abdominal cavity enclosing the abdominal organs, 392

adhesions to, 942-943

peritonitis: inflammation of the lining (peritoneum) of the abdominal cavity, 938, 1169

peritonsillar abscess/quinsy: abscess in the tissues adjoining a tonsil as a complication of tonsillitis

permanent wave, 784

pernicious: severe, destructive, and often fatal

pernicious anemia: severe, progressive anemia caused by lack of vitamin B12, formerly fatal but now controllable, 1116-1117

peroxyacetyl nitrate, 758

persecution, feelings of, 1323

personality area, in brain, *360*

personality changes, in multiple sclerosis, 1099

personality disorder/character disorder: any of a group of mental illnesses that apparently stem from an arrested development of the personality, 1326-1330

perspiration: *see* sweat

Pertolatum Rose Water Ointment USP XVI, 667

pertussis: *see* whooping cough

pessary:

1. device worn inside the vagina as a contraceptive or to support uterine prolapse, 1012

2. medicated suppository for use in the vagina

pessimism, undue, 1323

pesticides, in foods, 748, 769, *769*

pethidine/meperidine, 203

petit mal: minor epileptic seizure, with very brief loss of consciousness, 480, 1093-1094. Compare *grand mal*.

 medication for, 1096

petroleum derivatives, skin cancer and, 1274

pets, 514-515, *515*

 allergies and, 865, 1194

Peyer's patches: oval areas of lymphoid tissue in the intestine that manufacture lymphocytes, 372

peyote: the mescal cactus of Mexico or the powerful hallucinogenic drug obtained from its dried upper part (called buttons), 1375, *1375*

phalanges *(sing., phalanx)*: the bones of the fingers or toes, 337, *344*

pharmacist: one skilled in the compounding and dispensing of medicines

pharmacologist: expert in pharmacology

pharmacology: the science of the action of medicines, their nature, preparation, administration, and effects

pharmacy, *307*

pharyngitis: inflammation of the pharynx, commonly called a sore throat, 528, 830, 1255

pharynx: the part of the alimentary canal between the palate and the esophagus, serving as a passage for air and food, *379, 381, 382, 384, 396, 397, 962, 1156*

phenacetin (acetophenetidin), 207

phenazopyridine, 207

phenformin: *see* DBI

pheniramine, 207

phenmetrazine, 1366

phenobarbital/phenobarbitone, 207, 1096

phenol: *see* carbolic acid

phenothiazine, 1369

phentermine, 207

phenylalanine, 516

phenylbutazone, 207

phenylephrine, 208

phenylketonuria/PKU: inherited metabolic disorder that can cause mental retardation if not treated by a special diet soon after birth, 301, 516, 736, 1322

 genetic counseling and, 583

 mental retardation and, 509

phenyl-propanolamine, 208

phenytoin (formerly diphenylhydantoin), 208, 1096

phlebitis: inflammation of the inner membrane of a vein, 967-968, 1124

phlebotomy/bloodletting/venesection: the opening of a vein for letting blood

phlegm: viscid, stringy mucus secreted in abnormally large amounts, as in the air passages, 1182

phlegmatic disposition, 1329

phobia: intense anxiety irrationally felt for any of a variety of things or situations, such as closed or open places, animals of a particular kind, heights, etc., a manifestation of the phobic reaction, 486, 1323, 1325. *See also* fear of.

phobic reaction: neurosis characterized by displacement of anxiety of a conflict to a substitute, such as a particular domestic animal, closed places, etc., 1325

phonocardiogram: graph recording the sounds produced by the heart, used to evaluate heart murmurs and other abnormal sounds, 890

phosphates, water pollution by, *762, 763*

phosphorus

 in blood, 1219

in diet, 545-546

radioactive, 1119

photocoagulation, 286

physical dependence: accommodation of the body to continued use of a drug, such that withdrawing the drug causes pronounced physical reactions (withdrawal symptoms)

physical fitness: *see* fitness

physical medicine: branch of medicine utilizing physical procedures, such as heat, cold, massage, or mechanical devices, to diagnose disease or treat disabled patients, 216

and rehabilitation, 875

physical therapist: specialist in physical therapy, 217

physical therapy/physiotherapy: the treatment of disability, injury, or disease by external physical means, such as heat, massage, planned exercises, electricity, or mechanical devices, to restore function or aid rehabilitation

arthritis and, 308, 1054, *1057*, 1058-1059

cerebral palsy and, 1088

multiple sclerosis and, *1100*

muscular dystrophy and, 1106

poliomyelitis and, 1103, *1103*

stroke and, 1128, *1129*, *1141*

physician(s):

1. any authorized practitioner of medicine, 872

2. one trained in medicine, as distinguished from surgery, 872

emergency services, 158

physician-patient relationship, 279-285, 897-899

and nurse, in home care, 1037-1038

physiotherapy: *see* physical therapy

pia mater: the delicate, vascular, innermost membrane of the three membranes that envelop the brain and spinal cord

pica: appetite for substances unfit to eat, 515-516

piebald skin: vitiligo, 666

pies, nutrients in, 715

pigeon breast/pectus carinatum: congenital deformity in which the sternum protrudes, 296

pigeon toes, 487

piggy banks, 510

pigment: substance that imparts coloring to tissue

pigmentation, skin, 777, 778

loss of, 666, 804

in leprosy, *1315*

piles: *see* hemorrhoids

"pill, the": contraceptives, oral

pill-popping, 1365

pills

over-the-counter, 622, 1359-1360

reducing, 730

pilocarpine, 208

pimple/papule: small, usu. inflamed swelling on the skin, 543-544, 800-801

pinch test for obesity, 640, 719, *721*

pineal body: *see* pineal gland

pineal gland/pineal body: small, coneshaped body of rudimentary glandular structure located at the base of the brain and having no known function, 408

pineapple juice, nutrients in, 708

pinkeye: acute, contagious conjunctivitis, marked by redness of the eyeball, 855-856

pins, in repair of fractures, 970, *1078*, 1079

pinworm: parasitic worm of the lower intestines and rectum, esp. of children, causing intense itching in the anal area, 1171

pitch, hearing loss and, 772

pituitary body: *see* pituitary gland

pituitary gland/hypophysis cerebri/pituitary body: small endocrine gland situated at the base of the brain, consisting of anterior and posterior lobes whose hormonal secretions stimulate the production of hormones in other glands and regulate vital body functions such as growth and metabolism, *360, 401,* 402-404, *403,* 1211, *1212*

anterior lobe of, 402-403, *403,* 1213

posterior lobe of, 402, *403,* 1218-1219

tumor of, 974

pituitary replacement therapy, 287

pit vipers, 189-190

pityriasis rosea: skin disease, esp. of children, marked by a rash, 521

PKU: *see* phenylketonuria

placebo: any harmless substance given to humor a patient or as a test in controlled experiments on the effects of drugs

allergic reaction to, 866

placenta: the vascular structure in pregnant women that unites the fetus with the uterus, and through which the fetus is nourished via the umbilical cord, usu. expelled naturally immediately following birth (when it is called the *afterbirth*), 400, 599

Placidyl: ethchlorvynol, 1368

plague:

1. any epidemic disease that is contagious and often deadly

2. contagious, often fatal disease caused by a bacterium transmitted by fleas from infected rats, and characterized by fever, chills, prostration, and often by buboes (hence the name *bubonic plague*), 1294-1297, *1295, 1296*

Planned Parenthood Federation of America, 316-317

plantar warts: warts on the soles of the feet, caused by a virus, 799

plaque: mucus containing bacteria that collects on teeth, 657, 813, 814

plasma: the clear fluid portion of the blood, 369, 1111, *1113*

plasma proteins, 1112

plasmodium (*pl. plasmodia*), 1302

plaster cast, 1077

plastic surgeon: physician specializing in plastic or cosmetic surgery, 875, 977

plastic surgery: surgery that deals with the restoration or healing of lost, injured, or deformed parts of the body, mainly by the transfer of tissue, and with the improvement of appearance (cosmetic surgery), 667, 875, 903-904, 976-982, 1081

costs of, 977

platelet/thrombocyte: small, disk-shaped body found in blood that aids in clotting, *368,* 370, 1111, 1112

deficiency of, 1114

plates, metal

in hip fracture, *1078,* 1079

in radius fracture, 970, *971*

play, 440-441, *482, 483, 497*

playground, 481

play therapy: psychotherapy, esp. for patients who are children, in which toys or other playthings are made available for the patient to play with in the presence of the therapist

playthings: *see* toys

pleura: serous membrane that enfolds the lungs and lines the chest cavity, 396

inflammation of: *see* pleurisy

pleural cavity: the space between the two pleuras lining the lungs and chest cavity, 396-398

pleural membranes, 396-398

pleurisy: inflammation of the pleura, characterized by fever, chest pain, and difficulty in breathing, 398, 1059, 1185-1186, 1209

plexus: interlacement of cordlike body structures, such as blood vessels or nerves, 363-364

plexus block: *see* nerve block

plucking, of unwanted hair, 790

plums, nutrients in, 708

pneumococcus: bacterium that can cause pneumonia, *1181,* 1183, 1185

pneumoconiosis: any of various lung disorders, such as silicosis or black lung disease, resulting from the inhalation of dust or other minute particles, 1207-1209, *1209*

pneumoencephalogram: X-ray picture of the brain taken after air or gas has been injected to partially replace the cerebrospinal fluid, 890

pneumoencephalography: technique of producing pneumoencephalograms and interpreting them, 1086

pneumonia: inflammation of the lungs, usu. bacterial in origin and acute in course, characterized by high fever, chills, breathing difficulty, and cough, 1183-1186

 aspiration: pneumonia caused by inhaling particles of foreign matter, as food, 1160

pneumonic plague, 1295

pneumothorax: accumulation of air or gas in the pleural cavity, causing the lung to collapse, as from injury or disease, or by injection (artificial pneumothorax) in the treatment of tuberculosis, 397, 1210

podiatrics, 858, 859, 860

podiatrist/chiropodist: one who specializes in the treatment of the foot, 215, 674, 858, 859, 860

 Medicare coverage for, 677

podiatry/chiropody: the study and treatment of disorders of the feet, 214

Poison Control Centers, 149, 150, 150, 158, 517

 directory of, 151-156

poisoning, 150, 158

 children and, 516-517

 food, 168-169, 181, 1172

poison ivy, 188-189, 792-793, 793, 867-868, 867

poison oak, 188-189, 793, 831, 867-868, 867

poisons

 hemolytic anemia and, 1115

 hemotoxic, 189

 neurotoxic, 189

 safe storage of, 516-517

poison sumac, 188-189, 793, 867-868, 867

polio: see poliomyelitis

poliomyelitis/infantile paralysis/Heine-Medin disease: acute viral disease of the central nervous system characterized by fever, headache, sore throat, stiffness of the neck and back, and sometimes by paralysis and eventual atrophy of muscles, 433, 501, 517, 1101-1103, 1102

politeness, 504

pollen, 863, 1193-1194

pollen count, 1194

pollutant: something that pollutes the air, water, or soil

pollution, environmental, 753-775, 764

 kinds of, 753-756, 755, 759, 763, 769, 770

polychlorinated biphenyls, 767

polycystic: characterized by numerous cysts

polycystic kidney disease, 935, 1250

polycythemia: condition characterized by too many red blood corpuscles, 1119

polycythemia vera/erythremia: condition characterized by abnormally high number and proportion of red blood corpuscles

polyethylene socket, for joint, 1054

polymenorrhea: abnormally frequent menstruation, 992-993

polymorphonuclear leukocyte: see neutrophil

polymyositis: inflammation of a number of muscles and connective tissue, characterized by pain, swelling, and weakness, 1109

polyp: smooth growth or tumor found in the mucous membranes, as of the nose, bladder, uterus, or rectum

 in female reproductive system, 1016-1017

 miscarriage and, 585

 in stomach, 1277

"polypharmacy," 330

polyunsaturated: (of fats) tending to lower the cholesterol content of the blood, 697

 and blood cholesterol, 278

polyuria: escessive urination, 1249

polyvinyl chloride adhesive, respiratory allergy and, 865

pomade, 784, 839

pons: mass in the brain containing fibers that connect the medulla oblongata, the cerebellum, and the cerebrum, 360, *360*

pontic: in dentistry, a part of a bridge serving as a substitute for a missing tooth

popliteal: pertaining to the back part of the leg behind the knee

population, U.S., over age 65, *655*

pores in skin, 777

pork

    chart, *714*

    nutrients in, 701

    undercooked, danger in, 1171

portal vein: vein that conveys blood from the intestines and stomach to the liver

"port wine stain": hemangioma, 804

positive pressure breathing: breathing of air or other gas mixture at pressure greater than the surrounding atmospheric pressure

positron-emission tomography (PET), *1087*

posterior: toward the rear

posterior lobe hypophysis: the posterior part of the pituitary gland that produces hormones regulating kidney function and other vital processes, 402, *403*

posterior urethra: prostatic urethra

postmenopausal: being or occurring after menopause

postpartum: after childbirth

postural drainage: the loosening and draining of lung secretions by assuming a prone position with the head lower than the feet, 470

posture

    arthritis and, 1058

    backbone stress, 346-347, 352

    children's, 517-518

    as diagnostic clue, 881

    hemorrhoids, 950

    varicose veins, 966, 1125

pot *(slang):* marihuana

potassium, 208

dietary sources of, 922-923

loss of, in surgery, 922

teenagers' need for, 547

potassium permanganate, 1008

potatoes, nutrients in, 703

Pott's disease: tuberculosis or tissue destruction of the spinal vertebrae, causing angular, spinal curvature, 1067-1068

pox, great, 999, *1000. See also* syphilis.

PPD: purified protein derivative test for 894

Prader-Willi syndrome, 296

praise, effectiveness of, 476

precocity, 446

predaisone, 1293

prediabetic condition: diabetes, chemical

prednisolone, 208

prednisone, 209, 1100

pre-eclampsia: disorder of late pregnancy or following childbirth, 579. *See also* toxemia of pregnancy

preemie/premie: premature infant

pregnancy: condition or time of being pregnant, 575-591

    allergies during, 868

    anemia and, 846, 1118

    dental care in, 811, 812

    diabetes and, 1232

    diet during, 717

    ectopic, 585-586

    hair loss in, 630

    hiatus hernia and, 941-942, 1159

    medical checkups in, 426, 577

    periodontal disease in, 820

    spinal curvature in, 1066

    syphilis and, 1002, 1264

    unwanted, fear of, 605

    urinary infections and, 1257

    varicose veins and, 580-581

pregnant: carrying developing offspring in the uterus

preinvasive: before spreading to other tissues: said of malignant growths

prejudice, 518, 560

Preludin: phenmetrazine, 1366

premature: of a newborn baby, weighing less than 5 pounds, 589, 590

respiratory distress syndrome in, 499

premature ejaculation: ejaculation of semen during sexual intercourse before the female has had time to respond

premenopausal: being or occurring before menopause

premolar: *see* bicuspid

prenatal: before birth

prenatal care programs, 329

prenatal diagnosis: amniocentesis

preop: *see* preoperative

preoperative/preop: performed or occurring before a surgical operation, as shaving of the affected area, administration of certain drugs, etc., 904-908

prep: preparation of a patient for surgery, usu. including cleansing and shaving of the affected area

prepuce: the loose skin covering the head of the penis or the clitoris

presbyopia: farsightedness caused by aging of the lens or the muscles that expand and contract it, 1237, 1237

preschool child, 441-443

pressor: tending to raise blood pressure, as certain hormones, 422

pressure and hearing disorder, 1245

pressure points, 142, 143

pressure, sensation of, 354, 409, 777

pressurized aircraft and ear discomfort, 285

pretzels, nutrients in, 715

preventive measures, periodic checkups and, 876

preventive medicine: the branch of medical science concerned with preventing disease, as through immunological methods, 875

prickly heat/heat rash/miliaria: itchy rash of small red pimples caused by excessive sweating in hot weather, 521, 795

primaquine, 1302

primary:
1. not produced as a secondary effect or complication of another condition
2. original and not resulting from metastasis or other means of transmission, as a tumor or infection

primary teeth: *see* baby teeth

primidone, 1096

primipara: woman who is pregnant for the first time or who has borne one child

privacy, in family, 519

probenecid, 209

procarbazine, 1293

process: in anatomy, any outgrowth or projecting part of a larger structure, as the knobby portion of a vertebra, 340

proctologist: physician specializing in proctology, 215, 892

proctology: the branch of medicine that deals with the diagnosis and treatment of diseases of the lower colon, rectum, and anus, 214, 874, 892

proctoscope: surgical instrument for examining the interior of the rectum and part of the colon, 1273

proctoscopy: examination of the rectum and colon with the aid of a proctoscope, 1273

proctosigmoidoscope, 893

proctosigmoidoscopy: examination of the rectum and a portion of the colon (sigmoid) with the aid of a sigmoidoscope, 1273

prodrome: symptom resembling a premonition that signals the onset of a disease or of an epileptic seizure, 1093

profibrinolysin: the inactive precursor of fibrinolysin, an agent in the process of dissolving blood clots, 1112

profile, health, 622

progesterone: hormone of the ovary that prepares the uterus for receiving the fertilized ovum, 404, 407-408, 540, 1217

and corpus luteum cysts, 1015

prognathism:the condition of having a protruding jaw, esp. the lower

prognosis:prediction made by a doctor as to the probable course of a disease

Prohibition, 1339

prolactin: lactogenic hormone, 601

prolapse: move or slip forward or downward, as a displaced organ

prolapsed:slipped or moved from the usual place

promethazine, 209

pronate: turn, as the hand or foot, in a movement of pronation

pronation:

1. rotation of the hand or forearm so that the palm of the hand faces downward or backward

2. movement of the foot, as in improper walking, in which the sole is raised along the outer side and the toes turned out, often with an inward leaning of the ankle

prone: lying on the chest, with the face downward

proof: strength of alcohol in an alcoholic beverage, indicated by a proof number equal to twice the percentage of alcohol by volume (100 proof = 50% alcohol)

proof spirits, 1341

propantheline, 209

prophylactic: tending to ward off or prevent, as disease or conception

prophylactic therapy, in tuberculosis, 1190

prophylaxis: treatment intended to prevent disease, as the cleaning of teeth

dental, 809-810

propoxyphene, 209

propranolol: drug that causes blood vessels to dilate, used in the treatment of angina pectoris, 1134

prostate: partly muscular gland in males at the base of the bladder around the urethra that releases a fluid to convey

spermatozoa, *423*, 424, *424*, 425, 565, *565*, 926, *927*

cancer of, 929, 1260, 1280

sex hormones and, 675

disorders of, 674-675, 857, 926-927, 928-929, 1259-1260

impotence and, 688

enlarged benign:enlargement of the prostate gland resulting in difficulty in voiding and retention of urine in the bladder

examination of, 674-675, 1281

biopsy, 896

smear, 1281

hyperplasia of (enlarged), 674-675, 926-927, 1249

inflammation of: prostatitis

surgery of, 674, 927-929

prostatectomy: surgical removal of all or part of the prostate gland, 675, 927-929, *928*

prostatic urethra/posterior urethra: the part of the male urethra that passes across the prostate gland, 425

prostatitis: inflammation of the prostate gland, characterized by painful and excessive urination, 857

acute: severe, relatively uncommon form of prostatitis, marked by painful and excessive urination, high fever, and a discharge of pus from the penis, 857

prosthesis *(pl.,   prostheses)*/**prosthetic device:** artificial substitute for a missing or amputated part, as an arm or leg

prosthetic device: prosthesis

protein(s): any of a class of highly complex organic compounds, composed principally of amino acids, that occur in all living things and form an essential part of animal food requirements

in composition of body, 696

deprivation of, 718

dietary sources of, 696

digestion of, 386

and pregnancy, 717

rheumatoid arthritis and, 1059

synthesis of, by liver, 389

proteinuria: excretion of protein through the urine, 579

prothrombin: the inactive precursor of thrombin, an agent in the process of forming blood clots, 1112

protozoa (*sing., protozoon*): microscopic animal organisms that exist in countless numbers, including one-celled organisms and parasitic forms that cause malaria, sleeping sickness, and other diseases

protozoa, pathogenic, 996, 1300, 1302-1303, *1302*, 1304, 1305, 1306, *1306*

proud flesh: *see* granulation tissue

proximal: relatively near the center of the body or near a point considered as central. Compare *distal.*

proximal muscles: those muscles closest to the trunk of the body, such as the shoulder-arm and hip-thigh muscles

prunes, nutrients in, 708

pruritus: localized or general itching

anal: intense itching in the area of the anus

pseudoephedrine (isoephedrine), 209

pseudohypertrophic muscular dystrophy/Duchenne's muscular dystrophy: disease characterized by the enlargement and apparent over-development (hypertrophy) of certain muscles, esp. of the shoulder girdle, which subsequently atrophy

pseudoneoplasm: *see* pseudotumor

pseudotumor/pseudoneoplasm: condition that has the appearance of a tumor but is not a tumor, such as an inflammation, 1277-1278

psilocin, 1375

Psilocybe mexicana, 1375

psilocybin: derivative of the mushroom *Psilocybe mexicana*, which produces hallucinations in the user, 1375

psittacosis/parrot fever: infectious disease of parrots and other birds that can be transmitted to humans and cause symptoms like those of influenza

psoralen: chemical derived from a plant that is used in the treatment of psoriasis, 803

psoriasis: a noncontagious chronic condition of the skin, marked by bright red patches covered by silvery scales, 296, 801-803, *802*

arthritis and, 1064

and gout, 1061

and nails, loss of, 294

psoriatic arthropathy, 1064

Psychiatric Foundation, 319

psychiatrist: physician specializing in psychiatry, 217, 875

"board certified," 1331

psychiatry: the branch of medicine that treats disorders of the mind (or psyche), including psychoses and neuroses, 216, 875

psychic determinism, 1319-1321

psychoanalysis: system of psychotherapy originated by Sigmund Freud for treating emotional disorders by bringing to the attention of the conscious mind the repressed conflicts of the unconscious, 1319-1321, 1332-1333

psychoanalyst: one who practices psychoanalysis

psychodrama: psychotherapy in which a patient or group of patients act out situations centered about their personal conflicts in the presence of the therapist, 1334

psychogenic: caused by or contributed to by psychological factors

psychogenic symptoms, 1326

psychological counseling, 296

psychological dependence: emotional desire or need to continue using a drug

psychological evaluation, pre-operative, 905

psychologist: specialist in psychology, 1331

psychology: the science dealing with the mind, mental phenomena, consciousness, and behavior

psychomimetic: having properties capable of producing changes in behavior that mimic psychoses

drugs, 555

psychomotor: having to do with muscular movements resulting from mental processes

seizure, 480-481, 1094

psychomotor convulsion/temporal lobe convulsion: epileptic convulsion characterized by compulsive and often repetitious behavior of which the patient later has no memory

psychoneurosis: neurosis, 1323

psychopathic: *see* sociopathic

psychopharmacology, 297

psychophysiological/psychosomatic: pertaining to a class of disorders in which psychological factors contribute substantially to the physiological condition

psychophysiological disorders, 1326

psychosis (*pl., psychoses*): severe mental disorder often involving disorganization of the total personality, with or without organic disease, 1327-1330

LSD and, 1374

tranquilizers and, 1369

psychosomatic: pertaining to the effects of the emotions on body processes, esp. with respect to initiating or aggravating disease

complaints, 281, 1326

psychotherapist: specialist in psychotherapy, 1331

psychotherapy: the treatment of emotional and mental disorders by psychological methods, such as psychoanalysis, 1331, 1332-1334

alcoholism and, 1355

heroin addiction and, 1373

psychotic: one suffering from a psychosis

psychotropic: affecting the mind: said of certain drugs

ptomaine: substance derived from decomposing or putrefying animal or vegetable protein, rarely the cause of food poisoning, which is usu. caused by bacteria such as Salmonella

ptosis: drooping of the upper eyelid, 1108, 1110

ptyalin: enzyme in saliva that begins the chemical breakdown of starch, 380

puberty: period during which a person reaches sexual maturity and becomes functionally capable of reproduction, 297, 407, 444-445, 537-542, 1213

precocious: early menarche (first occurrence of menstruation), before the age of eight or nine

starvation diet and, 504

pubic: in the region of the lower abdomen

fracture, 1079

pubis: the lower anterior part of the hip bone, *341, 342*

Public Health Service, 1098

public housing, 692

puffed rice, nutrients in, 715

pulmonary: of or relating to the lungs, 214

pulmonary artery: artery, pulmonary

pulmonary emphysema: emphysema of the lungs; *see* emphysema

pulmonary tree, *393*

pulmonary tuberculosis: *see* tuberculosis

pulmonary vein: *see* vein, pulmonary

pulp:(of teeth) the soft tissue of blood vessels and nerves that fills the central cavity of a tooth, *339, 339, 807,* 808

pulp capping, 818

pulpotomy: surgical removal of the pulp of a tooth, 818

pulse: rhythmic pressure in the arteries due to the beating of the heart, 882, 918-919

measuring, in home care, 1038-1039

puncture wound: wound caused by an object that pierces the skin, as a nail or tack, involving increased danger of tetanus

punishment, 450, 519

pupil: contractile opening in the iris of the eye through which light reaches the retina, *409-410, 410,* 412-413, *412, 957*

purified protein derivative/PPD, 894

purine: one of a group of chemicals occurring naturally in certain foods and formerly implicated as a contributing cause of gout, 1062

purpura: blood disease characterized by hemorrhaging into the skin and mucous membranes, 1114

purulent: consisting of or secreting pus

pus: secretion from inflamed and healing tissues, usu. viscid or creamy, and containing decaying leukocytes, bacteria, and other tissue debris, 370

pustule: pus-filled bump on the skin, inflamed at the base

pyelitis: pyelonephritis

pyelogram: visualization of the kidney and ureter by X ray, 896, 1279

pyelonephritis/pyelitis: infection and inflammation of the kidneys, 1257-1258

pyloric sphincter: the ring of muscle surrounding the pylorus that acts as a valve, allowing food to pass from the stomach to the duodenum, 379, 383, 384, 937, 1156

pyloric stenosis: congenital condition in which the pylorus is too narrow to allow the stomach's contents to empty normally

pylorus: the opening between the stomach and the duodenum, 383

pyorrhea: discharge of pus, esp. when applied to the progressive inflammation of the gingival (gum) tissue, which may lead to loosening and loss of teeth, 849

pyrexia: *see* fever

pyrilamine/mepyramine, 210

pyrogenic: causing or inducing fever

pyrogenic arthritis, 1054, 1062

Q fever: infectious disease (rickettsial disease) transmitted by sheep and cattle and characterized by high fever, chills, and muscle pains

quacks, checklist on, 679

quadriplegia: paralysis of both arms and both legs

quadriplegic: one suffering from paralysis of both arms and both legs

quarrels, children's, 487-488

quinidine, 210

quinine: bitter substance obtained from the bark of the cinchona tree, used to treat malaria and myotonia, 1302

quinsy: *see* peritonsillar abscess

rabbit fever, 1093-1094

rabies/hydrophobia: acute viral disease of the central nervous system transmitted to humans by the bite or saliva of an infected animal, as a dog, bat, or squirrel, invariably fatal unless treated before symptoms appear, 163-164, *164*

racketball, *647*

radiation, exposure to, 755

and leukemia, 1291

and thyroid cancer, 1288

radiation sickness: illness caused by the body's absorption of excess radiation, marked by fatigue, nausea, vomiting, and sometimes internal hemorrhage and tissue breakdown

radiation therapy/radiotherapy: treatment of disease by radiation, as by X rays or other radioactive substances

in breast cancer, 1036, *1036*

with linear accelerator, *1026*, *1288*

in lymphoma, 1293

with radioactive iodine, 1214

with radioactive phosphorus, 1119

with radium needles, 1279

surgery and, *1239*, 1273

radical: of or involving procedures or treatment intended to go to the root of a disease and thereby eliminate it, as by excising an entire organ or part that is diseased

radiograph: X-ray photograph

radiography: X-ray photography

radioisotopes, in diagnosis, 892

radiologist: physician specializing in radiology, 875

radiology: the branch of medical science that deals with radiant energy, such as X rays and energy produced by radium, cobalt, and other radioactive substances, esp. in the diagnosis and treatment of disease, 875

radiopaque: impervious to X rays

radiotherapy: *see* radiation therapy

radishes, nutrients in, 703

radium needles, 1279

radius *(pl., radii):* the bone of the forearm on the same side as the thumb, thicker and shorter than the ulna bone, *341,* 344

rafampin, 210

ragweed, *1193,* 1194

rainy days, children's activities for, 454-455, *455*

raisins, nutrients in, 708

rale: abnormal sound heard in the chest with the aid of a stethoscope, indicating the presence of disease

rash(es)

allergic reactions and, 792-794

childhood, 520-521

symptomatic

of chicken pox, 461

of measles, 461, 504

of rheumatoid arthritis, 1059

of Rocky Mountain spotted fever, 502

of secondary syphilis, 1299

raspberries, nutrients in, 711

rats, plague and, 1294

rattlesnake bites, 189-190

Raynaud's disease: Raynaud's syndrome

Raynaud's syndrome/Raynaud's disease: condition characterized by spasms of small blood vessels when exposed to cold, esp. the fingers and toes, which become cyanotic (bluish) and then red, 297

razors, types of, 787-789

RBC: red blood cell; *see* erythrocyte

RBC (red blood cell) count, normal range, 886

Reach to Recovery program, 311, *311, 1035*

reaction time, aging and, 620

reading

children and, 522

in later years, 681

receptors, sense, *354,* 408

balance, 415-416

record players, noise level of, 519-520

records, medical

in home care, 1038-1041

transfer of, 283

recovery room: hospital room or section for patients immediately following surgery, where their post-operative conditions can be closely monitored, *916,* 917-918

rectocele: hernia in which part of the rectum protrudes through the wall of the vagina, 1012, *1012*

rectum: the terminal portion of the large intestine, extending from the sigmoid bend of the colon to the anus, *379, 384,* 391, *937*

cancer of, 944-946, 1272-1273

hernia of vagina and, 1012, *1012*

rectus abdominals, 248

red blood cells/erythrocytes/red blood corpuscles, *368,* 369, 371-373, *1113*

diseases of, 1114-1121

excess: *see* polycythemia

and malaria, 1302

red corpuscle: *see* erythrocyte

red marrow: marrow

reduce: move back into proper position, as a herniating bowel or the fragments of a broken bone

reducing: *see* weight reduction

reduction: manipulation back into proper position to restore normal function, as a fracture, dislocation, or herniated part

reduction of fractures, 970, 1076

referred pain: pain felt in one part of the body though originating in another part, as pain of the left shoulder and arm caused by a heart attack

reflex: involuntary response to a stimulus

spinal, 364

reflux: a flowing back, as of urine from the bladder up into the ureter

symptoms of, 961-963

voluntary agencies, 322-323

respiratory distress syndrome: *see* hyaline membrane disease

respiratory system, 392-402, *397*, *962*

diagnostic procedures for, 894

responsibilities

children and, 522

parental, 617-618

rest, 626

in arthritis, 671

restorations, dental, 810-811

resuscitation: mouth-to-mouth respiration

retardation, mental: *see* mental retardation

retention cyst: *see* cyst, follicular

reticulum: network of cells or cellular tissue

retina: the inner membrane at the back of the eyeball, containing light-sensitive rods and cones which receive the optical image, 410, *410*, *957*

blood vessels of, 1145

detached, 961, 1239-1240

retinoblastoma: tumor of the eye, found esp. in children, 458

retinopathy: diseased condition of the retina of the eye, *960*, 961

diabetic: *see* diabetic retinopathy

retinoscope: special device for examining the retina, 895

Retired Senior Volunteer Program, 684

retirement

activities in, 680-689

attitude toward, 656

and relocation, 690-691

retirement communities, 692

retirement housing, 689-693

Reye's syndrome, 297

Rh disease, 1120-1121

rhesus factor: Rh factor

rheumatic fever: acute infectious disease chiefly affecting children and young adults, characterized by painful inflammation around the joints, intermittent fever, and inflammation of the pericardium and valves of the heart, 523-524, 1065, 1132, 1146-1150

and delayed puberty, 539

prevention of, 1147

rheumatic heart disease: impairment of heart function as a result of rheumatic fever, 1132, 1148

rheumatism: painful inflammation and stiffness of muscles, joints, or connective tissue, 1051

rheumatoid arthritis: chronic disease characterized by swelling and inflammation of one or more joints, often resulting in stiffness and eventual impairment of mobility, 275, 671, 1051, 1054-1059, *1056*

voluntary agency, 307-309, *309*

rheumatoid arthritis, juvenile/Still's disease: form of rheumatoid arthritis affecting children, often characterized by fever, rash, pleurisy, and enlargement of the spleen as well as rheumatoid joint symptoms, *308*

rheumatoid spondylitis: *see* spondylitis, rheumatoid

rheumatologist: physician specializing in rheumatology, 873

rheumatology: subspecialty of internal medicine concerned with the study, diagnosis, and treatment of rheumatism and other diseases of the joints and muscles, 873, 887

Rh factor/rhesus factor: protein present in the blood of most people (called Rh-positive) and absent from others (called Rh-negative). Under certain conditions the blood of a pregnant Rh-negative woman may be incompatible with the blood of her fetus, 370-371, 509, 582, 1120-1121

rhinencephalon/"nose brain": the part of the brain controlling the sense of smell, 418

rhinitis: inflammation of the mucous membranes of the nose, 1192

rhinoplasty: plastic surgery of the nose, 630, 977-979, *978*

mental retardation and, 509

pregnancy and, 524-525, 581

rubbing alcohol, 1338

rubeola: measles

Rubin's test: tubal insufflation, 574

rudeness, 1323

rum, 1342

running, stress fracture and, 1075. *See also* jogging.

rupture:

1. any breaking apart, as of a blood vessel

2. hernia

Sabin vaccine: live polio vaccine taken orally to immunize against polio, 433, 436, 516, 1103

saccule, *416*

sacral: pertaining to the sacrum

sacroiliac: pertaining to the sacrum or the ilium, or to the places on either side of the lower back where they are joined

sacroiliac joint, 344, 1069

sacrum: bone in the lower spine formed by the fusing of five vertebrae, constituting the rear part of the pelvis, *341, 342*

saddle block: form of anesthesia used esp. for childbirth, in which the patient is injected in the lower spinal cord while in a sitting position, 595-596

safety glass: glass strengthened by any of various methods to reduce the likelihood of the glass shattering upon impact

St. Vitus's dance: chorea, 1147

sake, 1341

salad dressings, nutrients in, 716

salicylic acid preparations, foot care and, 674, 843

saline amniocentesis/salting out: technique of inducing abortion by injecting a saline solution into the amniotic fluid

saliva: fluid secreted by the salivary glands in the mouth that lubricates food and contains an enzyme (ptyalin) that begins to break down starch, 378-380, 418, 848, 1155

dental caries and, 380, 815

salivary glands: glands located in the mouth which secrete saliva, 378-380, *379, 381,* 400, 1156

disorders of, 1157

Salk Institute, 329

Salk vaccine: dead polio virus taken by injection to immunize against polio, 517, 1103

Salmonella: genus of aerobic bacteria that cause food poisoning and other diseases, including typhoid fever, *852*

Salmonella food poisoning, 1172

Salmonella typhosa: rod-shaped bacteria that cause typhoid fever, 1163

salmon, nutrients in, 701

salpingitis:

1. inflammation of a Fallopian tube, a potential cause of sterility, 1004

2. inflammation of a Eustachian tube

salt: sodium chloride

salt-free diets, 737-740, 1256

saltines, nutrients in, 713

saltiness: taste of, 380-381

salting out: the injection of a saline solution into the amniotic fluid to induce labor and thus terminate a pregnancy, 587

salt, iodized, 1214

salt-restricted diet, 737-740, 1256

salt, table: *see* sodium chloride

salt tablets, 837

sanatorium rest cure, 1188

sandfly, 1304-1305

sanguine disposition, *1329*

saphenous vein: either of two large, superficial veins of the leg, a common site of varicosity

sarcoid: *see* sarcoidosis

sarcoidosis/Boeck's sarcoid/sarcoid: disease of unknown cause with symptoms resembling those of tuberculosis, marked by the formation of nodules, esp. on the skin, lungs, and lymph nodes, 1190

sarcoma: malignant tumor that arises in the connective tissue (bones, cartilage, tendons), 1268

sarcoma, Ewing's: *see* Ewing's sarcoma

sardines, nutrients in, 701

saturated: (of fats) tending to increase the cholesterol content of the blood

saucerization: procedure of forming a shallow depression by scraping away tissue to assist healing, 933-934

sausage, nutrients in, 701

scabies/the itch: contagious inflammation of the skin caused by a mite and characterized by a rash and intense itching, 797

scag *(slang):* heroin

scalp, 359

scan: to measure for diagnostic purposes the concentration in a particular area of a radioactive material that has been introduced into the body. *See also* CAT scan.

scapula: shoulder blade, 340, *341*

scarlet fever: contagious disease caused by streptococci and characterized by a scarlet rash and high fever, 525, 1146

scar reduction, 982

Schistosoma, life cycle of, 1312-1313, *1312, 1313*

schistosomiasis/bilharziasis: tropical disease caused by a fluke worm (trematode) whose larvae penetrate the skin and invade the circulatory system, 1312-1314, *1314*

and bladder cancer, 1280

schizoid:

1. describing a personality disorder in which the individual is withdrawn from and indifferent to other people, 1327

2. pertaining to or resembling schizophrenia

schizophrenia: 1327-1328

catatonic: schizophrenia marked by motor disturbances, such as maintenance of fixed, often awkward, position with muscles rigid, 1327-1328

hebephrenic: schizophrenia marked by delusions, hallucinations, and regressed or childish behavior, 1327

paranoid: schizophrenia marked by variable delusions of persecution or grandeur, often with hallucinations and behavioral deterioration, 1328

schizophrenic: of or pertaining to schizophrenia

schizophrenic reaction/schizophrenia: psychosis characterized by withdrawal from external reality and a retreat into a fantasy life, with deterioration of behavior, 1327

Schlemm, canals of, 414

school, 525-526, *525*

reports, 489

schoolboy *(slang):* codeine

sciatica: pain along the sciatic nerve, 189, 836, 1067, 1068

sciatic nerve: nerve of the lower spine that traverses the hips and runs down the back of the thigh of each leg

SCID, 291

sclera: the firm outer coat of the eye continuous with the cornea, visible as the white of the eye, *410*, 413, *957*

sclerose: to harden and thicken, as tissue

sclerosis: abnormal thickening and hardening of tissue, as of the lining of arteries

amyotrophic lateral/Lou Gehrig's disease: disease characterized by increasing muscle weakness (atrophy) or paralysis, caused by the progressive degeneration of motor nerve cells in the brain and spinal cord, 363

multiple, 320-321, 363, 364, 1098-1101

scoliosis: spine, lateral curvature, 969, *1066*, 1067

scopolamine, 594

scorpion stings, 189

scratch test: skin test for allergic response to different substances by applying suspected allergens in diluted form to scratches, 869-870

screw(s), metal, in fractures, 970, *971*, 1076, *1077*

scrofula: tuberculosis of the lymph nodes, esp. of the neck

scrotum: pouch that contains the testicles, 424, 541

cancer of, 754, 929

scrub nurse: operating room nurse authorized to handle sterilized equipment in assisting the surgeon, 910-911, *933*

scurvy: disease characterized by livid spots under the skin, swollen and bleeding gums, and prostration, caused by lack of vitamin C

seasickness: motion sickness

seat belt(s), *1081*

sebaceous cyst: hard, round, movable mass contained in a sac, resulting from accumulated oil from a blocked sebaceous gland duct

sebaceous gland: gland within the dermis that secretes oil (sebum) for lubricating the skin and hair, *354*, 355, 357, 400, 777, *777*

and chapped skin, 839, *839*

overactive, 543

skin condition and, 780

seborrhea: abnormal increase of secretion from the sebaceous skin glands.

sebum: fatty lubricating substance secreted by the sebaceous glands, 357

secobarbital, 210

secondary: produced as an effect or complication of another condition, as distinguished from *primary*

secondary disease: disorder of a target gland caused by an excess or deficiency of a stimulating hormone supplied by the anterior pituitary gland

security, need for, 680

sedation: reduction of sensitivity to pain, stress, etc., by administering a sedative

pre-operative, 908

sedative: medicine for allaying irritation or nervousness, 195, 626, 905, 1334

sedentary activity, calorie expenditure in, 721

sedentary habits, and heart attacks, 219

seizure: *see* convulsion

self-expression, need for, 646, 680

self-medication, 622, 640, 1360

in diabetes, 1225, *1225*, *1230*

semen: thick, whitish fluid containing spermatozoa that is ejaculated by the male at orgasm, 565

examination of, 573

and nocturnal emission, 541-542

semicircular canals: three fluid-filled tubes of the inner ear that govern the sense of balance and communicate with the vestibular nerve, 415, *416*, *417*, *955*

seminal fluid: *see* semen

seminal vesicle: one of two small pouches on either side of the prostate gland that serve to store spermatozoa temporarily, 404, *424*, 425, *565*, 565-566, 610

seminiferous tubules, *424*, 927

senile macula degeneration: visual defect affecting the elderly, 672

senile psychosis/senile dementia: mental disorder of the aged characterized by progressive deterioration of the personality, irritability, loss of memory, etc.

senile purpura: small hemorrhages in the skin of older people, 666

senility: state of being senile

nerve cell loss and, 363

sensation, and skin, 354, 409

loss of, in leprosy, *1315*, 1316

sense(s), 354, 356, 408-418

aging and, 654

sense organs, diagnostic procedures, 895-896

sense receptor cells, 408

sensory area in brain, 358-359, *360*, *361*

sensory messages, 1074

sensory neuron, *363*

separated retina: retina, detached

separation

fear of, 438, *441*

marital, 649-652

sepsis: infection of the blood by disease-causing microorganisms

septicemia: blood poisoning

septic shock: shock resulting from infection of the blood by disease-causing microorganisms, 144

muscles of, 350, *350*

shouting, and hard-of-hearing, 669

shower bath, 780

shrimp, nutrients in, 701

shunt, aortal-pulmonary, 965

siblings

as baby sitters, *613*

rivalry of, 446, 456-457, *512*

sick headache: *see* migraine

sickle-cell anemia:hereditary disease occurring most commonly among Negro men and women, in which many or a majority of the red blood cells are sickle-shaped, producing chronic anemia, 1117-1118

genetic counseling and, 583

sickle-cell trait/sicklemia: trait in the genetic make-up of an individual that could cause sickle-cell anemia in his offspring if the other parent also has the trait, 1117-1118

sickle cells, 373, 1117

sickroom, equipment for, 1046, 1047-1048

side effects of drugs, 195, 1075, 1361-1362

SIDS (sudden infant death syndrome), 529-530

sigmoid:

1. *(adj.)* shaped like the letter S

2. *(n.)* (sigmoid colon/sigmoid flexure) S-shaped fold in the colon of the large intestine just above the rectum, *379*, 391, *937*, 1156

sigmoid colon: *see* sigmoid 2

sigmoid flexure: *see* sigmoid 2

sigmoidoscope: surgical instrument for examining the interior of the sigmoid, 1273

sign (of disease): observable or objective manifestation, as distinguished from symptoms reported by the patient, 878

silica: extremely hard mineral, the chief constituent of quartz and sand

silica dust, lung disease and, 1207

silicone, in mammoplasty, 979-980

silicosis: lung disorder, a form of pneumoconiosis, caused by inhaling silica dust, as of stone or sand, 755

silver nitrate solution, eyes of newborn and, 316

simple fracture: closed fracture

Simultaneous Multiple Analyzer tests

(SMA-12), 898

(SMA-24), 898

sinoatrial node: sinus node

sinus: opening or cavity, as in bone, or a channel or passageway, as for blood

sinuses, paranasal, 399-400

sinusitis:inflammation of a sinus, 275, 1182-1183

sinus node/sinoatrial node: small mass of nerve tissue in the right atrium of the heart that triggers heart contractions and regulates heartbeat, thus serving as cardiac pacemaker, 376

sitz bath:hot bath taken in a sitting position, 794

6-Mercoptopurine, 1292

skating, 624

skeletal muscle/voluntary muscle: striated muscle attached to bones and joints, used chiefly in voluntary action, 347, 350-351. Compare *smooth muscle.*

trouble spots in, 353

skeletal system

diagnostic procedures for, 887-888

diseases of, 1049-1083

friction in, 352

trouble spots in, 346-347

skeleton, 337-347, *341*

appendicular: the bones of the arms, hands, legs, and feet, 342-344

axial: the bones of the head and the trunk, 338-339, 342

skiing, 624

skin/integument: the outer, membranous covering of the body, consisting of an outer layer (epidermis) and inner layer (dermis), 353-356, *354*, 408, 409, 776-782

aging of, 629-630, 665-667, 778-779

speech
babies and, 438-439, 531
brain area of, 277, *360*
deafness and, 470-471, 669, 1247
defects, 528-529
disorders of, 478, 528-529
slurred, in cerebral palsy, 1088
stroke and, 1128
speech reading: lip reading
speech therapy, *321*, 528-529, 1088, *1287*
speed *(slang):* methamphetamine
speed freak *(slang):* heavy user of methamphetamine (speed), esp. by intravenous injection, to induce altered mental state
sperm: spermatozoa
spermatozoa *(sing., spermatozoon)/***sperm/sperm cells:** male reproductive cells or gametes, one of which must fertilize an ovum to produce an embryo, 424, 565-566, 1215
fertility tests on, 573
temperature and, 424-425
sperm banks, 931
sperm cell: the male reproductive cell, one of the spermatozoa
sperm cells: spermatozoa
sperm ducts: vas deferens
spermicide: contraceptive substance that destroys sperm, 609
sphincter(s): ringlike muscle surrounding an opening or tube that serves to narrow or close it
of digestive tract, *379*, 382-383, *384*, 1155, *1156*, 1159, 1160
urinary, 422
sphygmomanometer: device for measuring arterial blood pressure, *377*, 881-882, *881*, *882*, 1144
spiders
black widow, 166
brown house (recluse), 169
spinach, nutrients in, 703, 704
spinal: *see* spinal anesthesia

spinal anesthesia/spinal: form of anesthesia in which the patient is injected in the region of the spinal cord, 916
spinal arthritis: arthritis of the spine, found esp. in the elderly, 1054
spinal column/backbone/spine: the series of segmented bones (vertebrae) which enclose the spinal cord and provide support for the ribs, 338, 339-340
curvatures of, 1066-1067
fracture of, 165, 970, 1082-1083
fusion of
pathological, 1059-1060
therapeutic, 969, 970, 1069
infection of, 1064, 1068
injury to, 1082-1083
musculature of, 352
stresses on, 346-347, 352
tumors of, 1068
spinal cord: the part of the central nervous system enclosed within the spinal column, 340, 359
spinal erectors, 348
spinal fluid: *see* cerebrospinal fluid
spinal fluid exam: spinal tap
spinal meningitis, 1101
spinal nerves, 362
spinal puncture: spinal tap
spinal reflex: reaction to an outside stimulus that originates in the spinal cord and bypasses the brain, 364
spinal tap/lumbar puncture/spinal fluid exam/spinal puncture: needle puncture and withdrawal of cerebrospinal fluid from the lower spinal column for diagnostic examination, 359, 888, 1085
spine: *see* spinal column
spirochete: any of various spiral-shaped bacteria, some of which cause syphilis and yaws, 999, *1001*, 1261
spleen: vascular, ductless organ located near the stomach that produces red blood cells in infancy and modifies blood composition, 372, 1121
enlargement of, 1119

splint: appliance for supporting or immobilizing a part of the body, as a fractured bone, 182, 1077

splinters, 190

spondylitis: inflammation of the vertebrae of the spine

    rheumatoid/ankylosing spondylitis: chronic disease characterized by inflammation of the spine and resulting in the fusing (ankylosing) of the spinal joints, 1059-1060

spondylolisthesis: forward displacement of one of the lower vertebrae over the vertebra below it or over the sacrum, causing severe pain in the lower back, 969, 1069

sponge baths, 779-780

spontaneous abortion: miscarriage

spoon-feeding of bedridden patient, 1044

sporadic: characterized by scattered cases, as of a disease, rather than by concentration in one area

spore: single-celled reproductive body of a flowerless plant, capable of developing into an independent organism

sports

    in later years, 662-663

    in middle years, 623-625

    in teens, *548*, 548-550

sprain: the stretching or rupturing of ligaments, usu. accompanied by damage to blood vessels, 190-191, *191*

spur, bone, 1054

sputum: expectorated matter, as saliva, sometimes mixed with mucus, 895, 1182, 1188

sputum cup, 1048

sputum exam: bacteriological, chemical, and microscopic testing of sputum for presence of disease, 894

squabbles, children's, 487-488

squamous cell

    cancer, 666

    sunlight and, 666

squash (food), 704

squash (sport), 624

squint/strabismus, 467, 511

stapedius: small muscle in the tympanum of the middle ear whose function is to dampen loud sounds, 1089

stapes: stirrup, 414, *417*, 955, *955*

staph: *see* staphylococcus

staphylococcus (*pl., staphylococci*)/**staph:** parasitic bacterium that can cause boils and other infections

    aureus: bacterium that causes food poisoning

    infections and, 798, *852*, 1072

starches, 380, 696-697

startle reflex: *see* startle response

startle response/startle reflex: complex involuntary reaction to sudden noise occurring esp. in infancy, where it is marked by a sudden jerk of the arms and legs, 426

State Commission on Aging, 685

static exercises: isometrics, 236-237

statis dermatitis, 666

status, children and, 464, 561

status epilepticus: series of epileptic seizures, occurring virtually without interruption, 1093

steak, nutrients in, 690

stealing, by children, 477

steam inhalation, 854

steam inhalators (vaporizers), 536, 1046, 1205

    improvised, 175, 187, 1046

    types of, 1205-1206

stenosis: the narrowing of a duct or canal in the body

    valvular, 289, 1148

stepchildren, 447, 651-652

stepparents, 651-652

sterile:

    1. being incapable of producing offspring

    2. being free of germs

sterility:

    1. condition of being incapable of producing offspring

2. condition of being free of germs

gonorrhea and, 1004

mumps and, 510

tight clothing and, 541

sterilization: the process of destroying reproductive capacity by surgical means, as by tying the Fallopian tubes of a woman (tubal ligation) or by tying the seminal duct of a man (vasectomy)

voluntary

female, 610

male: *see* vasectomy

voluntary agencies, 316, 324-325

sternum, 340, *341,* 395

fractures of, 1081-1082

steroid(s): any of a group of organic compounds occurring naturally and produced synthetically, including the sex hormones, the bile acids, oral contraceptives, and many drugs, 195, 390

in arthritis, 1054, 1058

and patchy baldness, 631

in purpura, 1114

side effects of, 195

See also cortisone.

stethoscope: diagnostic device that conducts sounds produced within the body, as the heartbeat, to the ear of the examiner, *879,* 880, 881, *881, 882*

stiffness, arthritic, 1055, *1056*

exercise and, 1058

stiff toe: pain and stiffness in the joint of the big toe, 628

stilbestrol: *see* diethylstilbestrol

Still's disease: *see* rheumatoid arthritis, juvenile

stimulant: drug or other substance that increases or agitates the physiological processes of body or mind, 195, 300, 551-556. Compare *depressant*

stimulus (*pl., stimuli*): that which initiates an impulse or affects the activity of an organism

sting ray, sting of, 191

stirrup/stapes: the innermost of the three ossicles of the middle ear, the bone

between the anvil and the cochlea, 414, 416, *417,* 955, *955*

stitch in the side, 300

stockings, elastic, 581, 846, 1125

Stokes-Adams syndrome: sudden unconsciousness and sometimes convulsions caused by heart block, 1154

stoma: small opening in a surface, as in a membrane or wall of a blood vessel

stomach, 352, *379,* 383-385, *384, 386,* 1155, *1156,* 1157

diseases of, 1160-1165, 1275-1278

disorders of, 529, 736

aspirin and, 275

laxatives and, 292

displacement of, 941-942, 1159

gas in, 292, 1160

lining, inflammation/gastritis, 1168

surgery of, 940-941, 943-944

tumors of, 943-944, 1267, 1275-1278, *1276*

ulcers of: *see* peptic ulcer

stomach (region), exercises to relax, 625-626

stones

gallstones, 390, 947-948

in prostate, 929

in salivary glands, 1157

urinary, 932-933, 1010

stool/feces

blood in, 1273

in celiac disease, 459

See also feces.

stool exam: laboratory analysis of feces, as for presence of blood or parasitic organisms, 893

STP: DOM, 1376

stabismus/squint: disorder of the eye muscles in which one eye drifts so that its position is not parallel with the other, 467, 957-958

strain: excessive stretching of a muscle, tendon, or ligament, *191,* 191-192

stratum corneum: the outermost layer of the epidermis, consisting of horny, lifeless cells, 356 strawberries, nutrients in, 711

strawberry mark, 804

strep throat: streptococcal infection of the throat, 524, 528, 533, 1065

streptococcal: of or relating to the streptococcus bacterium

streptococcus: kind of bacteria including some forms that cause diseases, as pneumonia and scarlet fever, *816*

and impetigo, 798

and nephritis, 1254-1255

and rheumatic fever, 523-524, 1065, 1146, 1147

and scarlet fever, 525

stress, emotional

aging and, 620, 621

angina and, 289

asthma and, 451

bedwetting and, 1261

hyperthyroidism and, 1214

indigestion and, 1160

infertility and, 570-571

in middle age, 620, 642

nausea and, 511

stress fracture: tiny crack in a bone caused by repeated stress, 1075

stress, mechanical and skeletal system, *345*, 346-347, *351*, 352

stretchers, 159, *160*, 161

stretch marks, 590

striated: striped, as certain muscle

striated muscle: *see* skeletal muscle

striped muscle: *see* skeletal muscle

stripping: surgical removal of lengths of varicosed veins, esp. one of the saphenous veins of the leg, 967

stroke/apoplexy: attack of paralysis caused by the rupture of an artery and hemorrhage into the brain, or by an obstruction of an artery, as from a blood clot, 670-671, 1127-1130

emergency treatment for, 192

rehabilitation, *244*, 670-671, 1128

STS test, 1003

study groups, 649

stupor: condition in which the senses and faculties are suspended or greatly dulled, as from shock, drugs, etc.

stuttering, 528-529

sty: small, inflamed swelling of a sebaceous gland on the edge of the eyelid, 192, 855

subacute: intermediate between *acute* and *chronic*: said of a disease

subarachnoid: situated or occurring between the middle layer (arachnoid) and the innermost layer (pia mater) of the brain

subconscious, 1319, 1321

subcutaneous: situated or applied beneath the skin

subcutaneous injection: an injection given in the subcutaneous tissue beneath the skin

subcutaneous tissue: layer of fatty tissue below the skin (dermis) which acts as an insulator against heat and cold and as a shock absorber against injury, *354*, *355*, *777*, *778*

swelling of, 866

subdural: situated or occurring between the outermost layer (dura mater) and the middle layer (arachnoid) of the brain

subdural hematoma: *see* hematoma, subdural

subjective: (of symptoms) of a kind that only the patient is aware of. Compare *objective.*

sublingual gland: either of a pair of salivary glands located beneath the tongue, 378

submandibular gland: submaxillary gland, 378

submaxillary gland/submandibular gland: either of a pair of salivary glands located under each side of the lower jaw, 378

subtotal: less than total, as a surgical procedure involving the excision of an organ or part

sucking, 437, 514, 601

sudden infant death syndrome/crib death/ SIDS: death of an infant, usu. between one and six months of age and without any preceding sign of distress and of undetermined cause, 529-530

sudoriferous gland: *see* sweat gland

sugar

blood: *see* glucose

food, 696, 716

and tooth decay, 473, 812, 815

suicide, 300, 1328

sulfa drug: any of a group of organic compounds used in the treatment of a variety of bacterial infections, 195, 1005, 1006

sulfamethoxazole, 210

sulfisoxazole, 210

sulfonamide(s):any of a group of chemical compounds including the sulfa drugs, used in the treatment of bacterial infections

allergic reaction to, 865

sulfone drugs, 1317

sulfonylurea: drug used to treat diabetes, 1228

sulfur, in teenage diet, 546

sulfur dioxide

as air pollutant, 757-758, 1202

headache and, 832

respiratory tract and, 758

sulindac (Clinoril), 1057

sunburn, *192*, 192-193, 837-838

sunlight

and aging of skin, 665

and cancer of skin, 779, 1273-1275

and psoriasis, 802

and vitamin D, 1072

sunstroke/heatstroke: condition marked by an acutely high fever and the cessation of perspiration, caused by prolonged exposure to heat and sometimes leading to convulsions and coma, 185, 839

suntan, 356

suntan lotions, 837-838

superego/conscience: largely unconscious element of the personality, regarded as dominating the ego, for which it acts

principally in the role of conscience and critic, 1320

superficial: of, situated near, or on the surface

Superintendent of Documents, U.S. Government Printing Office, 722, 1028

superior vena cava: the large vein that brings blood from the upper part of the body to the heart

supination: rotation of the hand or forearm so that the palm of the hand faces upward or forward

supine: lying on the back, with the face upward

suppository: solid, usu. cylindrical medicated preparation that liquefies from heat after insertion in a body cavity, as the rectum or the vagina

contraceptive, 609

suppuration: the formation of pus

suppurative: characterized by the formation of pus; pussy

suramin, 1308

surgeon: physician who specializes in the diagnosis and treatment of disease by means of surgery, *907*, *943*

surgery: the branch of medicine dealing with the correction of disorders or other physical change by operation or manipulation, 872, 900-987

for accidental amputation, repair of, 986-987

advances in, 924

for aging skin, 667, 976-980

for appendicitis, 391, 938-939

authorization for, 907-908

for breast cancer, 1033-1035

for cervical cancer, 1023

for colitis, 1168-1169

for colon-rectum cancer, 892, 944-946, 1272-1273

and congenital heart disease, 965, 1132, 1152

coronary artery, *917*, 1134-1137

cosmetic, 631, 976-980

for diverticulosis, 1167

surgical: of or relating to surgery

surgical diathermy: electrosurgery

suture:

1. to sew together cut or separated edges, as of a wound, to promote healing

2. the thread, wire, gut, etc., used in this process

suture line: line formed by the edges of the separate bones of a baby's skull, 339

sweat gland/sudoriferous gland: any of numerous glands that secrete sweat, found almost everywhere in the skin except for the lips and a few other areas, 354, 357-358

swimmer's itch: mild form of schistosomiasis in which parasitic fluke worm larvae invade the skin of swimmers, causing dermatitis, 1314

sycosis/barber's itch: bacterial infection of the hair follicles, marked by inflammation, itching, and the formation of pus-filled pimples, 798

sympathetic nervous system: the part of the autonomic nervous system that controls such involuntary actions as the dilation of pupils, constriction of blood vessels and salivary glands, and increase of heartbeat, 362. Compare *parasympathetic nervous system*.

symptom: change in one's normal feeling or condition of well-being, indicating the presence of disease, 878

symptomatic: having observable symptoms of a disease or condition. Compare *asymptomatic*.

symptomatology: the combined symptoms of a disease

Synanon: organized live-in community of drug addicts in which group psychotherapy is used to encourage rehabilitation, 1373

synapse: the junction point between two neurons, across which a nerve impulse passes from the axon of one neuron to the dendrite of another, *363*, 363-364

syncope: temporary loss of consciousness; fainting

syndrome: set of symptoms occurring at the same period and indicating the presence or nature of a disease

synovia/synovial fluid: viscid, transparent fluid secreted as a lubricating agent in the interior of joints and elsewhere, 888

synovial aspiration/synovial fluid exam: laboratory analysis of synovia, withdrawn from joints by needle, in order to diagnose gout or certain forms of arthritis, 888

synovial fluid: synovia

synovial fluid exam: synovial aspiration, 888

synthetic chemicals, occupational hazards of, 755

syphilis: contagious venereal disease transmitted by sexual contact and congenitally to offspring of infected mothers, 999-1003, 1261-1264

and arteritis, 1124

and arthritis, 1064-1065

free clinics for, 1003

congenital, 1002, 1264

and mental retardation, 509

and teenagers, 568

test for, 898

voluntary agencies, 323-324

syringes, insulin, *1225*

syrup, nutrients in, 716

systemic: pertaining to or affecting the body as a whole

systole: the instant of peak pumping action of the heart, when the ventricles contract and blood is impelled outward into the arteries, followed immediately by relaxation (diastole), 377

systolic pressure: measure of blood pressure taken when the heart is contracting, the higher of the two figures in a reading, 881, 1144-1145

tabes dorsalis/locomotor ataxia: form of syphilis involving demyelination of spinal nerves and other destructive changes in the spinal cord, 1002

table tennis, 624

tachycardia: abnormally rapid heartbeat

paroxysmal: attacks of abnormally rapid heartbeat (tachycardia) that begin and end abruptly, 847, 1119

Tagamet: cimetidine, 1166

talc particles, lung disease and, 1207

tampon: plug of absorbent material for insertion in a body cavity or wound to stop bleeding or absorb secretions

T and A operation: *see* adenotonsillectomy

tangerines, nutrients in, 711

tankers and oil pollution, 763-765

tapeworm/cestode: any of various worms with segmented, ribbonlike bodies; often of considerable length, that are parasitic on the intestines of humans and other vertebrates, 1169-1170, *1170*

target gland: any of the endocrine glands that function when stimulated by hormones secreted by the anterior pituitary, as the thyroid, adrenal cortex, testicles, or ovaries

tar medications

dandruff and, 786

psoriasis and, 803

tarsal: any of the bones of the tarsus, or ankle, *344*

tarsus: ankle, *344*

tartar (dental calculus), 815

tartar emetic, 1313

Task Force on Research Planning in Environmental Health Science, 753, 755-756, 769

taste bud: one of the clusters of cells in the tongue that contain receptors for discriminating salt, sweet, sour, or bitter tastes, 380-381, *1156*

taste, sense of, *361*, 409, 417-418

aging and, 273

and food acceptance, 378

loss of, in Bell's palsy, 1089

receptors: *see* taste buds

Tay-Sachs disease, 293

TD (tetanus-diphtheria toxoid) immunization schedule, 500

tea, caffeine in, 638

teacher(s)

as authority figures, 525-526

and sex education, 564

tears, 413-414

teenagers, 537-569, *560*

alcohol and, 553, 1340

as baby sitters, 615-616

and barbiturate abuse, 1367-1368

daily food requirements of, *546*, 705

progressive exercises for, 252-263

rhinoplasty and, 978

smoking and, 1198

and venereal disease, 568

teeth, 805-827

artificial: *see* dentures

broken, 194

cleaning of, 812-814, *814*, 1158

development of, 441

and diet, 435, 1158

and digestion, 378, *379*, 380, *1156*

extraction of, 817-818

grinding of, 821, 825

permanent, 441, 805-806, *807*

primary, 441, 805, 806

structure of, 339, *339*, 806-808, *807*

See also dental care; orthodontics; tooth decay.

teething: process by which new teeth break (erupt) through the gums in infants and young children, 435, 531-532, 805

earache and, 479

teething biscuits, 435

television

audibility level of, 519

children and, 443, 448, 520

and eyestrain, 856

temperament, and body humors, *1329*

temperance movement, 1338

temperature, body, 1039-1040

basal, 573

control of, 354, 357

measurement of, 486, *1038*, 1039-1040

normal, 919, 1039-1040

of skin, effect of smoking on, 552, 1197

in sunstroke, 185, 839

of tumors, 1030, *1030*

variation of, 276, 919

tempered glass: safety glass that has high resistance to blunt objects and breaks by crumbling into small fragments instead of shattering

temper tantrum, 449-450, 489

temporal lobe: the portion of each cerebral hemisphere of the brain in back of and partly below the frontal lobes, the centers for hearing, 360

temporal lobe convulsions: convulsions, psychomotor

tendinitis: inflammation of a tendon, 844

tendon: band of tough, fibrous connective tissue that binds a muscle to another part, as a bone, and by means of which muscular force can be exerted on other parts of the body, *351*, 351-352

shortened, in rheumatoid arthritis, 1055

inflammation of, 844-845

tendon sheath, inflammation of: tenosynovitis

tennis, 229, 623

heart patients and, 296

tennis elbow: pain in the outer side of the elbow joint, usu. caused by a too vigorous twisting motion of the hand that strains a tendon or inflames a bursa, 844

tenosynovitis: inflammation of the sheath that covers a tendon, 844-845

tension

and backache, 673

exercises for, 625-626

and food, 752-753

and infertility, 570-571

in middle age, 642-643

premenstrual, 993-994

tension headache: severe headache induced by tension, which causes unconscious constriction of head and neck muscles, 834

terminal illness, 279, 693-694

and the hospice, 330-331

Terramycin: trade name for the antibiotic tetracycline, 195

testes: testicles

testicle(s)/testis (*pl., testes*): one of a pair of male reproductive glands (gonads) that produce spermatozoa and male sex hormones, situated in a pouch (scrotum) at the base of the penis, 407-408, *424*, 424-425, 1215-1217, *1216*

inflammation of, 510

tumor of, 929, 1216

undescended, 541, 930, 1216, 1217

testicular failure, 636

testis: *see* testicle

testosterone: male sex hormone manufactured in the testicles, 407, 1215

tests, diagnostic

admission lab, 898

batteries, 897-898

tetanus/lockjaw: acute bacterial infection usu. introduced through a puncture wound, leading to muscle spasms, esp. of the jaw muscles, and often fatal, 302, 433, 500, 532

in pregnancy, 582

tetanus-diphtheria toxoid: 500

booster, 301

tetany: nerve disorder characterized by muscle spasms and sometimes convulsions, caused by too little calcium in the blood, 407

tetracycline: crystalline powder isolated from a soil bacillus that forms the base of several antibiotics, including Aureomycin and Terramycin, 195.

tetrahydrocannabinol/THC: principal compound of cannabis (hashish or marihuana), believed to be the active ingredient, 1577

thalamus: round mass of gray matter at the base of the brain that transmits sensory impulses to the cerebral cortex

thalassemia/Cooley's anemia: form of anemia caused by inherited abnormality of red blood cells, often fatal in utero

thalidomide, 577, 583

THC: tetrahydrocannabinol, 1377

theophylline (aminophylline, oxtriphylline), 211

therapeutic: designed or tending to heal or to cure disease

therapist: *see* psychotherapist

therapy: treatment of a disease by a prescribed method or medicine

thermogram: measurement of the surface temperature of a region of the body, such as the breast, with an infrared sensing device, 1030, *1030*

thermography: technique of measuring the surface temperature of a region of the body, such as the breast, with an infrared sensing device, 1030, *1032*

thermometer(s), 1039-1040, 1048

thiamine/vitamin B₁: vitamin found in cereal grains, green peas, liver, egg yolk, and other sources, and also made synthetically, that protects against beriberi

thighbone

fracture of, *1078*

slipped epiphysis of, 1070

thighs, exercises for, 242-243, 271, *271*

"Thinking About Drinking" (pamphlet), 1357

thiopental/Pentothal, 914, 1367

thiotepa, 1279

thiourea, 1317

thirst, as symptom, 672, 1223

thoracic: of or relating to the thorax, or chest cavity

thoracic cage: see rib cage

thoracic cavity: see chest cavity

thoracic lymph duct, 374

thoracic spine: see vertebrae, thoracic

thoracic surgeon: surgeon specializing in thoracic surgery, having to do with the chest cavity, 875, 890, 894

thoracic surgery: branch of surgery having to do with the chest cavity and its organs, the heart and lungs, and large blood vessels

thoracic vertebrae, 340, 341

thorax: chest, 1178

Thorazine/chlorpromazine: trademark for a commonly used tranquilizer, 195, 199, 639

threadworm, 1171

throat: see pharynx

throat-clearing, habit of, 511

throat, sore: see pharyngitis

thrombin: enzyme present in the blood that reacts with fibrinogen to form fibrin in the process of clotting, 1112

thrombocytes: platelets

thromboembolism: obstruction of a blood vessel by a blood clot (thrombus) that has broken away from the place where it was formed, 607

thrombophlebitis: formation of a blood clot (thrombus) in the wall of an inflamed vein (phlebitis), 1124, 1209, 1210

thromboplastin: substance found in blood platelets that helps to convert prothrombin into thrombin in the clot-ting process, 1112

thrombosis: formation of a blood clot (thrombus) in a blood vessel, resulting in the partial or complete blocking of circulation, 1126

coronary, 1137

thrombus: stationary blood clot within a blood vessel, 1127, 1137

thrush: fungus infection in the mouth, esp. of infants, characterized by white patches that become sores, 1158

thumb-sucking, 511, 825

thymectomy: surgical removal of the thymus, 1110

thymus: glandlike lymphoid organ located near the base of the neck, believed to play a role in the body's immunological responses, 401, 408, 1212

tumor of, 1110

thyroid gland: endocrine gland located at the neck just below the larynx, extending around the front and to either side of the trachea (windpipe), and secreting the hormone thyroxin, which is vital to growth and metabolism, 401, 406, 954, 1211, 1212

cancer of, 1287-1288

disorders of, 406-407, 954, 1213-1214

pregnancy and, 584

thyroid hormone: see thyroxin

thyroid pills, 407, 730

thyroid (thyroid preparations), 211, 407, 730

thyroid-stimulating hormone/TSH: hormone secreted by the anterior lobe of the pituitary gland which stimulates the production of hormones in the thyroid gland, 403

thyrotrophin, 403

thyroxin: hormone secreted by the thyroid gland, vital to growth and metabolism, 403, 406-407, 1213-1214

thyroxine (T-4), 211

tibia: the shin bone, the inner and larger of the two bones of the lower leg, 341

degeneration of, 295

fractured, 1077

tic: involuntary, recurrent muscle twitch or spasm

tic douloureux: see trigeminal neuralgia

tick fever: see Rocky Mountain spotted fever

tickle, sensation of, 409

toxic:

1. caused by or having to do with a toxin or poison

2. poisonous

toxic psychosis: psychosis caused by a toxic agent, such as lead or alcohol

toxic substances, liver function and, 390

toxin(s): any of a group of poisonous compounds produced by animal, vegetable, or bacterial organisms,

food poisoning and, 1172

toxoplasmosis, 302

toy(s), 533-534, *534*

complicated, 489

guns, 448

putting away, 522

trabecula (*pl., trabeculae*): strand of connective tissue, as in a bone, *345*

trachea/windpipe: the passageway for air from the larynx to the lungs, *381*, 382, 396, *1156*

obstruction in, 147-150, *147, 148*, 538

reconstruction of, 1287

tracheostomy/tracheotomy: emergency surgical procedure of cutting into the trachea, 468, 1164

tracheotomy: *see* tracheostomy

traction: subjection of muscle or a fractured part to a pulling force, as by a system of weights and pulleys, 970, 1051, 1077, 1079

sensation of, 409

tranquilizer: drug with a calming or sedative effect, 195, 278, 1334-1335, 1355, 1369

transaminase, 301

transference: in psychoanalysis, the redirection of repressed childhood emotions to the analyst, 1333

transistor radios, 519-520

transplant: tissue or an organ transferred from its original site to another part of the body or to another individual, 982-986

See also under specific organs.

transsexual: person who is genetically and physically of one sex but who identifies psychologically with the other and may seek treatment by surgery or with hormones to bring the physical sexual characteristics into conformity with the psychological preference

transudate: fluid passing through pores or tissues, as of a membrane

transurethral resection, 927

transverse colon: the section of the colon leading from the ascending colon and extending horizontally across the abdomen beneath the liver and stomach, 391

transvestism: practice of wearing the clothes of the opposite sex

transvestite: one who wears the clothes of the opposite sex

trapezius, 248

trauma:

1. any injury or wound to the body

2. severe emotional shock

travel

jet, 273, 292

in later years, 680

in middle years, 649

trees, allergic reaction to, 274

trematode: any of a class of parasitic flatworms, as the flukes, causing various diseases such as schistosomiasis

tremor: any involuntary quivering or trembling, as of a muscle, 364, 1090

trench foot: foot condition resembling frostbite, due to exposure to continued dampness and cold, 286

trench mouth/Vincent's angina/Vincent's disease: painful infection of the gums (called necrotizing ulcerative gingivitis) and sometimes of the pharynx and palate, characterized by the formation of ulcers and necrosis, 820

trephine, 973

triceps muscle, 248, 352, *352*

trichina: Trichinella spiralis

Trichinella spiralis/trichina: the parasitic worm that causes trichinosis, 1171

trichinosis: disease caused by a parasitic worm (Trichinella spiralis) that enters the body via under-cooked or raw meat, esp. pork, invading the intestines and muscles and provoking gastrointestinal symptoms initially and muscle stiffness and pain later, 1171

trichomonas: genus of protozoa that cause vaginal infections in women, 996

trichomoniasis: vaginal infection by the trichomonas organism, 996-997

tridihexethyl, 212

trigeminal nerve, *361*

trigeminal neuralgia, 302, 972-973

triglyceride: glycerol compound containing one to three acids

trimester: period of three months, used to identify the progress of a pregnancy, which consists of three such periods

trimethadione, 1096

trimethoprim, 212

trip *(slang):* hallucinogenic experience, 1373-1374

triplets, 535

triprolidine, 212

trivalent: pertaining to a form of the Sabin polio vaccine in which each dose gives protection against three strains of polio, 517. Compare *monovalent.*

trochlear nerve, *361*

trophoblast: layer of cells developing around a fertilized ovum and contributing to the formation of the placenta, 586

trophoblastic disease: disease of the trophoblast in a pregnant woman, marked by the degeneration of the placenta into a mass of grapelike cysts *(hydatidiform mole),* 586-587

tropical diseases, 1163, 1299-1317

true skin: dermis

trypanosomiasis: sleeping sickness, 1306-1309

African: *see* sleeping sickness

American: *see* Chagas' disease

trypsin: enzyme in the pancreatic juice that breaks up proteins for digestion

tsetse fly, *1306,* 1307

TSH: throid-stimulating hormone, 403-404

tubal insufflation/Rubin's test: the injection of carbon dioxide gas, or sometimes ordinary air, into the uterus to check for obstructions in the Fallopian tubes, 574

tubal ligation: the tying or binding of a tube, especially of the Fallopian tubes as a method of sterilization

tubercle: small nodule or tumor formed within an organ, as that produced by the bacillus causing tuberculosis

tubercle bacillus: rod-shaped bacterium that causes tuberculosis, *1187*

tuberculin: liquid containing substances extracted from weakened (attenuated) tubercle bacilli, used as a test for tuberculosis

tuberculin test: skin test for determining whether tuberculosis bacteria are present, used esp. for children, 436, 500, *1189,* 1189-1190

tuberculoid: of or resembling a tubercle or tuberculosis

tuberculoid leprosy, 1316-1317

tuberculosis: infectious, communicable disease caused by the tubercle bacillus and characterized by the formation of tubercles within some organ or tissue, often the lungs (pulmonary tuberculosis), 961-962, 1186-1190

of skeletal system, 1063, 1067-1068, *1067*

test for: *see* tuberculin test

voluntary agencies, 322-323

tuberculous arthritis, 1063

tubule(s): very narrow, minute tube or duct

of kidney, *420, 421, 1254*

tularemia: acute bacterial infection that can be transmitted to humans from infected rabbits, squirrels, or other animals, by the bite of certain flies, or by direct contact, 194, 1297-1298

tumor: mass of tissue growing independently of surrounding tissue and having no physiological function, sometimes confined to the area of origin (benign) and sometimes invading other cells and tissue and causing their degeneration (malignant)

fibroid: benign tumor composed of fibrous tissue, usu. attached to the wall of the uterus

tuna, nutrients in, 701

tunica albuginea, *424*, *927*

turbinate: one of the thin, curved bones on the walls of the nasal passages, 399

turnips, nutrients in, 704

tweezers, hair removal with, 790

twilight sleep, 594

twins, 535

tissue compatibility of, 983

twist-grip exerciser, 236

tympanum:

1. the cavity in the middle ear lined with the tympanic membrane (eardrum) and containing the ossicles

2. eardrum

tympanic membrane: *see* eardrum

typhoid fever/enteric fever: acute, infectious disease caused by a Salmonella bacterium and characterized by diarrhea, fever, eruption of bright red spots on the chest and abdomen, and physical prostration, 1163-1164

sewage and, 765

typhus: acute disease caused by a rickettsial microorganism that is transmitted to humans by the bite of certain lice and fleas, and is characterized by high fever, severe headaches, and a red rash, 298

ulcer(s): open sore with an inflamed base on an external or internal body surface,

diabetic, 673, 859

of gastrointestinal tract: *see* peptic ulcers

new drugs for, 1166

surgery for, 940-941, *940*, 1166

varicose veins and, 966, 1125

ulcerative colitis: colitis accompanied by ulcerated lesions on the colon, characterized by bloody diarrhea and abdominal pain, 1168-1169

diet and, 736

ulcer diets, 731, 732-735, 922, 1165

ulna: the bone of the forearm on the same side as the little finger, longer and thinner than the radius bone, *341*, 344

ultrasonic examination, in pregnancy, *586*

ultraviolet radiation

psoriasis and, 803

vitamin D and, 1072

umbilical: pertaining to the middle part of the abdomen

umbilical cord: the ropelike tissue connecting the navel of the fetus with the placenta, 427, *596*

umbilical hernia, 496

umbilicus: navel

unconsciousness: loss of consciousness, having the appearance of sleep, usu. caused by injury, shock, or serious physical disturbance, 194, 364

See also coma; fainting.

underachievement, 489, 1323

underskin: tissue, subcutaneous

underweight, 730-731

undulant fever: *see* brucellosis

United Cerebral Palsy Association, 313

United Ostomy Association, 1273

universal donor, 371

unsaturated: (of fats) not tending to increase the cholesterol content of the blood, 697

ups/uppers/pep pills *(slang):* drugs or compounds that have a stimulating effect on the central nervous system, such as amphetamines, 195, 556, 1362-1367

urate: salt of uric acid

urea: soluble compound containing nitrogen, found in urine and in small amounts in the blood

uremia: toxic condition of the blood caused by the failure of the kidneys to function normally in filtering out and excreting waste products, such as urea, 1250-1252

ureter: either of two narrow, muscular ducts which convey urine from the kidneys to the bladder, *419*, 420, *423*, *931*, 1248, *1249*

stones in, 932

tumors of, 934

vaccination:

1. act or process of vaccinating, 1138

2. scar produced at the site of inoculation with a vaccine

See also immunization.

vaccine: preparation of live, attenuated, or dead microorganisms injected or administered orally to create immunity against a specific disease

Rocky Mountain spotted fever, 1299

3-in-1 (measles, mumps, and rubella), 499-500

yellow fever, 1304

vacuum aspiration: technique of inducing abortion in early pregnancy by utilizing suction to draw out embryo tissue

vagina: canal in the female leading from the external genital orifice below the pubis to the uterus, 566, *566*, 996, *996*

cysts of, 1013

hernia of, 1011-1013, *1012*

vaginitis: inflammation of the vagina

vagotomy: surgical procedure of cutting the vagus nerves, 941

vagus: the tenth cranial nerve, which originates in the brain and extends branches to the lungs, heart, stomach, and intestines, *361*

in peptic ulcer, 941

Valium/diazepam: trademark for commonly used tranquilizer, 195, 1369

valley fever (coccidioidomycosis), 1192

Valmid: ethinamate, 1368

valve: membranous structure inside a vessel or other organ, as the heart, allowing fluid to flow in one direction only

valves of heart, 289, 374-375

artificial, *1132*, *1148*

disease of: endocarditis, 1150

in rheumatic fever, 1147, 1148

vanishing creams, 782

vaporizers: *see* steam inhalators

varices, of esophagus, 1158-1159

varicose: abnormally dilated, as veins

varicose ulcer: ulcer resulting from varicose veins, usu. on the inner side of the leg above the ankle

varicose vein/varix: swollen and contorted vein, often in the leg, 632, 846, 966-967, *1124*, 1124-1125

and pulmonary embolism, 1209, 1210

in pregnancy, 580-581, 1013

stasis dermatitis and, 666

surgical procedures for, 967

varicosity:

1. condition of being varicose

2. *see* varicose vein

variola: smallpox

varix *(pl., varices)*: varicose vein

vascular: of, involving, or supplied with vessels, as blood vessels

vascular disease, smoking and, 1197

vascularization: process of becoming vascular

vascular surgeon: surgeon specializing in vascular surgery, having to do with the blood vessels, 890

vascular surgery: branch of surgery having to do with the operative treatment of diseases of the blood vessels, 966-968

vas deferens: duct in males that conveys semen from the testicles to the seminal vesicles, *424*, *425*, *565*

vasectomy: surgical removal of part of the vas deferens or sperm duct of the male, thus rendering him sterile by preventing semen from reaching the seminal vesicles, 610, 930-931

clinics, 317

voluntary agencies, 316, 324-325

vasoconstrictor: medicine that causes the blood vessels to contract, thus restricting blood flow

vasodilator: medicine that causes the blood vessels to dilate, thus producing greater blood flow

vasomotor: producing contraction or dilation of the blood vessels

vasopressin: hormone secreted by the posterior lobe of the pituitary gland that raises blood pressure and increases peristalsis, known also as antidiuretic hormone because of its action on the kidneys to stimulate the reabsorption of water, 402, *403*, 1218

VD: *see* venereal disease

veal, nutrients in, 701

vectorcardiogram: graph indicating the magnitude and direction of the electrical currents of the heart, 890

vegetable fat, nutrients in, 716

vegetables, nutrients in, 702, 703, 704

vein(s): any of a large number of muscular, tubular vessels conveying blood from all parts of the body to the heart, 142, 366, *366*

axillary, *367*

basilic, *367*

brachial, *367*

cephalic, *367*

coronary, 375

femoral, *367*

iliac, *367*

inflammation of/phlebitis, 1124

jugular, *367*

peroneal, *367*

popliteal, *367*

pulmonary: vein that delivers oxygen-rich blood from the lungs to the heart, 374-375, *965*

renal, *367*

saphenous, *367*, 966, *967*

subclavian, *367*

tibial, *367*

velum: soft palate

vena cava: either of two large veins that bring blood to the heart from the upper part of the body (superior vena cava) and lower part of the body (inferior vena cava), 367, 374, *374*, *965*

venereal disease: any of those diseases transmitted by sexual intercourse, such as syphilis and gonorrhea, 999-1006, 1261-1264

clinics, 1003

education about, 323

teenagers and, 568

voluntary agencies, 323, *323*

venereal maladies, external, 1006-1008

venereal wart/condyloma acuminatum: wart caused by a virus and occurring in the anal and genital areas, transmitted by sexual contact and by other means, 1006

venesection: *see* phlebotomy

venom: poison secreted by certain reptiles, insects, etc., transferred to a victim by a bite or sting

venous: having to do with or carried by the veins

ventral: toward, near, or in the abdomen. Compare *dorsal.*

ventricle(s): any of various body cavities, as of the brain, or chambers, esp. either of the two lower chambers of the heart, which receive blood from the atria and pump it into the arteries

brain, 1086

heart, *374*, 374-375, *965*

ventricular fibrillation, 1139-1140

ventriculography: technique of X-raying the brain after the removal of cerebrospinal fluid and the injection of air into the ventricles, 1085-1086

venule: small vein continuous with a capillary, 366, *366*

vermiform appendix/appendix vermiformis: the worm-shaped appendage attached to the cecum of the large intestine; *see* appendix vermiformis

vermifuge: any drug or remedy that destroys intestinal worms, 1169

vernix caseosa: cheesy substance sometimes covering a newborn baby's skin, 426

vertebra *(pl., vertebrae):* one of the segmented bones that make up the spinal column, 340, *341*, 342

disorders of, 968-970

injury to, 1082-1083

thoracic/thoracic spine: the vertebrae to which the ribs are attached, 342

vertebral disk, herniated, 968-969

vertebrate: any animal having a backbone

vertigo: disorder in which a person feels as if he or his surroundings are whirling around, 176, 1246

vesical: of or pertaining to the bladder

vesical stones, 932-933

vesicle: small bladderlike cavity, or a small sac containing fluid

vestibular nerve: the part of the auditory nerve leading from the vestibule of the inner ear to the brain, controlling equilibrium, 416, *417*, *955*

vestibule: space or cavity, as within the labyrinth of the inner ear, 416

vestigial: of the nature of a remnant of an organ that is no longer functional

Veterans Administration

hearing aids and, 668-669

nursing homes and, 679

viable: capable of living and developing normally, as a newborn infant

vibrissae *(sing., vibrissa)*: hairs that grow in the nasal cavity, 399

villi *(sing., villus)*: minute, hairlike structures on the mucous membrane of the small intestine that absorb nutrients, 386-387, 392

vinblastine, 1293

vinca alkaloid, 1292, 1293

Vincent's angina: *see* trench mouth

Vincent's disease: *see* trench mouth

vincristine, 1292, 1293

vinegar, nutrients in, 716

virulent:

1. severe and rapid in its progress, as a disease

2. highly infectious, as a disease-causing microorganism

virus *(pl., viruses)*: any of a large group of particles too small to be seen by an ordinary microscope, that are typically inert except when in contact with certain living cells, and that can cause a variety of infectious diseases

in cancer, 1269

Hodgkin's disease, 1290

in leukemia, 1122, 1292

in diseases of the nervous system, 1101

in respiratory diseases, 830, *1180*, 1181

in yellow fever, 1303-1304

viscera:

1. the internal organs of the body, as the stomach, lungs, heart, etc.

2. the intestines

visceral: pertaining to the viscera

viscid: sticky or adhesive

viscous: semifluid or gluelike in texture

vision

area of brain for, *360*, 411

color, 410-411

cranial nerve for, *360*

disturbances of, 672, 1099, 1242

peripheral, 410-411

Visiting Nurse Association, 334-335, 675

Visiting Nurse Service, 334-335, *1047*

visiting nurses, 334-335, 675

visiting patient in hospital, 280

VISTA, 684

visual purple: reddish purple protein found in the rods of the retina, esp. important to night vision, 411

visual radiations: smaller nerve bundles that split off from the optic nerve and enter the occipital lobes of the brain, 411

vitalometer: device for measuring sensitivity of a tooth

vital signs: measurement of body temperature, pulse rate, and respiration, 918-919

vitamin(s): any of a group of complex organic substances found in minute quantities in most natural foods and closely associated with the maintenance of normal physiological functions, 390, 659, 697, *707*, 1158

vitamin A: vitamin found in green and yellow vegetables, dairy products, liver, and fish liver oils, that prevents atrophy of epithelial tissue and protects against night blindness, 411, 630, 697, 1158

vitamin B₁: thiamine

vitamin B₂: riboflavin

vitamin B₁₂: vitamin extracted from liver and believed to protect against pernicious anemia, 1116, 1117

vitamin B complex: group of water-soluble vitamins including thiamine and riboflavin, 697, 1158

vitamin C: *see* ascorbic acid

vitamin D: vitamin that protects against rickets, found in fish liver oils, butter, egg yolks, and specially treated cow's milk, and also produced in the body on exposure to sunlight, 354, 407, 697, 703, 717, 1158

vitamin E: vitamin found in whole grain cereals, legume seeds, corn oil, egg yolks, meat, and milk, sometimes called the anti-sterility vitamin because its absence in rats causes sterility, 697

vitamin K: vitamin that promotes the clotting of blood and is found in green leafy vegetables, 697, 1112

vitamin supplements, 433, 622, 640, 659

vitiligo/piebald skin: skin disorder characterized by a loss of pigment in sharply defined areas, 666, 804

vitreous humor: the transparent, jellylike tissue that fills the posterior chamber or ball of the eye and is enclosed by the hyaloid membrane, *410, 957*

vocal cords/vocal folds: two bands of ligaments extending across the larynx which, when tense, are made to vibrate by the passage of air, thereby producing voice, 396

vocal folds: *see* vocal cords

vocational therapy, 1088

vodka, 1342

voice box: larynx

void: excrete waste, esp. urine

voiding cystometrics, 896

voluntary muscle: *see* skeletal muscle

volunteer work, *326*, 647, 683-684, *684, 925, 1045*

Volunteers in Service to America, 684

volvulus: obstruction of the intestines caused by twisting, 1161, *1161*

vomitus: vomited substance

vulva: the external genitals of the female, located beneath the front part of the pelvis

waffles, nutrients in, 715

waist, exercises for, 270, *270*

walking

beginning, 434, *438, 501,* 1051

and fitness, 628, 662, 722

in parkinsonism, 1090

walking pneumonia: mild viral pneumonia that does not confine the patient to bed

walleye: strabismus characterized by a tendency of the eyes to turn outward away from the nose. Compare *crossed eyes.*

war clubs, 236

warm-up exercises, 230

weight-lifting, 235

wart: small, usu. hard, benign growth formed on and rooted in the skin, caused by a virus, 300, 799

venereal, 1006

wasp, stings of, 185-186, 866, *866*

Wasserman test: blood test for the presence of the organism causing syphilis, 1003

water, 696, 698, 700

loss of, in surgery, 923

need for, 660, 673, 698, 700

storage of, in large intestine, 391-392

water blister: blister beneath the epidermis that contains lymph, 842

watermelon, nutrients in, 711

"water-pills": diuretics

water pollution, *762,* 762-767

water-salt balance, 405

wax, ear, 1244

waxing, for hair removal, 790

WBC (white blood cell) count, normal ranges of, 887

weather, discomforts due to, 794-796, 837-840

weaver's bottom, 1051

weaving, as physical therapy, *1100*

Medical Emergencies

Anyone attempting to deal with a medical emergency will do so with considerably more confidence if he has a clear notion of the order of importance of various problems. Over and above all technical knowledge about such things as tourniquets or cardiac massage is the ability of the rescuer to keep a cool head so that he can make the right decisions and delegate tasks to others who wish to be helpful.

Cessation of Breathing

The medical emergency which requires prompt attention before any others is cessation of breathing. No matter what other injuries are involved, artificial respiration must be administered immediately to anyone suffering from respiratory arrest.

To determine whether a person is breathing naturally, place your cheek as near as possible to the victim's mouth and nose. While you are feeling and listening for evidence of respiration, watch the victim's chest and upper abdomen to see if they rise and fall. If respiratory arrest is indicated, begin artificial respiration immediately.

Time is critical; a human body has only about a four-minute reserve supply of oxygen in its tissues, although some persons have been revived after being submerged in water for 10 minutes or more. Do not waste time moving the victim to a more comfortable location unless his position is life-threatening.

If more than one person is available, the second person should summon a doctor. A second rescuer can also assist in preparing the victim for artificial respiration by helping to loosen clothing around the neck, chest, and waist, and by inspecting the mouth for false teeth, chewing gum, or other objects that could block the flow of air. The victim's tongue must be pulled forward before artificial respiration begins.

Normal breathing should start after not more than 15 minutes of artificial respiration. If it doesn't, you should continue the procedure for at least two hours, alternating, if possible, with other persons to maintain maximum efficiency. Medical experts have defined normal breathing as 8 or more breaths per minute; if breathing resumes but slackens to a rate of fewer than 8 breaths per minute, or if breathing stops suddenly for more than 30 seconds, continue artificial respiration.

Mouth-to-Mouth and Mouth-to-Nose Artificial Respiration

Following is a description of the techniques used to provide mouth-to-mouth or mouth-to-nose artificial respiration. These are the preferred methods of artificial respiration because they move a greater volume of air into a victim's lungs than any alternative method.

After quickly clearing the victim's mouth and throat of obstacles, tilt the victim's head back as far as possible, with the chin up and neck stretched to insure an open passage of air to the lungs. If mouth-to-mouth breathing is employed, pull the lower jaw of the victim open with one hand, inserting your thumb between the victim's teeth, and pinch the nostrils with the other to prevent air leakage through the nose. If using the mouth-to-nose technique, hold one hand over the mouth to seal it against air leakage.

Next, open your own mouth and take a deep breath. Then blow forcefully into the victim's mouth (or nose) until you can see the chest rise. Quickly remove your mouth and listen for normal exhalation sounds from the victim. If you hear gurgling sounds, try to move the jaw higher because the throat may not be stretched open properly. Continue blowing forcefully into the victim's mouth (or nose) at a rate of once every three or four seconds. (For infants, do not blow forcefully; blow only small puffs of air from your cheeks.)

If the victim's stomach becomes distended, it may be a sign that air is being blown into the stomach; press firmly with one hand on the upper abdomen to push the air out of the stomach.

If you are hesitant about direct physical contact of the lips, make a ring with the index finger and thumb of the hand being used to hold the

MOUTH-TO-MOUTH RESPIRATION

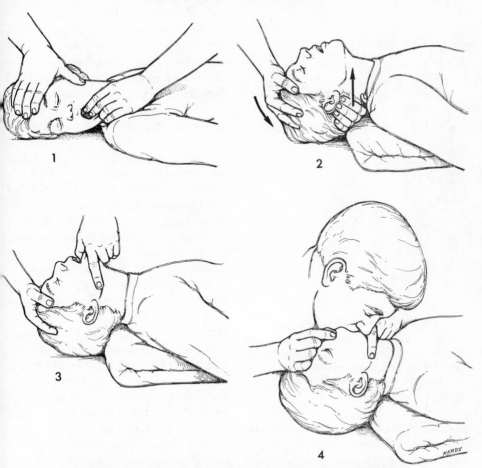

(1) Clear the victim's mouth and throat of obstructions. (2) Tilt the head back as far as possible, with the chin up and neck stretched taut. (3) Insert your thumb between the victim's teeth to pull his lower jaw open. Keep his head pushed back. (4) Pinch the nostrils shut. Open your mouth, take a deep breath, and, placing your mouth firmly against the victim's, blow forcefully. Repeat every 3 or 4 seconds.

victim's chin in position. Place the ring of fingers firmly about the victim's mouth; the outside of the thumb may at the same time be positioned to seal the nose against air leakage. Then blow the air into the victim's mouth through the finger-thumb ring. Direct lip-to-lip contact can also be avoided by placing a piece of gauze or other clean porous cloth over the victim's mouth.

Severe Bleeding

If the victim is not suffering from respiration failure or if breathing has been restored, severe bleeding is the second most serious emergency to attend to. Such bleeding occurs when either an artery or a vein has been severed. Arterial blood is bright red and spurts rather than flows from the body, sometimes in

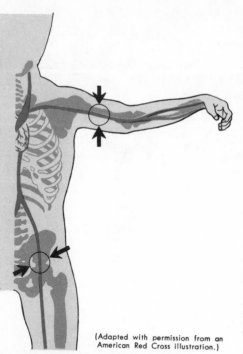

(Adapted with permission from an American Red Cross illustration.)

Two major pressure points: in the arm, the brachial artery; in the leg, the femoral artery. Continue to apply direct pressure and elevate the wounded part while utilizing pressure points to stop blood flow.

very large amounts. It is also more difficult to control than blood from a vein, which can be recognized by its dark red color and steady flow.

EMERGENCY TREATMENT: The quickest and most effective way to stop bleeding is by direct pressure on the wound. If heavy layers of sterile gauze are not available, use a clean handkerchief, or a clean piece of material torn from a shirt, slip, or sheet to cover the wound. Then place the fingers or the palm of the hand directly over the bleeding area. The pressure must be *firm and constant* and should be interrupted only when the blood has soaked through the dressing. *Do not remove the soaked dressing.* Cover it as quickly as possible with additional new

layers. When the blood stops seeping through to the surface of the dressing, secure it with strips of cloth until the victim can receive medical attention. This procedure is almost always successful in stopping blood flow from a vein.

If direct pressure doesn't stop arterial bleeding, two alternatives are possible: pressure by finger or hand on the pressure point nearest the wound, or the application of a tourniquet. No matter what the source of the bleeding, if the wound is on an arm or leg, elevation of the limb as high as is comfortable will reduce the blood flow.

TOURNIQUETS: A tourniquet improperly applied can be an extremely dangerous device, and should only be considered for a hemorrhage that can't be controlled in any other way.

It must be remembered that arterial blood flows away from the heart, and that venous blood flows toward the heart. Therefore, while a tourniquet placed on a limb between the site of a wound and the heart may slow or stop arterial bleeding, it may actually increase venous bleeding. By obstructing blood flow in the veins beyond the wound site, the venous blood flowing toward the heart will have to exit from the wound. Thus, the proper application of a tourniquet depends upon an understanding and differentiation of arterial from venous bleeding. Arterial bleeding can be recognized by the pumping action of the blood and by the bright red color of the blood.

Once a tourniquet is applied, it should not be left in place for an excessive period of time, since the tissues in the limb beyond the site of the wound need to be supplied with blood.

Shock

In any acute medical emergency, the possibility of the onset of shock must always be taken into account, especially following the fracture of a large bone, extensive burns, or serious wounds. If untreated, or if treated too late, shock can be fatal.

Shock is an emergency condition in which the circulation of the blood is so disrupted that all bodily functions are affected. It occurs when

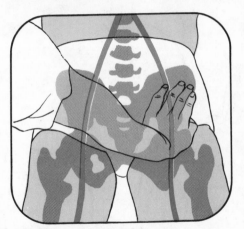

(Top) Use the femoral artery for control of severe bleeding from an open leg wound. Place the victim flat on his back, and put the heel of your hand directly over the pressure point. Apply pressure by forcing the artery against the pelvic bone. *(Bottom)* Use the brachial artery for control of severe bleeding from an open arm wound. Apply pressure by forcing the artery against the arm bone. Continue to apply direct pressure over the wound, and keep the wounded part elevated.

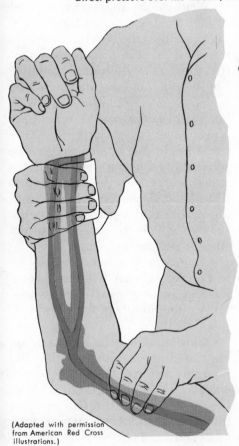

(Adapted with permission from American Red Cross illustrations.)

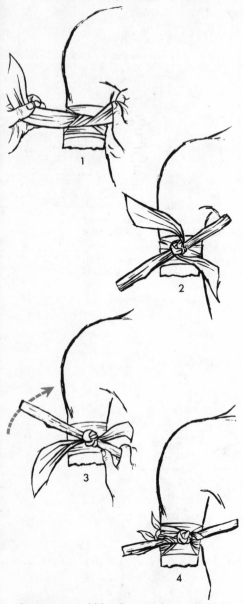

Severe arterial bleeding can be controlled by the correct application of a tourniquet. (1) A long strip of gauze or other material is wrapped twice around the arm or leg above the wound and tied in a half-knot. (2) A stick, called a windlass, is placed over the knot, and the knot is completed. (3) The windlass is turned to tighten the knot and finally, (4) the windlass is secured with the tails of the tourniquet. Improper use of a tourniquet can be very dangerous.

blood pressure is so low that insufficient blood supply reaches the vital tissues.

Types of Circulatory Shock and Their Causes

• *Low-volume shock* is a condition brought about by so great a loss of blood or blood plasma that the remaining blood is insufficient to fill the whole circulatory system. The blood loss may occur outside the body, as in a hemorrhage caused by injury to an artery or vein, or the loss may be internal because of the blood loss at the site of a major fracture, burn, or bleeding ulcer. Professional treatment involves replacement of blood loss by transfusion.

• *Neurogenic shock,* manifested by *fainting,* occurs when the regulating capacity of the nervous system is impaired by severe pain, profound fright, or overwhelming stimulus. This type of shock is usually relieved by having the victim lie down with his head lower than the rest of his body.

• *Allergic shock*, also called *anaphylactic shock*, occurs when the functioning of the blood vessels is disturbed by a person's sensitivity to the injection of a particular foreign substance, as in the case of an insect sting or certain medicines.

• *Septic shock* is brought on by infection from certain bacteria that release a poison which affects the proper functioning of the blood vessels.

• *Cardiac shock* can be caused by any circumstance that affects the pumping action of the heart.

SYMPTOMS: Shock caused by blood loss makes the victim feel restless, thirsty, and cold. He may perspire a great deal, and although his pulse is fast, it is also very weak. His breathing becomes labored and his lips turn blue.

EMERGENCY TREATMENT: A doctor should be called immediately if the onset of shock is suspected. Until medical help is obtained, the following procedures can alleviate some of the symptoms:

1. With a minimum amount of disturbance, arrange the victim so that he is lying on his back with his head somewhat lower than his feet. (*Exception:* If the victim's breathing is difficult, or if he has suffered a head injury or a stroke, keep his body flat but place a pillow or similar cushioning material under his head.) Loosen any clothing that may cause constriction, such as a belt, tie, waistband, shoes. Cover him warmly against possible chill, but see that he isn't too hot.

2. If his breathing is weak and shallow, begin mouth-to-mouth respiration.

3. If he is hemorrhaging, try to control bleeding.

4. When appropriate help and transportation facilities are available, quickly move the victim to the nearest hospital or health facility in order to begin resuscitative measures.

5. *Do not* try to force any food or stimulant into the victim's mouth.

Cardiac Arrest

Cardiac arrest is a condition in which the heart has stopped beating altogether or is beating so weakly or so irregularly that it cannot maintain proper blood circulation.

Common causes of cardiac arrest are heart attack, electric shock, hemorrhage, suffocation, and other forms of respiratory arrest. Symp-

Some people are so severely allergic to certain medications that exposure to them can produce unconsciousness and, if not treated promptly, even death. To alert others, emblems identifying the allergy are available for a slight charge from the nonprofit Medic Alert Foundation, Turlock, California 95380.

toms of cardiac arrest are unconsciousness, the absence of respiration and pulse, and the lack of a heartbeat or a heartbeat that is very weak or irregular.

Cardiac Massage

If the victim of a medical emergency manifests signs of cardiac arrest, he should be given cardiac massage at the same time that another rescuer is administering mouth-to-mouth resuscitation. Both procedures can be carried on in the moving vehicle taking him to the hospital.

It is assumed that he is lying down with his mouth clear and his air passage unobstructed. The massage is given in the following way:

1. The heel of one hand with the heel of the other crossed over it should be placed on the bottom third of the breastbone and pressed firmly

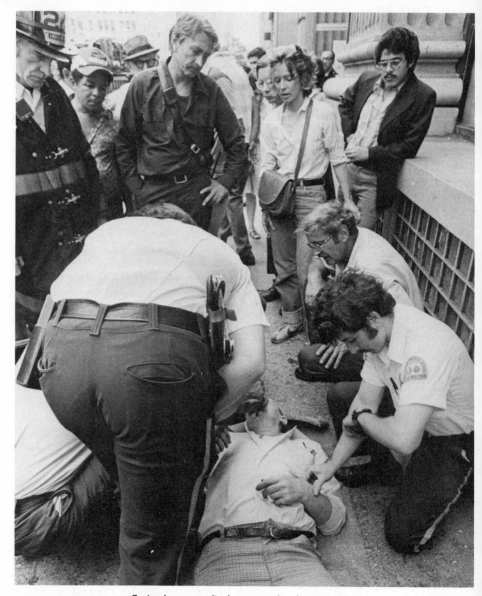

Trained paramedical personnel administer life-
giving first-aid treatment to a heart attack victim.

down with a force of about 80 pounds so that the breastbone moves about two inches toward the spine. Pressure should not be applied directly on the ribs by the fingers.

2. The hands are then relaxed to allow the chest to expand.

3. If one person is doing both the cardiac massage and the mouth-to-mouth respiration, he should stop the massage after every 15 chest compressions and administer two very quick lung inflations to the victim.

4. The rescuer should try to make the rate of cardiac massage simulate

restoration of the pulse rate. This is not always easily accomplished, but compression should reach 60 times per minute.

The techniques for administering cardiac massage to children are the same as those used for adults, except that much less pressure should be applied to a child's chest, and, in the case of babies or young children, the pressure should be exerted with the tips of the fingers rather than with the heel of the hand.

CAUTION: Cardiac massage can be damaging if applied improperly. Courses in emergency medical care offered by the American Red Cross and other groups are well worth taking. In an emergency in which cardiac massage is called for, an untrained person should seek the immediate aid of someone trained in the technique before attempting it himself.

Obstruction in the Windpipe

Many people die each year from choking on food; children incur an additional hazard in swallowing foreign objects. Most of these victims could be saved through quick action by nearly any other person, and without special equipment.

Food choking usually occurs because a bite of food becomes lodged at the back of the throat or at the opening of the trachea, or windpipe. The victim cannot breathe or speak. He may become pale or turn blue before collapsing. Death can occur within four or five minutes. But the lungs of an average person may contain at least one quart of air, inhaled before the start of choking, and that air can be used to unblock the windpipe and save the victim's life.

Finger Probe

If the object can be seen, a quick attempt can be made to remove it by probing with a finger. Use a hooking motion to dislodge the object. Under no circumstances should this method be pursued if it appears that the object is being pushed farther downward rather than being released and brought up.

BACK BLOWS FOR TREATMENT OF STRANGULATION

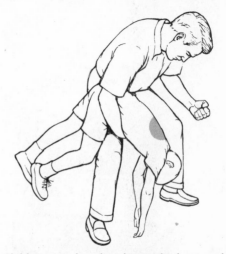

Children may be placed over the knee and struck sharply between the shoulders.

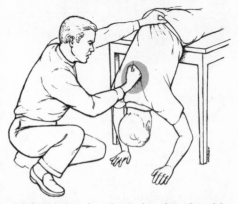

Adults may be placed over the edge of a table, supported by grasping the waist, and struck sharply between the shoulders with the fist.

Back Blows

Give the victim four quick, hard blows with the fist on his back between the shoulder blades. The blows should be given in rapid succession. If the victim is a child, he can be held over the knee while being struck; an adult should lie face down on a bed or table, with the upper half of his body suspended in the direction of the floor so that he can receive the same type of blows. A very small child or infant should be held upside down by the torso or legs and struck much more lightly than an adult.

The Heimlich Maneuver

If the back blows fail to dislodge the obstruction, the Heimlich ma-

THE HEIMLICH MANEUVER

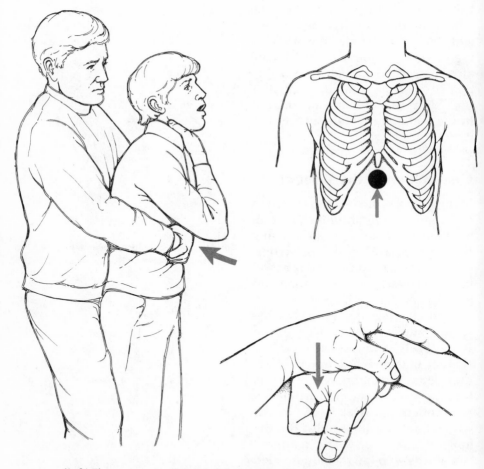

(Left) The rescuer stands behind the victim and grasps his hands firmly over the victim's abdomen just below the rib cage *(top right)*. The position of the rescuer's hands and the direction of thrust are shown at the bottom right.

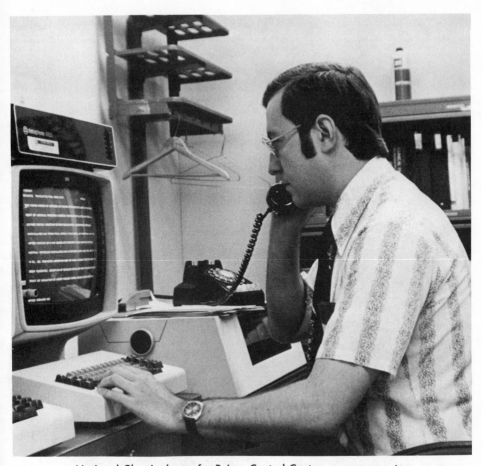

National Clearinghouse for Poison Control Centers uses a computer terminal for quick viewing of information about a particular product.

neuver should be given without delay. (Back blows may loosen the object even if they fail to dislodge it completely; that is why they are given first.) The lifesaving technique known as the *Heimlich maneuver* (named for Dr. Henry J. Heimlich) works simply by squeezing the volume of air trapped in the victim's lungs. The piece of food literally pops out of the throat as if it were ejected from a squeezed balloon.

To perform the Heimlich maneuver, the rescuer stands behind the victim and grasps his hands firmly over the victim's abdomen, just below the victim's rib cage. The rescuer makes a fist with one hand and places his other hand over the clenched fist. Then, the rescuer forces his fist sharply inward and upward against the victim's diaphragm. This action compresses the lungs within the rib cage. If the food does not pop out on the first try, the maneuver should be repeated until the air passage is unblocked.

When the victim is unable to stand, he should be rolled over on his back on the floor. The rescuer then kneels astride the victim and performs a variation of the Heimlich

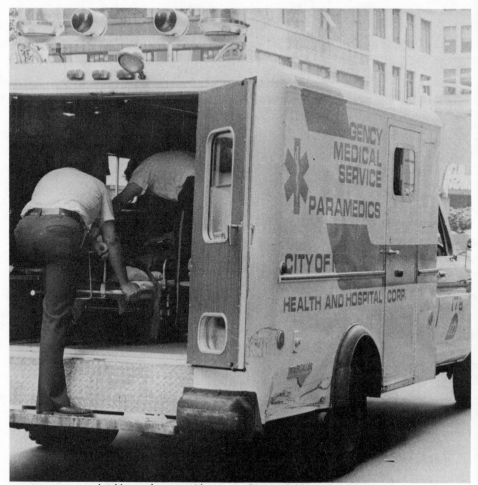

In cities and towns with paramedics available, technicians can speed poisoning victims to the nearest poison control center.

maneuver by placing the heel of one open hand, rather than a clenched fist, just below the victim's rib cage. The second hand is placed over the first. Then the rescuer presses upward (toward the victim's head) quickly to compress the lungs, repeating several times if necessary.

The Heimlich maneuver has been used successfully by persons who were alone when they choked on food; some pressed their own fist into their abdomen, others forced the edge of a chair or sink against their abdomen.

Poisoning

In all cases of poisoning, it is imperative to get professional assistance as soon as possible.

Listed below are telephone numbers for Poison Control Centers throughout the United States. These health service organizations are accessible 24 hours a day to provide information on how best to counteract the effects of toxic substances.

In the event of known or suspected poisoning, call the center nearest you immediately. Give the staff
(continued on p. 158)

TELEPHONE NUMBERS OF POISON CONTROL CENTERS*

ALABAMA

Anniston
205   237-5421

Auburn
205   826-4037;
Night: 887-6778,
3235

Birmingham
205   933-4050

Dothan
205   794-3131

Florence
205   764-8321

Gadsden
205   492-1240

Mobile
205   473-3325

Opelika
205   745-4611

ALASKA

Anchorage
907   277-6671

Fairbanks
907   456-6655

Juneau
907   586-2611

Ketchikan
907   225-5171

Sitka-Mt.
Edgecumbe
907   966-2411

ARIZONA

Douglas
602   364-8473

Flagstaff
602   744-5233

Ganado
602   755-3411

Kingman
602   757-2101

Nogales
602   287-2771

Phoenix
602   252-6611;
267-5011; 252-
5911; 277-6611;
258-7373

Prescott
602   445-2700

Tucson
602   624-2721;

622-5833; 327-
5461; 882-6300

Winslow
602   289-4691

Yuma
602   344-2000

ARKANSAS

El Dorado
501   863-2266

Fort Smith
501   782-3071;
441-4381

Harrison
501   365-6141

Helena
501   338-6411

Little Rock
501   664-5000

Osceola
501   563-2611

Pine Bluff
501   535-6800

CALIFORNIA

Fresno
209   233-0911

Los Angeles
213   664-2121

Oakland
415   652-8171;
654-5600

Orange
714   633-9393;
997-2722

Sacramento
916   453-3692,
3797

San Diego
714   294-6000

San Francisco
415   553-1574;
558-3881

San Jose
408   393-0262

CANAL ZONE

Balboa Heights
2-2600

COLORADO

Denver
303   893-7771

CONNECTICUT

Bridgeport
203   334-3566,
1081

Danbury
203   774-2300

Hartford
203   566-3456

Middletown
203   347-9471

New Britain
203   224-5672

New Haven
203   772-3900;
436-1960

Norwalk
203   838-3611

Waterbury
203   756-8351

DELAWARE

Wilmington
302   655-3389

DISTRICT OF COLUMBIA

Washington, DC
202   835-4080,
4081

FLORIDA

Apalachicola
904   653-3311

Bartow
813   533-1111

Bradenton
813   746-5111

Daytona Beach
904   255-0161

Ft. Lauderdale
305   525-5411

Fort Myers
813   334-5286

Ft. Walton Beach
904   242-1111

Gainesville
904   372-4321;
392-3261

Jacksonville
904   389-7751

Key West
305   294-5531

Lakeland
813   683-0411

Leesburg
904   787-7222

Melbourne
305   727-7000

Miami
305   325-7429

Miami Beach
305   674-2121,
2200

Naples
813   649-3131

Ocala
904   732-1111

Orlando
305   841-8411

Panama City
904   769-1511

Pensacola
904   434-4011

Plant City
813   752-1188

Pompano
305   941-8300

Punta Gorda
813   639-3131

Rockledge
305   636-2211

St. Petersburg
813   894-1161

Sarasota
813   955-1111

Tallahassee
904   599-5100

Tampa
813   253-0711

Titusville
305   269-1100

West Palm Beach
306   655-5511

Winter Haven
813   293-1121

GEORGIA

Albany
912   883-1800

Athens
404   549-9977

Atlanta
404   659-1212

*From the *National Clearinghouse for Poison Control Centers* Bulletin, July–August, 1976, U.S. Department of Health, Education, and Welfare

Augusta
404   724-7171

Columbus
404   324-4711

Macon
912   742-1122

Rome
404   232-1541

Savannah
912   355-3200

Thomasville
912   226-4121

Valdosta
912   242-3450

Waycross
912   283-3030

GUAM

Agana
746-9171

HAWAII

Honolulu
808   537-1831

IDAHO

Boise
208   376-1211

Idaho Falls
208   522-3620

Pocatello
208   232-2733

ILLINOIS

Alton
618   462-8851

Aurora
312   897-6021;
896-3911

Belleville
618   233-7750

Belvidere
815   547-5441

Berwyn
312   797-3159

Bloomington
309   828-5241;
662-3311

Cairo
618   734-2400

Canton
309   647-5240

Carbondale
618   549-0721

Carthage
217   357-3131

Centralia
618   532-6731

Champaign
217   337-2533

Chanute AFB
217   495-3133

Chester
618   826-4581

Chicago
312   942-5969;
649-4161; 633-
6542, 6543,
6544; 567-2017;
791-2810; 542-
2030; 774-8000;
770-2419; 978-
2000; 996-6885,
6886; 947-6231

Danville
217   443-5221;
442-6300

Decatur
217   877-8121;
429-2966

Des Plaines
312   297-1800

East St. Louis
618   874-7076;
274-1900

Effingham
217   342-2121

Elgin
312   695-3200;
742-9800

Elmhurst
312   833-1400

Evanston
312   492-6460,
2440

Evergreen Park
312   445-6000

Fairbury
815   692-2346

Freeport
815   235-4131

Galesburg
309   343-8131,
3161

Granite City
618   876-2020

Harvey
312   333-2300

Highland
618   654-2171

Highland Park
312   432-8000

Hinsdale
312   887-2600

Hoopeston
217   283-5531

Jacksonville
217   245-9541

Joliet
815   725-7133;
729-7563, 7565

Kankakee
815   933-1671;
939-4111

Kewanee
309   853-3361

Lake Forest
312   234-5600

La Salle
815   223-0607

Lincoln
217   732-2161

Macomb
309   833-4101

Mattoon
217   234-8881

Maywood
312   531-3000

McHenry
815   385-2200

Melrose Park
312   681-3000

Mendota
815   539-7461

Moline
309   762-3651

Monmouth
309   734-3141

Mt. Carmel
618   263-3112

Mt. Vernon
618   242-4600

Naperville
312   355-0450

Normal
309   829-7685

Oak Lawn
312   425-8000

Oak Park
312   383-6200

Olney
618   395-2131

Ottawa
815   433-3100

Park Ridge
312   696-5151

Pekin
309   347-1151

Peoria
309   672-5500,
4950; 691-4702;
672-2109, 2110,
2111

Peru
815   223-3300

Pittsfield
217   285-2113

Princeton
815   875-2811

Quincy
217   223-5811,
1200

Rockford
815   968-6861;
226-2041; 968-
6898

Rock Island
309   793-1000

St. Charles
312   584-3300

Scott Air Force
Base
618   256-7595

Springfield
217   528-2041;
544-6464

Spring Valley
815   663-2611

Streator
815   673-2311

Urbana
217   337-3311,
2131

Waukegan
312   688-4181,
6181

Winfield
312   653-6900

Woodstock
815   338-2500

Zion
312   872-4561

INDIANA

Anderson
317   649-2511

Angola
219   665-2141,
2166

Crown Point
219   738-2100

East Chicago
219   392-1700,
7203

Elkhart
219   294-2621

Evansville
812   426-3405;
477-6261;
426-8000

Fort Wayne
  219   484-6636;
  423-2614
Frankfort
  317   654-4451
Gary
  219   886-4710
Goshen
  219   533-2141
Hammond
  219   932-2300
Huntington
  219   356-3000
Indianapolis
  317   924-8355;
  639-6671
Kokomo
  217   453-0702
Lafayette
  317   742-0221
La Grange
  219   463-2144
La Porte
  219   362-7541
Lebanon
  317   482-2700
Madison
  812   265-5211
Marion
  317   662-4694
Mishawaka
  219   259-2431
Muncie
  317   747-3241
Portland
  317   726-7131
Richmond
  317   692-7010
Shelbyville
  317   392-3211
South Bend
  219   284-7458;
  234-2151
Terre Haute
  812   232-0361
Vincennes
  812   885-3348

IOWA

Des Moines
  515   283-6212
Dubuque
  319   588-8210
Fort Dodge
  515   573-3101
Iowa City
  319   356-1616

KANSAS

Atchison
  913   367-2131
Dodge City
  316   227-8133
Emporia
  316   342-7120
Fort Riley
  913   239-2323
Fort Scott
  316   223-2200;
  Night: 223-0476
Great Bend
  316   793-3523;
  Night: 792-2511
Hays
  913   628-8251
Kansas City
  913   831-6633;
  287-8881
Lawrence
  913   843-3680
Parsons
  316   421-4880
Salina
  913   827-5591
Topeka
  913   234-9961
Wichita
  316   685-2151

KENTUCKY

Ashland
  606   325-7755
Berea
  606   986-3061
Fort Thomas
  606   292-3215
Lexington
  606   278-3411;
  233-5320
Louisville
  502   589-8222
Murray
  502   753-7588
Owensboro
  502   683-3511
Paducah
  502   444-6361
Whitesburg
  606   633-2160

LOUISIANA

Bogalusa
  504   735-1322
Lake Charles
  318   478-1310

Monroe
  318   325-6454;
  Night: 325-2611
New Orleans
  504   524-3617,
  3618, 3619
Shreveport
  318   222-0709

MAINE

Portland
  207   871-0111

MARYLAND

Baltimore
  301   955-5000;
  528-7701;
  800   494-2414
Bethesda
  301   530-3880
Cumberland
  301   722-6677
Easton
  301   822-5555
Hagerstown
  301   797-2400

MASSACHUSETTS

Boston
  617   232-2120
Fall River
  617   674-5789
New Bedford
  617   997-1515
Springfield
  413   788-7321;
  787-3200
Webster
  617   943-2600
Worcester
  617   756-1551

MICHIGAN

Adrian
  517   263-2412
Ann Arbor
  313   764-5102
Battle Creek
  616   963-5521
Bay City
  517   895-8511
Berrien Center
  616   471-7761
Coldwater
  517   278-2359
Detroit
  313   494-5711;
  864-5400

Eloise
  313   722-3748,
  3749; Night:
  274-3000, 6232
Flint
  313   766-0111
Grand Rapids
  616   774-1774;
  247-7123; 774-
  6794, 7854
Hancock
  906   482-1122
Holland
  616   396-4661
Jackson
  517   783-2771
Kalamazoo
  616   383-7333,
  6401
Lansing
  517   372-5112
Marquette
  906   228-9440
Midland
  517   631-7700
Monroe
  313   241-6509
Petoskey
  616   347-7373
Pontiac
  313   858-3000
Port Huron
  313   987-5555
Saginaw
  517   755-1111
Traverse City
  616   947-6140

MINNESOTA

Bemidji
  218   751-5430
Brainerd
  218   829-2861
Crookston
  218   281-4682
Duluth
  218   727-6636,
  4551
Edina
  612   920-4400
Fergus Falls
  218   736-5475
Fridley
  612   786-2200
Mankato
  507   387-4031
Marshall
  507   532-9661

Minneapolis
612 332-0282;
347-3141; 296-
5276; 588-0616;
874-4233

Morris
612 589-1313

Rochester
507 285-5123;
282-4461

St. Cloud
612 251-2700

St. Paul
612 224-9121;
227-6521; 228-
3132; 291-3348,
3139; 298-8201;
222-4260

Virginia
218 741-3340

Willmar
612 235-4543

Worthington
507 372-2941

MISSISSIPPI

Brandon
601 825-2811

Columbia
601 736-6303

Greenwood
601 453-9751

Hattiesburg
601 544-7000

Jackson
601 968-1704;
982-0121; 354-
6650

Keesler AFB
Biloxi
601 377-2516,
6555, 6556

Laurel
601 649-4000

Meridian
601 483-6211

Pascagoula
601 762-6121

University
601 234-1522

Vicksburg
601 636-2131

MISSOURI

Cape Girardeau
314 334-4461

Columbia
314 882-8091

Hannibal
314 221-0414

Joplin
417 781-2727

Kansas City
816 471-0626;
421-8060

Kirksville
816 665-4611

Poplar Bluff
314 785-7721

Rolla
314 364-3100

St. Joseph
816 232-8461

St. Louis
314 865-4000;
367-6880

Springfield
417 836-3193;
881-8811

West Plains
417 256-3141

MONTANA

Bozeman
406 586-5431

Great Falls
406 761-1200

Helena
406 442-2480

NEBRASKA

Lincoln
402 483-3244

Omaha
402 553-5400

NEVADA

Las Vegas
702 385-1277

Reno
702 785-4129;
Night: 785-4140

NEW
HAMPSHIRE

Hanover
603 643-4000

NEW JERSEY

Atlantic City
609 344-4081

Belleville
201 751-1000

Boonton
201 334-5000

Bridgeton
609 451-6600

Camden
609 795-5554

Denville
201 627-3000

East Orange
201 672-8400

Elizabeth
201 527-5059

Englewood
201 568-3400

Flemington
201 782-2121

Livingston
201 992-5161

Long Branch
201 222-2210

Montclair
201 746-6000

Morristown
201 538-0900

Mount Holly
609 267-7877

Neptune
201 988-1818

Newark
201 926-7240,
7241, 7242, 7243

New Brunswick
201 828-3000;
545-8000

Newton
201 383-2121

Orange
201 678-1100

Passaic
201 473-1000

Perth Amboy
201 442-3700

Phillipsburg
201 859-1500

Point Pleasant
201 892-1100

Princeton
609 921-7700

Saddle Brook
201 843-6700

Somers Point
609 927-3501

Somerville
201 725-4000

Summit
201 522-2232

Teaneck
201 837-3070

Trenton
609 396-1077

Union
201 687-1900

Wayne
201 684-6900

NEW MEXICO

Alamogordo
505 437-3770

Albuquerque
505 843-2551

Carlsbad
505 887-3521

Clovis
505 763-4493

Las Cruces
505 522-8641

Roswell
505 622-8170

NEW YORK

Albany
518 445-3131

Binghamton
607 772-1100;
729-6521

Buffalo
716 878-7000

Dunkirk
716 366-1111

East Meadow
516 542-2323,
2324, 2325

Elmira
607 737-4194;
733-6541

Endicott
607 754-7171

Glens Falls
518 792-3151

Ithaca
607 274-4011,
4383, 4411

Jamestown
716 487-0141

Johnson City
607 773-6611

Kingston
914 331-3131

New York
212 340-4495

Niagara Falls
716 278-4511

Nyack
914 358-6200

Oswego
315 343-1920

Rochester
716 275-5151

Syracuse
315   476-3166;
473-5831

Watertown
315   788-8700

NORTH CAROLINA

Asheville
704   255-4660

Charlotte
704   372-5100

Durham
919   684-8111

Greensboro
919   379-4109

Hendersonville
704   693-6522

Hickory
704   328-2191

Jacksonville
919   353-1234

Wilmington
919   763-9021

NORTH DAKOTA

Bismarck
701   223-4700

Dickinson
701   225-6771

Fargo
701   237-8115

Grand Forks
701   775-4241

Jamestown
701   252-1050

Minot
701   838-0341

Williston
701   572-7661

OHIO

Akron
216   379-8562

Canton
216   452-9911

Cincinnati
513   872-5111

Cleveland
216   231-4455

Columbus
614   228-1323

Dayton
513   461-4790;
878-6623

Lorain
216   282-2220

Mansfield
419   522-3411

Springfield
513   325-0531

Toledo
419   382-7971

Youngstown
216   746-2222

Zanesville
614   454-4000

OKLAHOMA

Ada
405   332-2323

Ardmore
405   223-5400

Lawton
405   355-8620

McAlester
918   426-1800

Oklahoma City
405   271-5454

Ponca City
405   765-3321

Tulsa
918   584-1351

OREGON

Portland
503   225-8500

PENNSYLVANIA

Allentown
215   433-2311;
821-3252

Altoona
814   944-1681

Bethlehem
215   691-4141

Bloomsburg
717   784-7121

Bradford
814   368-4143

Bryn Mawr
215   527-0600

Carlisle
717   249-1212

Chambersburg
717   264-5171

Chester
215   494-0721

Clearfield
814   765-5341

Coaldale
717   645-2131

Coudersport
814   274-9300

Danville
717   275-6116

Doylestown
215   345-2281

Drexel Hill
215   259-3800

Du Bois
814   371-2200

East Stroudsburg
717   421-3194

Easton
215   258-6221

Erie
814   455-3961;
864-4031;
455-6711; 459-
4000

Gettysburg
717   334-2121

Greensburg
412   837-0100

Hanover
717   637-3711

Harrisburg
717   782-3639,
4141

Hershey
717   534-6111

Indiana
412   463-0261

Jeannette
412   527-3551,
1511

Jersey Shore
717   398-0100

Johnstown
814   536-6671;
535-7541; 536-
5353

Kittanning
814   542-5011

Lancaster
717   299-5511,
4546

Lansdale
215   368-2100

Latrobe
412   539-9711

Lebanon
717   272-7611

Lehighton
215   377-1300

Lewistown
717   248-5411

Muncy
717   546-8282

Nanticoke
717   735-5000

Oil City
814   644-1211

Paoli
215   647-2200

Philadelphia
215   823-8460

Philipsburg
814   342-3320

Pittsburgh
412   681-6669;
766-8300

Pittston
717   654-3341

Pottstown
215   327-1000

Pottsville
717   622-3400

Reading
215   376-4881;
378-6218

Sayre
717   888-6666

Scranton
717   346-3801;
961-4205; 343-
5566

Sellersville
215   257-3611

Sewickley
412   741-6600

Sharon
412   981-1700

Somerset
814   443-2626

State College
814   238-4351

Titusville
814   827-1851

Tunkhannock
717   836-2161

Uniontown
412   437-4531

Washington
412   225-7000

Wellsboro
717   724-1631

Wilkes-Barre
717   823-1121

Williamsport
717   322-7861

York
717   843-8623

PUERTO RICO

Arecibo
809   878-3535

Fajardo
809   863-0505

Mayaguez
809   832-8686

Ponce
809   842-8354,
2080

Rio Piedras
809   764-3515

RHODE ISLAND

Kingston
401   792-2775,
2762

Pawtucket
401   724-1230

Providence
401   277-4000;
521-5055

SOUTH CAROLINA

Charleston
803   792-4201

Columbia
803   765-7359

SOUTH DAKOTA

Aberdeen
605   225-5110

Sioux Falls
605   336-3894

TENNESSEE

Chattanooga
615   755-6100

Columbia
615   388-2320

Cookeville
615   528-2541

Jackson
901   424-0424

Johnson City
615   926-1131

Knoxville
615   971-3261

Memphis
901   522-3000

Nashville
615   322-3391

TEXAS

Abilene
915   677-3551

Amarillo
806   376-4431

Austin
512   478-4490

Beaumont
713   833-7409

Corpus Christi
512   884-4511

El Paso
915   544-1200

Fort Worth
817   336-5521,
6611

Galveston
713   765-1420,
1561

Grand Prairie
214   641-1313

Harlingen
512   423-1224

Laredo
512   722-2431

Lubbock
806   792-1011

Midland
915   684-8257

Odessa
915   337-7311

Plainview
806   296-9601

San Angelo
915   653-6741

San Antonio
512   223-1481

Tyler
214   597-0351

Waco
817   753-1412;
756-6111

Wharton
713   532-2440;
Night: 532-1440

Wichita Falls
817   322-6771

UTAH

Salt Lake City
801   581-3711

VIRGIN ISLANDS

St. Croix
809   773-1212,
1311; 772-0260,
0212

St. John
809   776-1469

St. Thomas
809   774-1321

VIRGINIA

Alexandria
703   370-9000

Arlington
703   558-6161

Blacksburg
804   951-1111

Charlottesville
804   296-9888

Danville
804   799-2100

Falls Church
703   698-3600,
3111

Hampton
804   722-1131

Harrisonburg
804   434-4421

Lexington
804   463-9141

Lynchburg
804   846-6511

Nassawadox
804   442-8000

Norfolk
804   489-5111

Petersburg
804   732-7220

Portsmouth
804   397-6541

Richmond
804   770-5123

Roanoke
703   981-7336

Staunton
703   885-0361

Waynesboro
703   942-8355

Williamsburg
804   229-1120

WASHINGTON

Aberdeen
206   533-0450

Bellingham
206   676-8400

Longview
206   636-5252

Madigan
206   967-6972

Olympia
206   491-0222

Richland
509   943-1283

Seattle
206   634-5252

Spokane
509   747-1077

Tacoma
206   272-1281

Vancouver
206   256-2064

Yakima
509   248-4400

WEST VIRGINIA

Beckley
304   252-6431

Belle
304   949-4314

Charleston
304   348-4211

Clarksburg
304   623-3177

Huntington
304   696-6160,
2224, 2573

Martinsburg
304   267-8981

Morgantown
304   293-5341

Parkersburg
304   424-2212,
4251

Pt. Pleasant
304   675-4340

Ronceverte
304   647-4411,
4412, 4413

Weirton
304   748-3232

Welch
304   436-3161

Weston
304   269-3000

Wheeling
304   243-3281

WISCONSIN

Eau Claire
715   835-1511

Green Bay
414   432-8621

Kenosha
414   656-2201

Madison
608   262-3702

Milwaukee
414   344-7100

WYOMING

Casper
307   577-7201

Cheyenne
307   634-3341

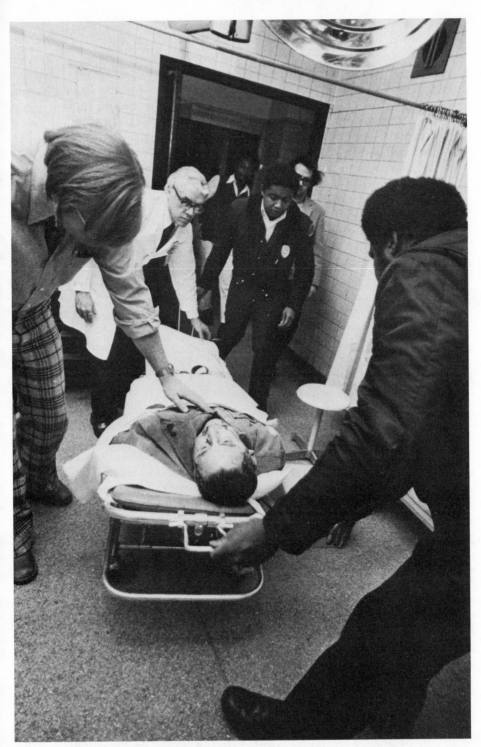

Each second counts in treating trauma cases; paramedics speed a patient
to a hospital emergency room specially equipped for such cases.

member to whom you speak as much information as possible: the name or nature of the poison ingested, if you know; if not, the symptoms manifested by the victim.

If for any reason it is impossible to telephone or get to a Poison Control Center (or a doctor or hospital), follow these two general rules:

1. If a strong acid or alkali or a petroleum product has been ingested, dilute the poison by administering large quantities of milk or water. Do not induce vomiting.

2. For methanol or related products such as window cleaners, antifreeze, paint removers, and shoe polish, induce vomiting—preferably with syrup of ipecac.

Calling for Help

Every household should have a card close by the telephone—if possible attached to an adjacent wall—that contains the numbers of various emergency services. In most communities, it is possible to simply dial the operator and ask for the police or fire department. In many large cities, there is a special three-digit number that can be dialed for reaching the police directly.

An ambulance can be summoned either by asking for a police ambulance, by calling the nearest hospital, or by having on hand the telephone numbers of whatever private ambulance services are locally available. Such services are listed in the classified pages of the telephone directory.

Practically all hospitals have emergency rooms for the prompt treatment of accident cases. If the victim is in good enough physical condition, he can be placed in a prone position in a family station wagon for removal to a hospital. However, under no circumstances should a person who has sustained major injuries or who has collapsed be made to sit upright in a car. First aid must be administered to him on the spot until a suitable conveyance arrives.

Every family should find out the telephone number of the nearest Poison Control Center (see p. 151) and note it on the emergency number card.

Reaching a Doctor

Emergencies are usually best handled in a hospital since they are likely to require oxygen, blood transfusions, or other services only a hospital can provide. However, there are many situations in which a doctor's guidance on the phone can be extremely helpful and reassuring.

Since there are times when the family physician may not be available by phone, it's a good idea to ask for the names and phone numbers of doctors who can be called when your own doctor can't be reached. In many communities, it is also possible to get the services of a physician by calling the County Medical Society.

A family on vacation in a remote area or on a cross-country trip by car can be directed to the nearest medical services by calling the telephone operator. If the operator can't provide adequate information promptly, ask to be connected with the nearest headquarters of the State Police.

Emergency Transport

In the majority of situations, the transfer of an injured person should

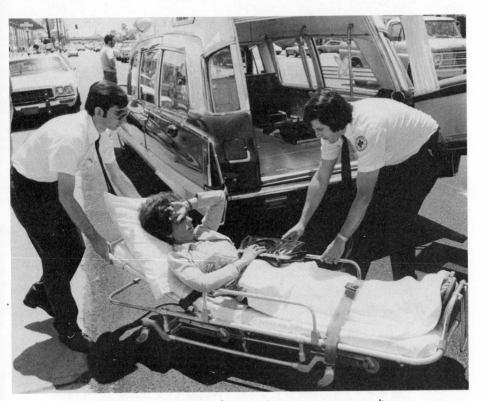

Trained ambulance technicians from a private company are an alternative to police and fire department paramedics for moving injury patients.

be handled only by experienced rescue personnel. If you yourself must move a victim to a doctor's office or hospital emergency room, here are a few important rules to remember:

1. Give all necessary first aid before attempting to move the victim. Do everything to reduce pain and to make the patient comfortable.

2. If you improvise a stretcher, be sure it is strong enough to carry the victim and that you have enough people to carry it. Shutters, doors, boards, and even ladders may be used as stretchers. Just be sure that the stretcher is padded underneath to protect the victim and that a blanket or coat is available to cover him and protect him from exposure.

3. Bring the stretcher to the vic-

tim, not the victim to the stretcher. Slide him onto the stretcher by grasping his clothing or lift him—if enough bearers are available—as shown in the illustration.

4. Secure the victim to the stretcher so he won't fall off. You may want to tie his feet together to minimize his movements.

5. Unless specific injuries prevent it, the victim should be lying on his back while he is being moved. However, a person who is having difficulty breathing because of a chest injury might be more comfortable if his head and shoulders are raised slightly. A person with a severe injury to the back of his head should be kept lying on his side. In any case, place the patient in a com-

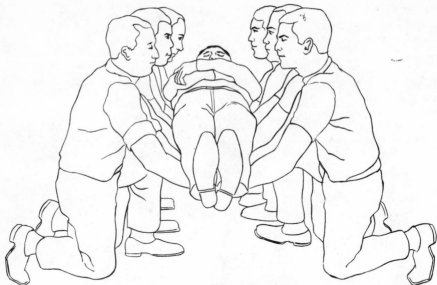

(Adapted with permission from American Red Cross illustrations.)

How to lift an injured or unconscious person to place him on a stretcher. Three bearers on each side of the victim kneel on the knee closer to the victim's feet. The bearers work their hands and forearms gently under the victim to about the midline of the back. On signal, they lift together as shown; on a following signal, they stand as a unit, if that is necessary. In lowering the victim to a stretcher or other litter, the procedure is reversed.

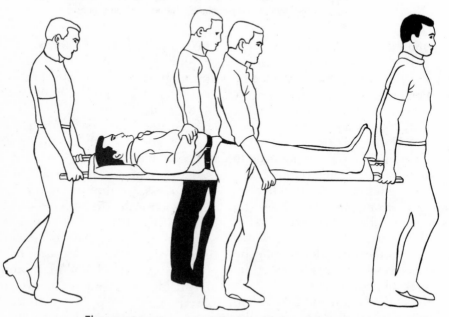

The proper way to carry a victim on a stretcher. One bearer is at the head, one at the foot, and one at either side of the stretcher. The victim should be carried feet first.

fortable position that will protect him from further injury.

6. Try to transport the patient feet first.

7. Unless absolutely necessary, don't try to put a stretcher into a passenger car. It's almost impossible to get the stretcher or injured person into a passenger car without further injuring him. If there is no ambulance, a station wagon or truck makes a good substitute.

8. When you turn the patient over to a doctor or take him to an emergency room of a hospital, give a complete account of the situation to the person taking charge. Tell the doctor what you've done for the patient and what you suspect might cause further problems.

ALPHABETIC GUIDE TO MEDICAL EMERGENCIES

Abdominal wound

Abdominal wounds can result from gunshots during hunting or working with firearms, from falling on a knife or sharp object at home or work, or from a variety of other mishaps ranging from automobile accidents to a mugging attack. Such a wound can be a major emergency requiring surgery and other professional care. Call a doctor or arrange for quick transportation to a hospital as quickly as possible.

EMERGENCY TREATMENT: If there is severe bleeding, try to control it with pressure. Keep the victim lying on his back with the knees bent; place a pillow, coat, or a similar soft object under the knees to help hold them in the bent position. If abdominal organs are exposed, do not touch them for any reason. Cover the wound with a sterile dressing. Keep the dressing moistened with sterile water or the cleanest water available. Boiled water can be used to moisten the dressing, but be sure it has cooled before applying.

If the victim is to be moved to a hospital or doctor's office, be sure the dressing over the wound is large enough and is held in place with a bandage. In addition to pain, you can expect the victim to experience nausea and vomiting, muscle spasms, and severe shock. Make the victim as comfortable as possible under the circumstances; if he complains of thirst, moisten his mouth with a few drops of water, but do not permit him to swallow the liquid.

Abrasions

EMERGENCY TREATMENT: Wash the area in which the skin is scraped or rubbed off with soap and water, using clean gauze or cotton. Allow the abrasion to air-dry, and then cover it with a loose sterile dressing held in place with a bandage. If a sterile dressing is not available, use a clean handerchief.

Change the dressing after the first 24 hours, using household hydrogen peroxide to ease its removal if it sticks to the abrasion because of clotted blood. If the skinned area appears to be accompanied by swelling, or is painful or tender to the touch, consult a doctor.

Acid burns

Among acids likely to be encountered at work and around the home are sulphuric, nitric, and hydrochloric acids. Wet-cell batteries, such as automobile batteries, contain acid powerful enough to cause chemical destruction of body tissues, and some metal cleaners contain powerful acids.

EMERGENCY TREATMENT: Wash off the acid immediately, using large amounts of clean, fresh, cool water. Strip off or cut off any clothing that may have absorbed any of the acid. If possible, put the victim in a shower bath; if a shower is not available, flood the affected skin areas with as much water as possible. However, do not apply water forcefully since this could aggravate damage already done to skin or other tissues.

After as much of the acid as possible has been eliminated by flooding with water, apply a mild solution of sodium bicarbonate or another mild alkali such as lime water. However,

caution should be exercised in neutralizing an acid burn because the chemical reaction between an acid and an alkali can produce intense heat that would aggravate the injury; also, not all acids are effectively neutralized by alkalis—carbolic acid burns, for example, should be neutralized with alcohol.

Wash the affected areas once more with fresh water, then dry gently with sterile gauze; be careful not to break the skin or to open blisters. Extensive acid burns will cause extreme pain and shock; have the victim lie down with the head and chest a little lower than the rest of the body. As soon as possible, summon a physician or rush the victim to the emergency room of a hospital.

Aerosol sprays

Although aerosol sprays generally are regarded as safe when handled according to directions, they can be directed accidentally toward the face with resulting contamination of the eyes or inhalation of the fumes. The pressurized containers may also contain products or propellants that are highly flammable, producing burns when used near an open flame. When stored near heat, in direct sunlight, or in a closed auto, the containers may explode violently.

EMERGENCY TREATMENT: If eyes are contaminated by spray particles, flush the eye surfaces with water to remove any particles of the powder mist. Then carefully examine eye surfaces to determine if chemicals appear to be imbedded in the surface of the cornea. If aerosol spray is inhaled, move the patient to a well-ventilated area; keep him lying down, warm, and quiet. If breathing fails, administer artificial respiration. Victims of exploding containers or burning contents of aerosol containers should be given appropriate emergency treatment for bleeding, burns, and shock.

The redness and irritation of eye injuries should subside within a short time. If they do not, or if particles of spray seem to be imbedded in the surface of the eyes, take the victim to an ophthalmologist. A doctor should also be summoned if a victim fails to recover quickly from the effects of inhaling an aerosol spray, particularly if the victim suffers from asthma or a similar lung disorder or from an abnormal heart condition.

Alkali burns

Alkalis are used in the manufacture of soap and cleaners and in certain household cleaning products. They combine with fats to form soaps and may produce a painful injury when in contact with body surfaces.

EMERGENCY TREATMENT: Flood the burned area with copious amounts of clean, cool, fresh water. Put the victim under a shower if possible, or otherwise pour running water over the area for as long as is necessary to dilute and weaken the corrosive chemical. Do not apply the water with such force that skin or other tissues are damaged. Remove clothing contaminated by the chemical.

Neutralize the remaining alkali with diluted vinegar, lemon juice, or a similar mild acid. Then wash the affected areas again with fresh water. Dry carefully with sterile gauze, being careful not to open blisters or otherwise cause skin breaks that could result in infection. Summon professional medical care as soon as possible. Meanwhile, treat the victim for shock.

Angina pectoris

Angina pectoris is a condition that causes acute chest pain because of interference with the supply of oxygen to the heart. Although the pain is sometimes confused with ulcer or acute indigestion symptoms, it has a distinct characteristic of its own, producing a feeling of heaviness, strangling, tightness, or suffocation. Angina is a symptom rather than a disease, and may be a chronic condition with those over 50. It is usually treated by placing a nitroglycerine tablet under the tongue.

An attack of acute angina can be brought on by emotional stress, overeating, strenuous exercise, or by any activity that makes excessive demands on heart function.

EMERGENCY TREATMENT: An attack usually subsides in about ten minutes, during which the patient appears to be gasping for breath. He should be kept in a semireclining position rather than made to lie flat, and should be moved carefully only in order to place pillows under his head and chest so that he can breathe more easily. A doctor should be called promptly after the onset of an attack.

Animal bites/rabies

Wild animals, particularly bats, serve as a natural reservoir of rabies, a disease that is almost always fatal unless promptly and properly treated. But the virus may be present in the saliva of any warm-blooded animal. Domestic animals should be immunized against rabies by vaccines injected by a veterinarian.

Rabies is transmitted to humans by an animal bite or through a cut or scratch already in the skin. The in-

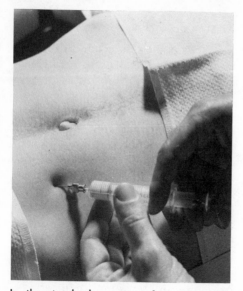

In the standard treatment for exposure to rabies, daily injections of vaccine are given in the abdomen for 14 to 21 days.

the patient is taken to a hospital or doctor's office. A tetanus injection is also indicated, and police and health authorities should be promptly notified of the biting incident.

If at all possible the biting animal should be identified—if a wild animal, captured alive—and held for observation for a period of 10 to 15 days. If it can be determined during that period that the animal is not rabid, further treatment may not be required. If the animal is rabid, however, or if it cannot be located and impounded, the patient may have to undergo a series of daily rabies vaccine injections lasting from 14 days for a case of mild exposure to 21 days for severe exposure (a bite near the head, for example), plus several booster shots. Because of the sensitivity of some individuals to the rabies vaccines used, the treatment itself can be quite dangerous.

Recent research, however, has established that a new vaccine called HDCV (human diploid cell vaccine), which requires only six or fewer injections, is immunologically effective and is not usually accompanied by any side effects. The new vaccine has been used successfully on people of all ages who had been bitten by animals known to be rabid.

fected saliva may enter through any opening, including the membranes lining the nose or mouth. After an incubation period of about ten days, a person infected by a rabid animal experiences pain at the site of infection, extreme sensitivity of the skin to temperature changes, and painful spasms of the larynx that make it almost impossible to drink. Saliva thickens and the patient becomes restless and easily excitable. By the time symptoms develop, death may be imminent. Obviously, professional medical attention should begin promptly after having been exposed to the possibility of infection.

EMERGENCY TREATMENT: The area around the wound should be washed thoroughly and repeatedly with soap and water, using a sterile gauze dressing to wipe fluid away from— not toward—the wound. Another sterile dressing is used to dry the wound and a third to cover it while

Appendicitis

The common signal for approaching appendicitis is a period of several days of indigestion and constipation, culminating in pain and tenderness on the lower right side of the abdomen. Besides these symptoms, appendicitis may be accompanied by nausea and a slight fever. Call a doctor immediately and describe the symptoms in detail; delay may result in a ruptured appendix.

EMERGENCY TREATMENT: While awaiting medical care, the victim may find some relief from the pain and discomfort by having an ice bag placed over the abdomen. Do not apply heat and give nothing by mouth. A laxative should not be offered.

Asphyxiation

See GAS POISONING.

Asthma attack

EMERGENCY TREATMENT: Make the patient comfortable and offer reassurance. If he has been examined by a doctor and properly diagnosed, the patient probably has an inhalant device or other forms of medication on his person or nearby.

The coughing and wheezing spell may have been triggered by the presence of an allergenic substance such as animal hair, feathers, or kapok in pillows or cushions. Such items should be removed from the presence of the patient. In addition, placing the patient in a room with high humidity, such as a bathroom with the shower turned on, may be helpful.

Asthma attacks are rarely fatal in young people, but elderly persons should be watched carefully because of possible heart strain. In a severe attack, professional medical care including oxygen equipment may be required.

Back injuries

In the event of any serious back injury, call a doctor or arrange for immediate professional transfer of the victim to a hospital.

EMERGENCY TREATMENT: Until determined otherwise by a physician, treat the injured person as a victim of a fractured spine. If he complains that he cannot move his head, feet, or toes, the chances are that the back is fractured. But even if he can move his feet or legs, it does not necessarily mean that he can be moved safely, since the back can be fractured without immediate injury to the spinal cord.

If the victim shows symptoms of shock, do not attempt to lower his head or move his body into the usual position for shock control. If it is absolutely essential to move the victim because of immediate danger to his life, make a rigid stretcher from a wide piece of solid lumber such as a door and cover the stretcher with a blanket for padding. Then carefully slide or pull the victim onto the stretcher, using his clothing to hold him. Tie the body onto the stretcher with strips of cloth.

Back pain

See SCIATICA.

Black eye

Although a black eye is frequently regarded as a minor medical problem, it can result in serious visual problems, including cataract or glaucoma.

EMERGENCY TREATMENT: Inspect the area about the eye for possible damage to the eye itself, such as hemorrhage, rupture of the eyeball, or dislocated lens. Check also for cuts around the eye that may require professional medical care. Then treat the bruised area by putting the victim to bed, covering the eye with a bandage, and applying an ice bag to the area.

If vision appears to be distorted or lacerations need stitching and antibiotic treatment, take the victim to a doctor's office. A doctor should also be consulted about continued pain and swelling about the eye.

Black widow spider bites

EMERGENCY TREATMENT: Make the victim lie still. If the bite is on the arm or leg, position the victim so that the bite is lower than the level of the heart. Apply a rubber band or similar tourniquet between the bite and the heart to retard venom flow toward the heart. The bite usually is marked by two puncture points. Apply ice packs to the bite. Summon a doctor or carry the patient to the nearest hospital.

Loosen the tourniquet or constriction band for a few seconds every 15 minutes while awaiting help; you should be able to feel a pulse beyond the tourniquet if it is not too tight. Do not let the victim move about. Do not permit him to drink alcoholic beverages. He probably will feel weakness, tremor, and severe pain, but reassure him that he will recover. Medications, usually available only to a physician, should be administered promptly.

Bleeding, internal

Internal bleeding is always a very serious condition; it requires immediate professional medical attention.

In cases of internal bleeding, blood is sometimes brought to the outside of the body by coughing from the lungs, by vomiting from the stomach, by trickling from the ear or nose, or by passing in the urine or bowel movement.

Often, however, internal bleeding is concealed, and the only symptom may be the swelling that appears around the site of broken bones. A person can lose three or four pints of blood inside the body without a trace of blood appearing outside the body.

SOME SYMPTOMS OF INTERNAL BLEEDING: The victim will appear ill and pale. His skin will be colder than normal, especially the hands and feet; often the skin looks clammy because of sweating. The pulse usually will be rapid (over 90 beats a minute) and feeble.

EMERGENCY TREATMENT: Serious internal bleeding is beyond the scope of first aid. If necessary treat the victim for respiratory and cardiac arrest and for shock while waiting for medical aid.

Bleeding, minor

Bleeding from minor cuts, scrapes, and bruises usually stops by itself, but even small injuries of this kind should receive attention to prevent infection.

EMERGENCY TREATMENT: The injured area should be washed thoroughly with soap and water, or if possible, held under running water. The surface should then be covered with a sterile bandage.

The type of wound known as a puncture wound may bleed very little, but is potentially extremely dangerous because of the possibility of tetanus infection. Anyone who steps on a rusty nail or thumbtack or has a similar accident involving a pointed object that penetrates deep under the skin surface should consult a physician about the need for anti-tetanus inoculation or a booster shot.

Blisters

EMERGENCY TREATMENT: If the blister is on a hand or foot or other easily accessible part of the body, wash the area around the blister thoroughly with soap and water. After carefully drying the skin around the blister, apply an antiseptic to the same area. Then sterilize the point and a substantial part of a needle by heating it in an open flame. When the needle has been thoroughly sterilized, use the point to puncture the blister along the margin of the blister. Carefully squeeze the fluid from the blister by pressing it with a sterile gauze dressing; the dressing should soak up most of the fluid. Next, place a fresh sterile dressing over the blister and fasten it in place with a bandage. If a blister forms in a tender area or in a place that is not easily accessible, such as under the arm, do not open it yourself; consult your doctor.

The danger from any break in the skin is that germs or dirt can slip through the natural barrier to produce an infection or inflammation. Continue to apply an antiseptic each day to the puncture area until it has healed. If it appears that an infection has developed or healing is unusually slow, consult a doctor. Persons with diabetes or circulatory problems may have to be more cautious about healing of skin breaks than other individuals.

Blood blisters

Blood blisters, sometimes called hematomas, usually are caused by a sharp blow to the body surface such as hitting a finger with a hammer while pounding nails.

EMERGENCY TREATMENT: Wash the area of the blood blister thoroughly with soap and water. Do not open it. If it is a small blood blister, cover it with a protective bandage; in many cases, the tiny pool of blood under the skin will be absorbed by the sur-

rounding tissues if there is no further pressure at that point.

If the blood blister fails to heal quickly or becomes infected, consult a physician. Because the pool of blood has resulted from damage to a blood vessel, a blood blister usually is more vulnerable to infection or inflammation than an ordinary blister.

Boils

Boils frequently are an early sign of diabetes or another illness and should be watched carefully if they occur often. In general, they result from germs or dirt being rubbed into the skin by tight-fitting clothing, scratching, or through tiny cuts made during shaving.

EMERGENCY TREATMENT: If the boil is above the lip, do not squeeze it or apply any pressure. The infection in that area of the face may drain into the brain because of the pattern of blood circulation on the face. Let a doctor treat any boil on the face. If the boil is on the surface of another part of the body, apply moist hot packs, but do not squeeze or press on the boil because that action can force the infection into the circulatory system. A wet compress can be made by soaking a wash cloth or towel in warm water.

If the boil erupts, carefully wipe away the pus with a sterile dressing, and then cover it with another sterile dressing. If the boil is large or slow to erupt, or if it is slow to heal, consult a doctor.

Bone bruises

EMERGENCY TREATMENT: Make sure the bone is not broken. If the injury is limited to the thin layer of tissue surrounding the bone, and the function of the limb is normal though painful, apply a compression dressing and an ice pack. Limit use of the injured limb for the next day or two.

As the pain and swelling recede, cover the injured area with a foam-rubber pad held in place with an elastic bandage. Because the part of the limb that is likely to receive a bone bruise lacks a layer of muscle

and fat, it will be particularly sensitive to any pressure until recovery is complete.

Botulism

The bacteria that produce the lethal toxin of botulism are commonly present on unwashed farm vegetables and thrive in containers that

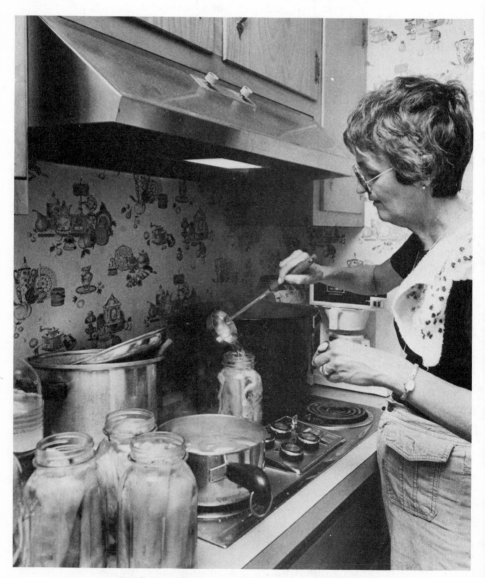

Botulism can be prevented by canning or preserving foods in jars that are properly sterilized and sealed.

are improperly sealed against the damaging effects of air. Home-canned vegetables, particularly string beans, are a likely source of botulism, but the toxin can be found in fruits, meats, and other foods. It can also appear in food that has been properly prepared but allowed to cool before being served. Examples are cold soups and marinated vegetables.

EMERGENCY TREATMENT: As soon as acute symptoms—nausea, diarrhea, and abdominal distress—appear, try to induce vomiting. Vomiting usually can be started by touching the back of the victim's throat with a finger or the handle of a spoon, which should be smooth and blunt, or by offering him a glass of water in which two tablespoons of salt have been dissolved. Call a doctor; describe all of the symptoms, which also may include, after several hours, double vision, muscular weakness, and difficulty in swallowing and breathing. Save samples of the food suspected of contamination for analysis.

Prompt hospitalization and injection of antitoxin are needed to save most cases of botulism poisoning. Additional emergency measures may include artificial respiration if regular breathing fails because of paralysis of respiratory muscles. Continue artificial respiration until professional medical care is provided. If other individuals have eaten the contaminated food, they should receive treatment for botulism even if they show no symptoms of the toxin's effects, since symptoms may be delayed several days.

Brown house (or recluse) spider bites

EMERGENCY TREATMENT: Apply an ice bag or cold pack to the wound area. Aspirin and antihistamines may be offered to help relieve any pain or feeling of irritation. Keep the victim lying down and quiet. Call a doctor as quickly as possible and describe the situation; the doctor will advise what further action should be taken at this point.

The effects of a brown spider bite frequently last much longer than the pain of the bite, which may be comparatively mild for an insect bite or sting. But the poison from the bite can gradually destroy the surrounding tissues, leaving at first an ulcer and eventually a disfiguring scar. A physician's treatment is needed to control the loss of tissue; he probably will prescribe drugs and recommend continued use of cold compresses. The victim, meanwhile, will feel numbness and muscular weakness, requiring a prolonged period of bed rest in addition to the medical treatments.

Bruises/contusions

EMERGENCY TREATMENT: Bruises or contusions result usually from a blow to the body that is powerful enough to damage muscles, tendons, blood vessels, or other tissues without causing a break in the skin.

Because the bruised area will be tender, protect it from further injury. If possible, immobilize the injured body part with a sling, bandage, or other device that makes the victim feel more comfortable; pillows, folded blankets, or similar soft materials can be used to elevate an arm or leg. Apply an ice bag or cold water dressing to the injured area.

A simple bruise usually will heal without extensive treatment. The swelling and discoloration are due to blood oozing from damaged tissues. However, severe bruising can be quite serious and requires medical attention. Keep the victim quiet and watch for symptoms of shock. Give aspirin for pain.

Bullet wounds

Bullet wounds, whether accidental or purposely inflicted, can range from those that are superficial and external to those that involve internal bleeding and extensive tissue damage.

EMERGENCY TREATMENT: A surface bullet wound accompanied by bleeding should be covered promptly with sterile gauze to prevent further infection. The flow of blood should be controlled as described on p. 141. *Don't* try to clean the wound with soap or water.

If the wound is internal, keep the patient lying down and wrap him with coats or blankets placed over and under his body. If respiration has ceased or is impaired, give mouth-to-mouth respiration and treat him for shock. Get medical aid promptly.

Burns, thermal

Burns are generally described according to the depth or area of skin damage involved. First-degree burns are the most superficial. They are marked by reddening of the skin and swelling, increased warmth, tenderness and pain. Second-degree burns, deeper than first-degree, are in effect open wounds, characterized by blisters and severe pain in addition to redness. Third-degree burns are deep enough to involve damage to muscles and bones. The skin is charred and there may be no pain because nerve endings have been destroyed. However, the area of the burn generally is more important than the degree of burn; a first or second-degree burn covering a large area of the body is more likely to be fatal than a small third-degree burn.

EMERGENCY TREATMENT: You will want to get professional medical help for treatment of a severe burn, but there are a number of things you can do until such help is obtained. If burns are minor, apply ice or ice water until pain subsides. Then wash the area with soap and water. Cover with a sterile dressing. Give the victim one or two aspirin tablets to help relieve discomfort. A sterile gauze pad soaked in a solution of two tablespoons of baking soda (sodium bicarbonate) per quart of lukewarm water may be applied.

For more extensive or severe burns, there are three first-aid objectives: (1) relieve pain, (2) prevent shock, (3) prevent infection. To relieve pain, exclude air by applying a thick dressing of four to six layers plus additional coverings of clean, tightly-woven material; for extensive burns, use clean sheets or towels. Clothing should be cut away —never pulled—from burned areas; where fabric is stuck to the wound, leave it for a doctor to remove later. Do not apply any ointment, grease, powder, salve, or other medication; the doctor simply will have to remove such material before he can begin professional treatment of the burns.

To prevent shock, make sure the victim's head is lower than his feet. Be sure that the victim is covered sufficiently to keep him warm, but not enough to make him overheated; exposure to cold can make the effects of shock more severe. Provide the

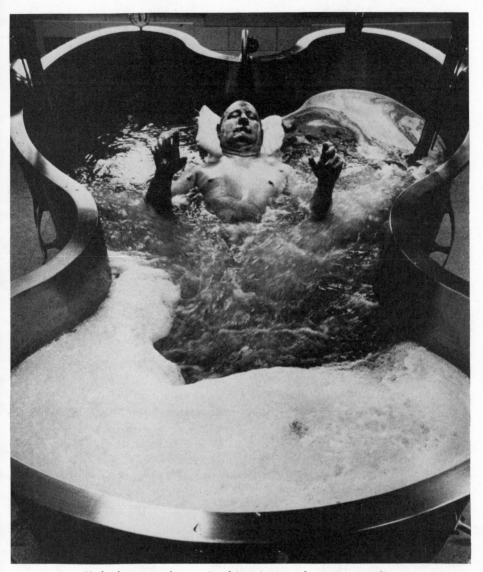

Hydrotherapy—therapy involving the use of water, as in this whirlpool bath—is one of the methods of treating burn patients.

victim with plenty of nonalcoholic liquids such as sweetened water, tea, or fruit juices, so long as he is conscious and able to swallow.

To prevent infection, do not permit absorbent cotton or adhesive tape to touch the wound caused by a burn. Do not apply iodine or any other antiseptic to the burn. Do not open any blisters. Do not permit any unsterile matter to contact the burn area. If possible, prevent other persons from coughing, sneezing, or even breathing toward the wound resulting from a burn. Serious infections frequently develop in burn victims from contamination by microorganisms of the mouth and nose.

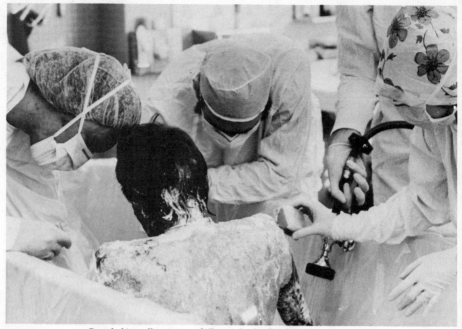

Dead skin cells are carefully washed off a burn victim, in order to prevent infection and provide a clear view of burn damage.

See also CHEMICAL BURNS OF THE EYE.

Carbuncles

Carbuncles are quite similar to boils except that they usually develop around multiple hair follicles and commonly appear on the neck or face. Personal hygiene is one factor involved in the development of carbuncles; persons apparently susceptible to the pustular inflammations must exercise special care in cleansing areas in which carbuncles occur, particularly if they suffer from diabetes or circulatory ailments.

EMERGENCY TREATMENT: Apply moist hot packs to the boil-like swelling. Change the moist hot packs frequently, or place a hot-water bottle on the moist dressing to maintain the moist heat application. Do not handle the carbuncle beyond whatever contact is necessary to ap-

ply or maintain the moist heat. The carbuncle should eventually rupture or reach a point where it can be opened with a sterile sharp instrument. After the carbuncle has ruptured and drained, and the fluid from the growth has been carefully cleaned away, apply a sterile dressing.

Frequently, carbuncles, must be opened and drained by a physician.

Cat scratch fever

Although the scratch or bite of a house cat or alley cat may appear at first to be only a mild injury, the wound can become the site of entry for a disease virus transmitted by apparently healthy cats. The inflammation, accompanied by fever, generally affects the lymph nodes and produces some aches and pains as well as fatigue. Although the disease is seldom fatal, an untreated case can spread to brain tissues and lead to other complications.

EMERGENCY TREATMENT: Wash the scratch thoroughly with water and either soap or a mild detergent. Apply a mild antiseptic such as hydrogen peroxide. Cover with a sterile dressing.

Watch the area of the scratch carefully for the next week or two. If redness or swelling develop, even after the scratch appears healed, consult your doctor. The inflammation of the scratch area may be accompanied by mild fever and symptoms similar to those of influenza; in small children, the symptoms may be quite serious. Bed rest and antibiotics usually are prescribed.

Charley horse

A charley horse occurs because a small number of muscle fibers have been torn or ruptured by overstraining the muscle, or by the force of a blow to the muscle.

EMERGENCY TREATMENT: Rest the injured muscle and apply an ice pack if there is swelling. A compression dressing can be applied to support the muscle. Avoid movement that stretches the muscle, and restrict other movements that make the victim uncomfortable. If pain and swelling persist, call a doctor.

During the recovery period, which may not begin for a day or two, apply local heat with a hot water bottle or an electric heating pad, being careful not to burn the victim. A return to active use of the muscle can begin gradually as pain permits.

Chemical burns of the eye

EMERGENCY TREATMENT: Flush the victim's eye immediately with large quantities of fresh, clean water; a drinking fountain can be used to provide a steady stream of water. If a drinking fountain is not available, lay the victim on the floor or ground with his head turned slightly to one side and pour water into the eye from a cup or glass. Always direct the stream of water so that it enters the eye surface at the inside corner and flows across the eye to the outside corner. If the victim is unable, because of intense pain, to open his eyes, it may be necessary to hold the lids apart while water pours across the eye. Continue flushing the eye for at least 15 minutes. (An alternate method is to immerse the victim's face in a pan or basin or bucket of water while he opens and closes his eyes repeatedly; continue the process for at least 15 minutes.)

When the chemical has been flushed from the victim's eye, the eye should be covered with a small, thick compress held in place with a bandage that covers both eyes, if possible; the bandage can be tied around the victim's head. NOTE: Apply nothing but water to the eye; do not attempt to neutralize a chemical burn of the eye and do not apply oil, ointment, salve, or other medications. Rush the victim to a doctor as soon as possible, preferably to an ophthalmologist.

Chemicals on skin

Many household and industrial chemicals, such as ammonia, lye, iodine, creosote, and a wide range of insecticides can cause serious injury if accidentally spilled on the skin.

EMERGENCY TREATMENT: Wash the body surface which has been affected by the chemical with large amounts of water. Do not try to neutralize the chemical with another substance; the reaction may aggravate the injury. If blisters appear, apply a sterile dressing. If the chemical is a refrigerant, such as Freon, or carbon dioxide under pressure, treat for frostbite.

If the chemical has splashed into the eyes or produces serious injury to the affected body surface, call a doctor. The victim should be watched closely for possible poisoning effects if the chemical is a pesticide, since such substances may be absorbed through the skin to produce internal toxic reactions. If there is any question about the toxicity of a chemical, ask your doctor or call the nearest poison control center.

Chigger bites

EMERGENCY TREATMENT: Apply ice water or rub ice over the area afflicted by bites of the tiny red insects. Bathing the area with alcohol, ammonia water or a solution of baking soda also will provide some relief from the itching.

Wash thoroughly with soap, using a scrub brush to prevent further infestation by the chiggers in other areas of the body. Rub alcohol over the surrounding areas and apply sulfur ointment as protection against mites that may not have attached themselves to the skin. Continue applications of ice water or alcohol to skin areas invaded by the insects. Clothing that was worn should be laundered immediately.

Chilblains

EMERGENCY TREATMENT: Move the victim to a moderately warm place and remove wet or tight clothing. Soak the affected body area in warm —but not hot—water for about 10 minutes. Then carefully blot the skin dry, but do not rub the skin. Replace the clothing with garments that are warm, soft, and dry.

Give the victim a stimulant such as tea or coffee, or an alcoholic beverage, and put him to bed with only light blankets; avoid the pressure of heavy blankets or heavy, tight garments on the sensitive skin areas. The victim should move the affected body areas gently to help restore normal circulation. If complications develop, such as marked discoloration of the skin, pain, or blistering and splitting of the skin, call a doctor.

Cold sores/fever blisters

EMERGENCY TREATMENT: Apply a soothing ointment or a medication such as camphor ice. Avoid squeezing or otherwise handling the blisters; moisture can aggravate the sores and hinder their healing. Repeated appearances of cold sores or fever blisters, which are caused by the herpes simplex virus, may require treatment by a physician.

Concussion

See HEAD INJURIES.

Contusions

See BRUISES.

Convulsions

EMERGENCY TREATMENT: Protect the victim from injury by moving him to a safe place; loosen any constricting clothing such as a tie or belt; put a pillow or coat under his head; if his mouth is open, place a folded cloth between his teeth to keep him from biting his tongue. Do not force anything into his mouth. Keep the patient warm but do not disturb him; do not try to restrain his convulsive movements.

Send for a doctor as quickly as possible. Watch the patient's breathing and begin artificial respiration if breathing stops for more than one minute. Be sure that breathing actually has stopped; the patient may be sleeping or unconscious after an attack but breathing normally.

Convulsions in a small child may signal the onset of an infectious disease and may be accompanied by a high fever. The same general precautions should be taken to prevent self-injury on the part of the child. If placed in a bed, the child should be protected against falling onto the floor. Place him on his side—not on his back or stomach—if he vomits. Cold compresses or ice packs on the back of the neck and the head may help relieve symptoms. Immediate professional medical care is vital because brain damage can result if treatment is delayed.

See also EPILEPTIC SEIZURES.

Cramps

See MUSCLE CRAMPS.

Croup

Croup is a breathing disorder usually caused by a virus infection and less often by bacteria or allergy. It is a common condition during childhood, and in some cases, may require brief hospitalization for proper treatment.

The onset of a croup attack is likely to occur during the night with a sudden hoarse or barking cough accompanied by difficulty in breathing. The coughing is usually followed by choking spasms that sound as though the child is strangling. There may also be a mild fever. A doctor should be called immediately when these symptoms appear.

EMERGENCY TREATMENT: The most effective treatment for croup is cool moist air. Cool water vaporizers are available as well as warm steam vaporizers. Another alternative is to take the child into the bathroom, close the door and windows, and let the hot water run from the shower and sink taps until the room is filled with steam.

It is also possible to improvise a croup tent by boiling water in a kettle on a portable hot plate and arranging a blanket over the back of a chair so that it encloses the child and an adult as well as the steaming kettle. A child should never be left alone even for an instant in such a makeshift arrangement.

If the symptoms do not subside in about 20 minutes with any of the above procedures, or if there is mounting fever, and if the doctor is not on his way, the child should be rushed to the closest hospital. Cold moist night air, rather than being a danger, may actually make the symptoms subside temporarily.

Diabetic coma and insulin shock

Diabetics should always carry an identification tag or card to alert others of their condition in the event of a diabetic coma—which is due to a lack of insulin. They also should advise friends or family members of their diabetic condition and the proper emergency measures that can be taken in the event of an onset of diabetic coma. A bottle of rapid-acting insulin should be kept on hand for such an emergency.

EMERGENCY TREATMENT: If the victim is being treated for diabetes, he probably will have nearby a supply of insulin and a hypodermic apparatus for injecting it. Find the insulin, hypodermic syringe, and needle; clean a spot on the upper arm or thigh, and inject about 50 units of insulin. Call a doctor without delay, and describe the patient's symptoms and your treatment. The patient usually will respond without ill effects, but may be quite thirsty. Give him plenty of fluids, as needed.

If the victim does not respond to the insulin, or if you cannot find the insulin and hypodermic syringe, rush the victim to the nearest doctor's office.

Insulin shock—which is due to a reaction to too much insulin and not enough sugar in the blood—can be treated in an emergency by offering a sugar-rich fluid such as a cola beverage or orange juice. Diabetics frequently carry a lump of sugar or candy which can be placed in their mouth in case of an insulin shock reaction. It should be tucked between the teeth and cheek so the victim will not choke on it.

If you find a diabetic in a coma and do not know the cause, assume the cause is an insulin reaction and treat him with sugar. This will give immediate relief to an insulin reaction but will not affect diabetic coma.

Diarrhea

EMERGENCY TREATMENT: Give the victim an antidiarrheal agent; all drugstores carry medications composed of kaolin and pectin that are useful for this purpose. Certain bismuth compounds also are recommended for diarrhea control.

Put the victim in bed for a period of at least 12 hours and withhold food and drink for that length of time. Do not let the victim become dehydrated; if he is thirsty, let him suck on pieces of ice. If the diarrhea appears to be subsiding, let him sip a mild beverage like tea or ginger ale; cola syrup is also recommended.

Later on the patient can try eating bland foods such as dry toast, crackers, gelatin desserts, or jellied consomme. Avoid feeding rich, fatty, or spicy foods. If the diarrhea fails to subside or is complicated by colic or vomiting, call a physician.

Dizziness/vertigo

Emotional upsets, allergies, and improper eating and drinking habits—too much food, too little food, or foods that are too rich—can precipitate symptoms of dizziness. The cause also can be a physical disorder such as abnormal functioning of the inner ear or a circulatory problem. Smoking tobacco, certain drugs such as quinine, and fumes of some chemicals also can produce dizziness.

EMERGENCY TREATMENT: Have the victim lie down with the eyes closed. In many cases, a period of simple bed rest will alleviate the symptoms. Keep the victim quiet and comfortable. If the feeling of dizziness continues, becomes worse, or is accompanied by nausea and vomiting, call a physician.

Severe or persistent dizziness or vertigo requires a longer period of bed rest and the use of medicines prescribed by a doctor. While recovering, the victim should avoid sudden changes in body position or turning the head rapidly. In some types of vertigo, surgery is required to cure the disorder.

Drowning

Victims of drowning seldom die because of water in the lungs or stomach. They die because of lack of air.

EMERGENCY TREATMENT: If the victim's breathing has been impaired, start artificial respiration immediately. If there is evidence of cardiac arrest, administer cardiac massage. When the victim is able to breathe for himself, treat him for shock and get medical help.

Drug overdose (barbiturates)

Barbiturates are used in a number of drugs prescribed as sedatives, although many are also available through illegal channels. Because the drugs can affect the judgment of the user, he may not remember having taken a dose and so may take additional pills, thus producing overdose effects.

EMERGENCY TREATMENT: If the drug was taken orally, try to induce vomiting in the victim. Have him drink a glass of water containing two tablespoons of salt. Or touch the back of his throat gently with a finger or a smooth blunt object like the handle of a spoon. Then give the victim plenty of warm water to drink. It is important to rid the stomach of as much of the drug as possible and to dilute the substance remaining in the gastrointestinal tract.

As soon as possible, call a doctor or get the victim to the nearest hospital or doctor's office. If breathing fails, administer artificial respiration.

Drug overdose (stimulants)

Although most of the powerful stimulant drugs, or pep pills, are available only through a doctor's prescription, the same medications are available through illicit sources. When taken without direction of a supervising physician, the stimulants can produce a variety of adverse side effects, and when used frequently over a period of time can result in physical and psychological problems that require hospital treatment.

EMERGENCY TREATMENT: Give the victim a solution of one tablespoon of activated charcoal mixed with a small amount of water, or give him a glass of milk, to dilute the effects of the medication in the stomach. Then induce vomiting by pressing gently on the back of the throat with a finger or the smooth blunt edge of a spoon handle. Vomiting also may be induced with a solution made of one teaspoonful of mustard in a half glass of water. Do not give syrup of ipecac to a victim who has been taking stimulants.

As soon as possible call a doctor or get the victim to the nearest hospital or doctor's office. If breathing fails, administer artificial respiration.

Earaches

An earache may be associated with a wide variety of ailments ranging from the common cold or influenza to impacted molars or tonsillitis. An earache also may be involved in certain infectious diseases such as measles or scarlet fever. Because of the relationship of ear structures to other parts of the head and throat, an infection involving the symptoms of earache can easily spread to the brain tissues or the spongy mastoid bone behind the ear. Call a doctor and describe all of the symptoms, including temperature, any discharge, pain, ringing in the ear, or deafness. Delay in reporting an earache to a doctor can result in complications that require hospital treatment.

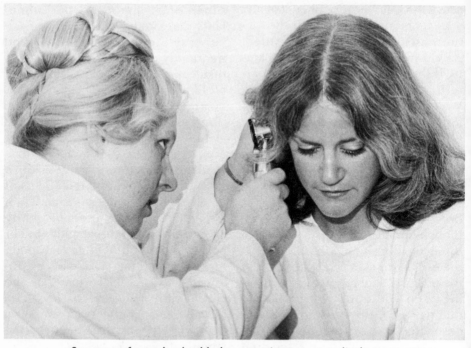

Symptoms of earache should always receive prompt medical attention. An ear infection can spread to the mastoid bone or to the brain.

EMERGENCY TREATMENT: This may include a few drops of warm olive oil or sweet oil held in the ear by a small wad of cotton. Aspirin can be given to help relieve any pain. Professional medical treatment may include the use of antibiotics.

Ear, foreign body in

EMERGENCY TREATMENT: Do not insert a hairpin, stick, or other object in the ear in an effort to remove a foreign object; you are likely to force the object farther into the ear canal. Instead, have the victim tilt his head to one side, with the ear containing the foreign object facing upward. While pulling gently on the lobe of the ear to straighten the canal, pour a little warmed olive oil or mineral oil into the ear. Then have the victim tilt that ear downward so the oil will run out quickly; it should dislodge the foreign object.

Wipe the ear canal gently with a cotton-tipped matchstick, or a similar device that will not irritate the lining of the ear canal, after the foreign body has been removed. If the emergency treatment is not successful, call a doctor.

Electric shocks

An electric shock from the usual 110-volt current in most homes can be a serious emergency, especially if the person's skin or clothing is wet. Under these circumstances, the shock may paralyze the part of the brain that controls breathing and stop the heart completely or disorder its pumping action.

EMERGENCY TREATMENT: It is of the utmost importance to break the electrical contact *immediately* by unplugging the wire of the appliance involved or by shutting off the house current switch. *Do not touch the victim of the shock while he is still acting as an electrical conductor.*

If the shock has come from a faulty wire out of doors and the source of the electrical current can't be reached easily, make a lasso of dry rope on a long sturdy dry stick. Catch the victim's hand or foot in the loop and drag him away from the wire. Another way to break the contact is to cut the wire with a dry axe.

If the victim of the shock is unconscious, or if his pulse is very weak, administer mouth-to-mouth respiration and cardiac massage until he can get to a hospital.

Epileptic seizures

Epilepsy is a disorder of the nervous system that produces convulsive seizures. In a major seizure or *grand mal*, the epileptic usually falls to the ground. Indeed, falling is in most cases one of the principal dangers of the disease. Then the epileptic's body begins to twitch or jerk spasmodically. His breathing may be labored, and saliva may appear on his lips. His face may become pale or bluish. Although the scene can be frightening, it is not truly a medical emergency; the afflicted person is in no danger of losing his life.

EMERGENCY TREATMENT: Make the person suffering the seizure as comfortable as possible. If he is on a hard surface, put something soft under his

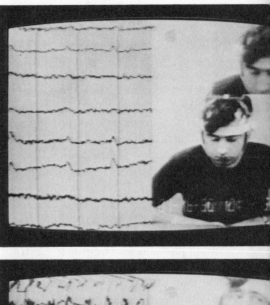

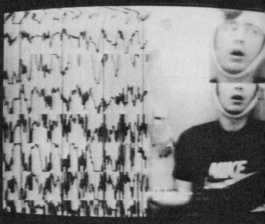

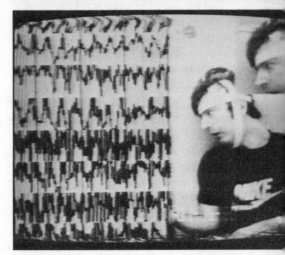

A severe epileptic seizure is recorded as it progresses (from top) on videotape. Images of the patient's electroencephalogram reading appear with the appropriate photo of the patient—clearly showing how his brain waves speeded up.

head, and move any hard or dangerous objects away from him. *Make no attempt to restrain his movements, and do not force anything into his mouth.* Just leave him alone until the attack is over, as it should be in a few minutes. If his mouth is already open, you might put something soft, such as a folded handerchief, between his side teeth. This will help to prevent him from biting his tongue or lips. If he seems to go into another seizure after coming out of the first, or if the seizure lasts more than ten minutes, call a doctor. If his lower jaw sags and begins to obstruct his breathing, support of the lower jaw may be helpful in improving his breathing.

When the seizure is over, the patient should be allowed to rest quietly. Some people sleep heavily after a seizure. Others awake at once but are disoriented or confused for a while. Treat the episode in a matter-of-fact way. If it is the first seizure the person is aware of having had, advise him to see his physician promptly.

Eye, foreign body in

EMERGENCY TREATMENT: Do not rub the eye or touch it with unwashed hands. The foreign body usually becomes lodged on the inner surface of the upper eyelid. Pull the upper eyelid down over the lower lid to help work the object loose. Tears or clean water can help wash out the dirt or other object. If the bit of irritating material can be seen on the surface of the eyeball, try very carefully to flick it out with the tip of a clean, moistened handkerchief or a piece of moistened cotton. Never touch the surface of the eye with dry materials. Sometimes a foreign body can be removed by carefully rolling the upper lid over a pencil or wooden matchstick to expose the object.

After the foreign object has been removed, the eye should be washed with clean water or with a solution made from one teaspoon of salt dissolved in a pint of water. This will help remove any remaining particles of the foreign body as well as any traces of irritating chemicals that might have been a part of it. Iron particles, for example, may leave traces of rust on the eye's surface unless washed away.

If the object cannot be located and removed without difficulty, a small patch of gauze or a folded handkerchief should be taped over the eye and the victim taken to a doctor's office—preferably the office of an ophthalmologist. A doctor also should be consulted if a feeling of irritation in the eye continues after the foreign body has been removed.

Fever

EMERGENCY TREATMENT: If the fever is mild, around 100° F. by mouth, have the victim rest in bed and provide him with a light diet. Watch closely for other symptoms, such as a rash, and any further increase in body temperature. Aspirin usually can be given.

If the temperature rises to 101° or higher, is accompanied by pain, headache, delirium, confused behavior, coughing, vomiting, or other indications of a severe illness, call a doctor. Describe all of the symptoms in detail, including the appearance of any rash and when it began.

Fever blisters

See COLD SORES.

Finger dislocation

EMERGENCY TREATMENT: Call a doctor and arrange for inspection and treatment of the injury. If a doctor is not immediately available, the finger dislocation may be reduced (put back in proper alignment) by grasping it firmly and carefully pulling it into normal position. Pull very slowly and avoid rough handling that might complicate the injury by damaging a tendon. If the dislocation cannot be reduced after the first try, go through the procedure once more. But do not try it more than twice.

Whether or not you are successful in reducing the finger dislocation, the finger should be immobilized after your efforts until a doctor can examine it. A clean flat wooden stick can be strapped along the palm side of the finger with adhesive tape or strips of bandage to hold it in place.

Fingernail injuries/hangnails

EMERGENCY TREATMENT: Wash the injured nail area thoroughly with warm water and soap. Trim off any torn bits of nail. Cover with a small adhesive dressing or bandage.

Apply petroleum jelly or cold cream to the injured nail area twice a day, morning and night, until it is healed. If redness or irritation develops in the adjoining skin area, indicating an infection, consult your doctor.

Fish poisoning

EMERGENCY TREATMENT: Induce vomiting in the victim to remove the bits of poisonous fish from the stomach. Vomiting usually can be started by pressing on the back of the throat with a finger or a spoon handle that is blunt and smooth, or by having the victim drink a solution of two tablespoons of salt in a glass of water.

Call a doctor as soon as possible. Describe the type of fish eaten and the symptoms, which may include nausea, diarrhea, abdominal pain, muscular weakness, and a numbness or tingling sensation that begins about the face and spreads to the extremities.

If breathing fails, administer mouth-to-mouth artificial respiration; a substance commonly found in poisonous fish causes respiratory failure. Also, be prepared to provide emergency treatment for convulsions.

Food poisoning

EMERGENCY TREATMENT: If the victim is not already vomiting, try to induce it to clear the stomach. Vomiting can be started in most cases by pressing gently on the back of the throat with a finger or a blunt smooth spoon handle, or by having the patient drink a glass of water containing two tablespoons of salt. If the victim has vomited, put him to bed.

Call a doctor and describe the food ingested and the symptoms which developed. If symptoms are severe, professional medical treatment with antibiotics and medications for cramps may be required. Special medications also may be needed for diarrhea caused by bacterial food poisoning.

Fractures

Any break in a bone is called a fracture. The break is called an *open* or *compound fracture* if one or both ends of the broken bone pierce the skin. A *closed* or *simple fracture* is one in which the broken bone doesn't come through the skin.

It is sometimes difficult to distinguish a strained muscle or a sprained ligament from a broken bone, since sprains and strains can be extremely painful even though they are less serious than breaks. However, when there is any doubt, the injury should be treated as though it were a simple fracture.

EMERGENCY TREATMENT: Don't try to help the injured person move around or get up unless he has slowly tested out the injured part of his body and is sure that nothing has been broken. If he is in extreme pain, or if the injured part has begun to swell, or if by running the finger lightly along the affected bone a break can be felt, *do not* move him. Under no circumstances should he be crowded into a car if his legs, hip, ribs, or back are involved in the accident. Call for an ambulance immediately, and until it arrives, treat the person for shock.

SPLINTING: In a situation where it is imperative to move someone who may have a fracture, the first step is to apply a splint so that the broken bone ends are immobilized.

Splints can be improvised from anything rigid enough and of the right length to support the fractured part of the body: a metal rod, board, long cardboard tube, tightly rolled newspaper or blanket. If the object being used has to be padded for softness, use a small blanket or any other soft material, such as a jacket.

The splint should be long enough so that it can be tied with a bandage, torn sheet, or neckties beyond the joint above and below the fracture as well as at the site of the break. If a leg is involved, it should be elevated with pillows or any other firm support after the splint has been applied. If the victim has to wait a considerable length of time before receiving professional attention, the splint bandaging should be checked from time to time to make sure it isn't too tight.

In the case of an open or compound fracture, additional steps must be taken. Remove that part of the victim's clothing which is covering the wound. Do not wash or probe into the wound, but control bleeding by applying pressure over the wound through a sterile or clean dressing.

Frostbite

EMERGENCY TREATMENT: Begin rapid rewarming of the affected tissues as soon as possible. If possible, immerse the victim in a warm bath, but avoid scalding. (The temperature should be between 102° and 105° F.) Warm wet towels also will help if changed frequently and applied gently. Do not massage, rub, or even touch the frostbitten flesh. If warm water or a warming fire is not available, place the patient in a sleeping bag or cover him with coats and blankets. Hot liquids can be offered if available to help raise the body temperature.

For any true frostbite case, prompt medical attention is important. The depth and degree of the frozen tissue cannot be determined without a careful examination by a physician.

Gall bladder attacks

Although gallstones can affect a wide variety of individuals, the most common victims are overweight persons who enjoy rich foods. The actual attack of spasms caused by gallstones passing through the duct leading from the gall bladder to the digestive tract usually is preceded by periods of stomach distress including belching. X rays usually will reveal the presence of gallstones when the early warning signs are noted, and measures can be taken to reduce the threat of a gall-bladder attack.

EMERGENCY TREATMENT: Call a doctor and describe in detail the symptoms, which may include colic high in the abdomen and pain extending to the right shoulder; the pain may be accompanied by nausea, vomiting, and sweating. Hot water bottles may be applied to the abdomen to help relieve distress while waiting for professional medical care. If the doctor permits, the victim may be allowed to sip certain fluids such as fruit juices, but do not offer him solid food.

Gas poisoning

Before attempting to revive someone overcome by toxic gas poisoning, the most important thing to do is to remove him to the fresh air. If this isn't feasible, all windows and doors should be opened to let in as much fresh air as possible.

Any interior with a dangerous concentration of carbon monoxide or other toxic gases is apt to be highly explosive. Therefore, gas and electricity should be shut off as quickly as possible. *Under no circumstances should any matches be lighted in an interior where there are noxious fumes.*

The rescuer needn't waste time covering his face with a handkerchief or other cloth. He should hold his breath instead, or take only a few quick, shallow breaths while bringing the victim to the out-of-doors or to an open window.

EMERGENCY TREATMENT: Administer artificial respiration if the victim is suffering respiratory arrest. Arrange for medical help as soon as possible, requesting that oxygen be brought to the scene.

Head injuries

Accidents involving the head can result in concussion, skull fracture, or brain injury. Symptoms of head injury include loss of consciousness, discharge of a watery or blood-tinged fluid from the ears, nose, or mouth, and a difference in size of the pupils of the eyes. Head injuries must be thought of as serious; they demand immediate medical assistance.

EMERGENCY TREATMENT: Place the victim in a supine position, and, if there is no evidence of injury to his neck, arrange for a slight elevation of his head *and* shoulders. Make certain that he has a clear airway and administer artificial respiration if necessary. If vomitus, blood, or other fluids appear to flow from the victim's mouth, turn his head gently to one side. Control bleeding and treat for shock. Do not administer stimulants or fluids of any kind.

Heart attack

A heart attack is caused by interference with the blood supply to the heart muscle. When the attack is brought on because of a blood clot in the coronary artery, it is known as *coronary occlusion* or *coronary thrombosis.*

The most dramatic symptom of a serious heart attack is a crushing chest pain that usually travels down the left arm into the hand or into the neck and back. The pain may bring on dizziness, cold sweat, complete

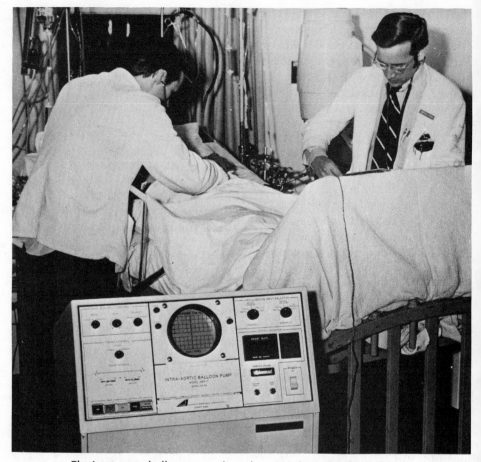

The intra-aorta balloon pump shown here is a device used to take over the major pumping action of the heart following an acute heart attack.

collapse, and loss of consciousness. The face has an ashen pallor, and there may be vomiting.

EMERGENCY TREATMENT: The victim *must not be moved* unless he has fallen in a dangerous place. If no doctor is immediately available, an ambulance should be called at once. No attempt should be made to get the victim of a heart attack into an automobile.

Until help arrives, give the victim every reassurance that he will get prompt treatment, and keep him as calm and quiet as possible. Don't give him any medicine or stimulants.

If oxygen is available, start administering it to the victim immediately, either by mask or nasal catheter, depending on which is available.

If the victim is suffering from respiratory arrest, begin artificial respiration. If he is suffering from cardiac arrest, begin cardiac massage.

Heat exhaustion

Heat exhaustion occurs when the body is exposed to high temperatures and large amounts of blood accumulate in the skin as a way of cooling it. As a result, there is a marked decrease in the amount of blood that circulates through the heart and to the brain. The victim becomes markedly pale and is covered with cold perspiration. Breathing is increasingly shallow and the pulse weakens. In acute cases, fainting occurs. Medical aid should be summoned for anyone suffering from heat exhaustion.

EMERGENCY TREATMENT: Place the victim in a reclining position with his feet raised about 10 inches above his body. Loosen or remove his clothing, and apply cold, wet cloths to his wrists and forehead. If he has fainted and doesn't recover promptly, smelling salts or spirits of ammonia should be placed under his nose. When the victim is conscious, give him sips of salt water (approximately one teaspoon of salt per glass of water), the total intake to be about two glasses in an hour's time. If the victim vomits, discontinue the salt solution.

Heatstroke/sunstroke

Heatstroke is characterized by an acutely high body temperature caused by the cessation of perspiration. The victim's skin becomes hot, dry, and flushed, and he may suffer collapse. Should the skin turn ashen gray, a physician must be called immediately. Prompt hospital treatment is recommended for anyone showing signs of sunstroke who has previously had any kind of heart damage.

EMERGENCY TREATMENT: The following measures are designed to reduce the victim's body temperature as quickly as possible and prevent damage to the internal organs:

Place him in a tub of very cold water, or, if this is not possible, spray or sponge his body repeatedly with cold water or rubbing alcohol. Take his temperature by mouth, and when it has dropped to about 100° F., remove him to a bed and wrap him in cold, wet sheets. If possible, expose him to an electric fan or an air conditioner.

Hiccups

EMERGENCY TREATMENT: Have the victim slowly drink a large glass of water. If cold water is not effective, have him drink warm water containing a teaspoonful of baking soda. Milk also can be employed. For babies and small children, offer sips of warm water. Do not offer carbonated beverages.

Another helpful measure is breathing into a large paper bag a number of times to raise the carbon dioxide level in the lungs. Rest and relaxation are recommended; have the victim lie down to read or watch television.

If the hiccups fail to go away, and continued spastic contractions of the diaphragm interfere with eating and sleeping, call your doctor.

Insect stings

Honeybees, wasps, hornets, and yellow jackets are the most common stinging insects and are most likely to attack on a hot summer day. Strongly scented perfumes or cosmetics and brightly colored, rough-finished clothing attract bees and should be avoided by persons working or playing in garden areas. It should also be noted that many commercial repellents do not protect against stinging insects.

EMERGENCY TREATMENT: If one is stung, the insect's stinger should be scraped gently but quickly from the skin; don't squeeze it. Apply Epsom salt solution to the sting area. Antihistamines are often helpful in reducing the patient's discomfort. If a severe reaction develops, call a doctor.

There are a few people who are critically allergic to the sting of wasps, bees, yellow jackets, or fire ants. This sensitivity causes the vocal cord tissue to swell to the point where breathing may become impossible. A single sting to a sensitive person may result in a dangerous drop in blood pressure, thus producing shock. Anyone with such a severe allergy who is stung should be rushed to a hospital immediately.

A person who becomes aware of having this type of allergy should consult with a physician about the kind of medicine to carry for use in a crisis.

Insulin shock

See DIABETIC COMA AND INSULIN SHOCK.

Jaw dislocation

The jaw can be dislocated during a physical attack or fight; from a blow on the jaw during sports activities; or from overextension of the joint during yawning, laughing, or attempting to eat a large mouthful of food. The jaw becomes literally locked open so the victim cannot explain his predicament.

EMERGENCY TREATMENT: Reducing a dislocated jaw will require that you insert your thumbs between the teeth of the victim. The jaw can be expected to snap into place quickly, and there is a danger that the teeth will clamp down on the thumbs when this happens, so the thumbs should be adequately padded with handkerchiefs or bandages. Once

the thumbs are protected, insert them in the mouth and over the lower molars, as far back on the lower jaw as possible. While pressing down with the thumbs, lift the chin with the fingers outside the mouth. As the jaw begins to slip into normal position when it is pushed downward and backward with the chin lifted upward, quickly remove the thumbs from between the jaws.

Once the jaw is back in normal position, the mouth should remain closed for several hours while the ligaments recover from their displaced condition. If necessary, put a cravat bandage over the head to hold the mouth closed. If difficulty is experienced in reducing a jaw dislocation, the victim should be taken to a hospital where an anesthetic can be applied. A dislocated jaw can be extremely painful.

Jellyfish stings

EMERGENCY TREATMENT: Wash the area of the sting thoroughly with alcohol or fresh water. Be sure that any pieces of jellyfish tentacles have been removed from the skin. Aspirin or antihistamines can be administered to relieve pain and itching, but curtail the use of antihistamines if the victim has consumed alcoholic beverages. The leg or arm that received the sting can be soaked in hot water if the pain continues. Otherwise, apply calamine lotion.

If the victim appears to suffer a severe reaction from the sting, summon a doctor. The victim may experience shock, muscle cramps, convulsions, or loss of consciousness. Artificial respiration may be required while awaiting arrival of a doctor. The physician can administer drugs to relieve muscle cramps and provide sedatives or analgesics.

Kidney stones

EMERGENCY TREATMENT: Call a doctor if the victim experiences the agonizing cramps or colic associated with kidney stones. Discuss the symptoms in detail with the doctor to make sure the pain is caused by kidney stones rather than appendicitis.

Comforting heat may be applied to the back and the abdomen of the side affected by the spasms. Paregoric can be administered, if available, while waiting for medical care; about two teaspoonsful of paregoric in a half glass of water may help relieve symptoms.

Knee injuries

EMERGENCY TREATMENT: If the injury appears to be severe, including possible fracture of the kneecap, immobilize the knee. To immobilize the knee, place the injured leg on a board that is about four inches wide and three to four feet in length. Place padding between the board and the knee, and between the board and the back of the ankle. Then use four strips of bandage to fasten the leg to the padded board—one at the ankle, one at the thigh, and one each above and below the knee.

Summon a doctor or move the patient to a doctor's office. Keep the knee protected against cold or exposure to the elements, but otherwise do not apply a bandage or any type of pressure to the knee itself; any rapid swelling would be aggravated by unnecessary pressure in that area. Be prepared to treat the patient for shock.

Laryngitis

Laryngitis is associated with colds and influenza and may be accompanied by a fever. The ailment can be aggravated by smoking, and it is possible that the vocal cords can be damaged if the victim tries to force the use of his voice while the larynx is swollen by the infection.

EMERGENCY TREATMENT: Have the victim inhale the warm moist air of a steam kettle or vaporizer. A vaporizer can be improvised in an emergency by pouring boiling water into a bowl and forming a "tent" over the steaming bowl with a large towel or sheet, or by placing a large paper bag over the bowl and cutting an opening at the closed end of the bag so the face can be exposed to the steam. The hot water can contain a bit of camphor or menthol, if available, to make the warm moist air more soothing to the throat, but this is not necessary.

Continue the use of the vaporizer for several days, as needed. The victim should not use the vocal cords any more than absolutely necessary. If the infection does not subside within the first few days, a doctor should be consulted.

Leeches

EMERGENCY TREATMENT: Do not try to pull leeches off the skin. They will usually drop away from the skin if a heated object such as a lighted cigarette is held close to them. Leeches also are likely to let go if iodine is applied to their bodies. The wound caused by a leech should be washed carefully with soap and water and an antiseptic applied.

Lightning shock

EMERGENCY TREATMENT: If the victim is not breathing, apply artificial respiration. If a second person is available to help, have him summon a doctor while artificial respiration is administered. Continue artificial respiration until breathing resumes or the doctor arrives.

When the victim is breathing regularly, treat him for shock. Keep him lying down with his feet higher than his head, his clothing loosened around the neck, and his body covered with a blanket or coat for warmth. If the victim shows signs of vomiting, turn his head to one side so he will not swallow the vomitus.

If the victim is breathing regularly and does not show signs of shock, he may be given a few sips of a stimulating beverage such as coffee, tea, or brandy.

Motion sickness

EMERGENCY TREATMENT: Have the victim lie down in a position that is most comfortable to him. The head should be fixed so that any view of motion is avoided. Reading or other use of the eyes should be prohibited. Food or fluids should be restricted to very small amounts. If traveling by car, stop at a rest area; in an airplane or ship, place the victim in an area where motion is least noticeable.

Drugs, such as Dramamine, are helpful for control of the symptoms of motion sickness; they are most effective when started about 90 minutes before travel begins and repeated at regular intervals thereafter.

Muscle cramps

EMERGENCY TREATMENT: Gently massage the affected muscle, sometimes stretching it to help relieve the painful contraction. Then relax the muscle by using a hot water bottle or an electric heating pad, or by soaking the affected area in a warm bath.

A repetition of cramps may require

medical attention.

Nosebleeds

EMERGENCY TREATMENT: Have the victim sit erect but with the head tilted slightly forward to prevent blood from running down the throat. Apply pressure by pinching the nostrils; if bleeding is from just one nostril, use pressure on that side. A small wedge of absorbent cotton or gauze can be inserted into the bleeding nostril. Make sure that the cotton or gauze extends out of the nostril to aid in its removal when the bleeding has stopped. Encourage the victim to breathe through the mouth while the nose is bleeding. After five minutes, release pressure on the nose to see if the bleeding has stopped. If the bleeding continues, repeat pressure on the nostril for an additional five minutes. Cold compresses applied to the nose can help stop the bleeding.

If bleeding continues after the second five-minute period of pressure treatment, get the victim to a doctor's office or a hospital emergency room.

Poison ivy/poison oak/poison sumac

EMERGENCY TREATMENT: The poison of these three plants is the same and the treatment is identical. Bathe the skin area exposed to poison ivy, poison oak, or poison sumac with soap and water or with alcohol within 15 minutes after contact. If exposure is not discovered until a rash appears, apply cool wet dressings. Dressings can be made of old bed sheets or soft linens soaked in a solution of one teaspoon of salt per pint of water. Dressings should be applied four times a day for periods of 15 to 60 minutes each time; during these periods, dressings can be removed and reapplied every few minutes. The itching that often accompanies the rash can be relieved by taking antihistamine tablets.

Creams or lotions may be prescribed by a doctor or supplied by a pharmacist. Do not use such folk remedies as ammonia or turpentine; do not use skin lotions not approved by a doctor or druggist. Haphazard application of medications on poison ivy blisters and rashes can result in complications including skin irritation, infection, or pigmented lesions of the skin.

Rabies

See ANIMAL BITES.

Sciatica/lower back pain

Although lower back pain is frequently triggered by fatigue, anxiety, or by strained muscles or tendons, it may be a symptom of a slipped or ruptured disk between the vertebrae, or of a similar disorder requiring extensive medical attention.

EMERGENCY TREATMENT: Reduce the pressure on the lower back by having the victim lie down on a hard flat surface; if a bed is used there should be a board or sheet of plywood between the springs and mattress. Pillows should be placed under the knees instead of under the head, to help keep the back flat. Give aspirin to relieve the pain, and apply heat to the back. Call a doctor if the symptoms do not subside overnight.

Scorpion stings

EMERGENCY TREATMENT: Apply ice to the region of the sting, except in the case of an arm or leg, in which event the limb may be immersed in ice water. Continue the ice or ice-water treatment for at least one hour. Try to keep the area of the sting at a position lower than the heart. No tourniquet is required. Should the breathing of a scorpion sting victim becomes depressed, administer artificial respiration. If symptoms fail to subside within a couple of hours, notify a physician, or transfer the victim to a doctor's office or hospital.

For children under six, call a physician in the event of any scorpion sting. Children stung by scorpions may become convulsive, and this condition can result in fatal exhaustion unless it receives prompt medical treatment.

Snakebites

Of the many varieties of snakes found in the United States, only four kinds are poisonous: copperheads, rattlesnakes, moccasins, and coral snakes. The first three belong to the category of pit vipers and are known as *hemotoxic* because their poison enters the bloodstream. The coral snake, which is comparatively rare, is related to the cobra and is the most dangerous of all because its venom is *neurotoxic*. This means that the poison transmitted by its bite goes directly to the nervous system and the brain.

HOW TO DIFFERENTIATE BETWEEN SNAKEBITES: Snakes of the pit viper family have a fang on each side of the head. These fangs leave characteristic puncture wounds on the skin in addition to two rows of tiny bites or scratches left by the teeth. A bite from a nonpoisonous snake leaves six rows—four upper and two lower—of very small bite marks or scratches and no puncture wounds.

The marks left by the bite of a coral

snake do not leave any puncture wounds either, but this snake bites with a chewing motion, hanging on to the victim rather than attacking quickly. The coral snake is very easy to recognize because of its distinctive markings: wide horizontal bands of red and black separated by narrow bands of yellow.

SYMPTOMS: A bite from any of the pit vipers produces immediate and severe pain and darkening of the skin, followed by weakness, blurred vision, quickened pulse, nausea, and vomiting. The bite of a coral snake produces somewhat the same symptoms, although there is less local pain and considerable drowsiness leading to unconsciousness.

If a doctor or a hospital is a short distance away, the patient should receive professional help *immediately*. He should be transported lying down, either on an improvised stretcher or carried by his companions—with the wounded part lower than his heart. He should be advised to move as little as possible.

EMERGENCY TREATMENT: If several hours must elapse before a doctor or a hospital can be reached, the following procedures should be applied promptly:

1. Keep the victim lying down and as still as possible.

2. Tie a constricting band *above* the wound between it and the heart and tight enough to slow but not stop blood circulation. A handkerchief, necktie, sock, or piece of torn shirt will serve.

3. If a snakebite kit is available, use the knife it contains; otherwise, sterilize a knife or razor blade in a flame. Carefully make small cuts in the skin where the swelling has developed. Make the cuts along the

length of the limb, not across or at right angles to it. The incisions should be shallow because of the danger of severing nerves, blood vessels, or muscles.

4. Use the suction cups in the snakebite kit, if available, to draw out as much of the venom as possible. If suction cups are not available, the venom can be removed by sucking it out with the mouth. Although snake venom is not a stomach poison, it should not be swallowed but should be rinsed from the mouth.

5. This procedure should be continued for from 30 to 60 minutes or until the swelling subsides and the other symptoms decrease.

6. You may apply cold compresses to the bite area while waiting for professional assistance.

7. Treat the victim for shock.

8. Give artificial respiration if necessary.

Splinters

EMERGENCY TREATMENT: Clean the area about the splinter with soap and water or an antiseptic. Next, sterilize a needle by holding it over an open flame. After it cools, insert the needle above the splinter so it will tear a line in the skin, making the splinter lie loose in the wound. Then, gently lift the splinter out, using a pair of tweezers or the point of the needle. If tweezers are used, they should be sterilized first.

Wash the wound area again with soap and water, or apply an antiseptic. It is best to cover the wound with an adhesive bandage. If redness or irritation develops around the splinter wound, consult a doctor.

Sprains

A sprain occurs when a joint is

wrenched or twisted in such a way that the ligaments holding it in position are ruptured, possibly damaging the surrounding blood vessels, tendons, nerves, and muscles. This type of injury is more serious than a strain and is usually accompanied by pain, sometimes severe, soreness, swelling, and discoloration of the affected area. Most sprains occur as a result of falls, athletic accidents, or improper handling of heavy weights.

EMERGENCY TREATMENT: This consists of prompt rest, the application of cold compresses to relieve swelling and any internal bleeding in the joint, and elevation of the affected area. Aspirin is recommended to reduce discomfort. If the swelling and soreness increase after such treatment, a physician should be consulted to make sure that the injury is not a fracture or a bone dislocation.

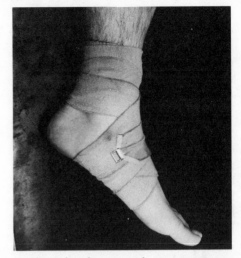

An elastic bandage provides temporary support for healing tendons or ligaments following a strain or sprain.

Sting ray

EMERGENCY TREATMENT: If an arm or leg is the target of a sting ray, wash the area thoroughly with salt water. Quickly remove any pieces of the stinger imbedded in the skin or flesh; poison can still be discharged into the victim from the sting-ray sheath. After initial cleansing of an arm or leg sting, soak the wound with hot water for up to an hour. Apply antiseptic or a sterile dressing after the soak.

Consult a physician after a sting-ray attack. The doctor will make a thorough examination of the wound to determine whether stitches or antibiotics are required. Fever, vomiting, or muscular twitching also may result from an apparently simple leg or arm wound by a sting ray.

If the sting occurs in the chest or abdomen, the victim should be rushed to a hospital as soon as possible because such a wound can produce convulsions or loss of consciousness.

Strains

When a muscle is stretched because of misuse or overuse, the interior bundles of tissue may tear, or the tendon which connects it to the bone may be stretched. This condition is known as strain. It occurs most commonly to the muscles of the lower back when heavy weights are improperly lifted, or in the area of the calf or ankle as the result of a sudden, violent twist or undue pressure.

EMERGENCY TREATMENT: Bed rest, the application of heat, and gentle massage are recommended for back strain. If the strain is in the leg, elevate the limb to help reduce pain and swelling, and apply cold compresses or an ice bag to the area. Aspirin may be taken to reduce discomfort.

In severe cases of strained back

muscles, a physician may have to be consulted for strapping. For a strained ankle, a flexible elastic bandage can be helpful in providing the necessary support until the injured muscle heals.

Stroke

Stroke, or apoplexy, is caused by a disruption of normal blood flow to the brain, either by rupture of a blood vessel within the brain or by blockage of an artery supplying the brain. The condition is enhanced by hardening of the arteries and high blood pressure, and is most likely to occur in older persons. A stroke usually occurs with little or no warning and the onset may be marked by a variety of manifestations ranging from headache, slurred speech, or blurred vision, to sudden collapse and unconsciousness.

EMERGENCY TREATMENT: Try to place the victim in a semi-reclining position, or, if he is lying down, be sure there is a pillow under his head. Avoid conditions that might increase the flow of blood toward the head. Summon a doctor immediately. Loosen any clothing that may be tight. If the patient wears dentures, remove them.

Before professional medical assistance is available, the victim may vomit or go into shock or convulsions. If he vomits, try to prevent a backflow of vomitus into the breathing passages. If shock occurs, do not place the victim in the shock position but do keep him warm and comfortable. If convulsions develop, place a handkerchief or similar soft object between the jaws to prevent tongue biting.

Sty on eyelid

Sties usually develop around hair follicles because of a bacterial infection. Like cold sores, they are most likely to develop in association with poor health and lowered resistance to infection.

EMERGENCY TREATMENT: Apply warm, moist packs or compresses to the sty for periods of 15 to 20 minutes at intervals of three or four hours. Moist heat generally is more penetrating than dry heat.

The sty should eventually rupture and the pus should then be washed carefully away from the eye area. If the sty does not rupture or is very painful, consult a doctor. Do not squeeze or otherwise handle the sty except to apply the warm moist compresses.

Sunburn

EMERGENCY TREATMENT: Apply cold wet compresses to help relieve the pain. Compresses can be soaked in whole milk, salt water, or a solution of corn starch mixed with water. The victim also may get some relief by soaking in a bathtub filled with

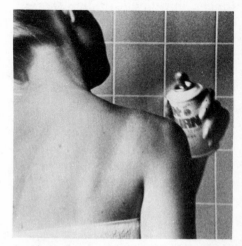

Avoid using topical anesthetics on sunburnt skin. They may cause allergic reactions. Use a soothing lotion such as baby oil.

plain water. Soothing lotions, such as baby oil or a bland cold cream, can be applied after carefully drying the skin. Don't rub the burn area while drying. Avoid the use of "shake" lotions, like calamine, which may aggravate the burn by a drying action. The victim should, of course, avoid further exposure to sunlight.

If pain is excessive, or extensive blistering is present, consult a physician. Avoid application of over-the-counter topical anesthetics that may cause allergic skin reactions.

A severe or extensive sunburn is comparable to a second-degree thermal burn and may be accompanied by symptoms of shock; if such symptoms are present the victim should be treated for shock. See also BURNS, THERMAL.

Sunstroke

See HEATSTROKE.

Tick bites

EMERGENCY TREATMENT: Do not try to scrape or rub the insect off the skin with your fingers; scraping, rubbing, or pulling may break off only part of the insect body, leaving the head firmly attached to the skin. Rubbing also can smear disease organisms from the tick into the bite. To make the tick drop away from the skin, cover it with a heavy oil, such as salad, mineral, or lubricating oil. Oil usually will block the insect's breathing pores, suffocating it. If oil is not readily available, carefully place a heated object against the tick's body; a lighted cigarette or a

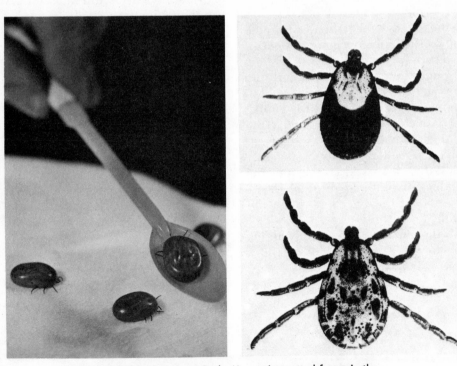

Wood ticks that cause Rocky Mountain spotted fever, in the engorged state (left), and in the unengorged state (right). The female is at the top right, the male at the bottom right.

match that has been ignited and snuffed out can serve as a hot object.

Carefully inspect the bite area to be sure that all parts of the tick have been removed. Use a pair of tweezers to remove any tick parts found. Then carefully wash the bite and surrounding area with soap and water and apply an antiseptic. Also, wash your hands and any equipment that may have come in contact with the tick. Consult a physician if symptoms of tick fever or tularemia, such as unexplained muscular weakness, occur following a bite.

Toothaches

EMERGENCY TREATMENT: Give an adult one or two aspirin tablets; a young child should be given no more than one-half of an adult tablet. The aspirin should be swallowed with plenty of water. Do not let it dissolve in the mouth or be held near the aching tooth. Aspirin becomes effective as a pain-killer only after it has gone through the digestive tract and into the bloodstream; if aspirin is held in the mouth, it may irritate the gums.

Oil of cloves can be applied to the aching tooth. Dip a small wad of cotton into the oil of cloves, then gently pack the oil-soaked cotton into the tooth cavity with a pair of tweezers. Do not let the tweezers touch the tooth.

If the jaw is swollen, apply an ice bag for periods of 15 minutes at a time, at intermittent intervals. Never apply heat to a swollen jaw when treating a toothache. Arrange to see your dentist as soon as possible.

Tooth, broken

EMERGENCY TREATMENT: Apply a few drops of oil of cloves to the injured tooth to help relieve pain. If oil of cloves is not available, give an adult one to two regular aspirin tablets. One-half of a regular tablet can be given to a young child.

Make an emergency filling from a wad of cotton containing a few drops of oil of cloves. An emergency filling also can be made from powdered chalk; it is important to protect the cavity from infection while providing pain relief.

If the tooth has been knocked out of the socket, retrieve the tooth, because it can be restored in some cases. Do not wash the tooth; ordinary washing can damage dental tissues. A dentist will take care of cleaning it properly. Wrap the tooth in a damp clean handkerchief or tissue or place the tooth in a container of slightly salty warm water for the trip to the dentist.

Unconsciousness

Unconsciousness is the condition which has the appearance of sleep, but is usually the result of injury, shock, or serious physical disturbance. A brief loss of consciousness followed by spontaneous recovery is called *fainting*. A prolonged episode of unconsciousness is a *coma*.

EMERGENCY TREATMENT: Call a doctor at once. If none is available, get the victim to the nearest hospital. If the loss of consciousness is accompanied by loss of breathing, begin mouth-to-mouth respiration. If the victim is suffering cardiac arrest, administer cardiac massage. Don't try to revive the victim with any kind of stimulant unless told to do so by a doctor.

Vertigo

See DIZZINESS.

CHAPTER 2

100 Commonly Prescribed Generic Drugs

The table that follows gives the names of 100 commonly prescribed generic drugs. These drugs are not patented, or the patents on them have expired. For that reason any drug company may manufacture and sell them under their generic names or under completely new brand names. The generic names are also called the "official" or "non-proprietary" names. They usually describe the chemical makeup or the class of the drug.

With each drug included in the table, several types of information are given. The table shows, for example, what the drug does, what its medical description is (anti-emetic, diuretic, and so on), and what illnesses, diseases, or disorders it is usually used to treat. Some, but not all, of each generic drug's trade-name equivalents are also shown.

It should be remembered that the list of 100 includes only some of the most commonly prescribed generic drugs. Hundreds of others, less widely used, might be listed. To save money, it's generally wise to ask your doctor when he writes a prescription whether the drug is available generically.

Name	Action	Prescribed for	Trade Names (CD = comb. drug)
ACETAMINOPHEN (Paracetamol)	Believed to reduce concentration of chemicals involved in production of pain, fever, and inflammation (analgesic; antipyretic)	Relief of mild to moderate pain; reduction of fever	Datril Tylenol Co-Tylenol (CD) Excedrin (CD) Sinarest (CD) Sinutab (CD)
AMITRIPTYLINE	Believed to restore to normal levels the constituents of brain tissue that transmit nerve impulses (antidepressant)	Relief of emotional depression; gradual improvement of mood	Elamil Etrafon (CD) Triavil (CD)
AMPICILLIN	Interferes with ability of susceptible bacteria to produce new protective cell walls as they grow and multiply (antibiotic)	Elimination of infections responsive to action of this drug	Amcill Pensyn Polycillin Principen

ANTACIDS (Aluminum Hydroxide) (Calcium Carbonate) (Sodium Bicarbonate)	Neutralizes stomach acid; reduces action of digestive enzyme pepsin (relief from gastric hyperacidity)	Relief of heartburn, sour stomach, acid indigestion, and discomfort associated with peptic ulcer, gastritis, esophagitis, hiatal hernia	Absorbable:
			Sodium bicarbonate:
			  Alka-Seltzer
			  Brioschi
			  Bromo-Seltzer
			Less absorbable:
			Aluminum hydroxide:
			  Amphojel
			Calcium carbonate:
			  Alka-2
			  Amitone

Name	Action	Prescribed for	Trade Names (CD = comb. drug)
ASPIRIN (Acetylsalicylic Acid)	Dilates blood vessels in skin, thus hastening loss of body heat (antipyretic); reduces tissue concentration of chemicals involved in production of inflammation and pain (analgesic; antirheumatic)	Reduction of fever; relief of mild to moderate pain and inflammation; prevention of blood clots, as in phlebitis, heart attack, stroke	Bayer Aspirin St. Joseph Children's Aspirin Preparations containing aspirin: (all CD) Alka-Seltzer Anacin A.P.C. Tablets Bufferin Empirin Compound 4-Way Tablets Vanquish
ATROPINE (Belladonna, Hyoscyamine)	Prevents stimulation of muscular contractions and glandular secretion in organ involved (antispasmodic [anticholinergic])	Relief of discomfort associated with excessive activity and spasm of digestive tract; irritation and spasm of lower urinary tract; painful menstruation	Donna Extendtabs Bellergal (CD) Donnagel-PG (CD) Donnatal (CD) Nembu-donna (CD)
BENDROFLUMETHIAZIDE	Increases elimination of salt and water (diuretic); relaxes walls of smaller arteries, allowing them to expand; combined effect lowers blood pressure (antihypertensive)	Elimination of excessive fluid retention (edema); reduction of high blood pressure	Naturetin Rautrax-N (CD) Rauzide (CD)
BROMPHENIRAMINE	Blocks action of histamine after release from sensitized tissue cells, thus reducing intensity of allergic response (antihistamine)	Relief of symptoms of hayfever (allergic rhinitis) and of allergic reactions of skin (itching, swelling, hives, rash)	Dimetane Veltane Dimetapp (CD)
BUTABARBITAL	Believed to block transmission of nerve impulses (hypnotic; sedative)	Low dosage: relief of moderate anxiety or tension (sedative effect); higher dosage: at bedtime to induce sleep (hypnotic effect)	Buticaps Butisol Butte Quiebar

Name	Action	Prescribed for	Trade Names (CD = comb. drug)
CAFFEINE	Constricts blood vessel walls; increases energy level of chemical systems responsible for nerve tissue activity (cardiac, respiratory, psychic stimulant)	Prevention and early relief of vascular headaches such as migraine; relief of drowsiness and mental fatigue	Nodoz Cafergot (CD) Cafermine (CD)
CARISOPRODOL	Believed to block transmission of nerve impulses and/or to produce a sedative effect (muscle relaxant)	Relief of discomfort caused by spasms of voluntary muscles	Rela Soma (CD) Soma Compound (CD)
CHLORAL HYDRATE	Believed to affect wake-sleep centers of brain (hypnotic)	Low dosage: relief of mild to moderate anxiety or tension (sedative effect); higher dosage: at bedtime to relieve insomnia (hypnotic effect)	Noctec Oradrate Somnos
CHLORAMPHENICOL	Prevents growth and multiplication of susceptible bacteria by interfering with formation of their essential proteins (antibiotic)	Elimination of infections responsive to action of this drug	Amphicol Chloromycetin Ophthochlor
CHLORDIAZEPOXIDE	Believed to reduce activity of some parts of limbic system (tranquilizer)	Relief of mild to moderate anxiety and tension without significant sedation	Libritabs Librium
CHLOROTHIAZIDE	Increases elimination of salt and water (diuretic); relaxes walls of smaller arteries, allowing them to expand; combined effect lowers blood pressure (antihypertensive)	Elimination of excessive fluid retention (edema); reduction of high blood pressure	Diuril Aldoclor (CD) Diupres (CD)
CHLORPHENIRAMINE	Blocks action of histamine after release from sensitized tissue cells, thus reducing intensity of allergic response (antihistamine)	Relief of symptoms of hayfever (allergic rhinitis) and of allergic reactions of skin (itching, swelling, hives, rash)	Chlor-Trimeton Polaramine Teldrin

Name	Action	Prescribed for	Trade Names (CD = comb. drug)
CHLORPROMAZINE	Believed to inhibit action of dopamine, thus correcting an imbalance of nerve impulse transmissions thought to be responsible for certain mental disorders (antiemetic; tranquilizer)	Relief of severe anxiety, agitation, and psychotic behavior	Klorazine Promapar Thorazine
CODEINE	Believed to affect tissue sites that react specifically with opium and its derivatives (antitussive; narcotic analgesic)	Relief of moderate pain; control of coughing	None as a single entity—many for combination products
DEXAMETHASONE	Believed to inhibit several tissue mechanisms that induce inflammation (adrenocortical steroid [anti-inflammatory])	Symptomatic relief of inflammation (swelling, redness, heat, pain)	Decadron Dexameth Hexadrol
DEXTROAMPHETAMINE (d-Amphetamine)	Increases release of nerve impulse transmitter (central stimulant); this may also improve concentration and attention span of hyperactive child (primary calming action unknown); alters chemical control of nerve impulse transmission in appetite control center of brain (appetite suppressant [anorexiant])	Reduction or prevention of sleep epilepsy (narcolepsy); reduction of symptoms of abnormal hyperactivity (as in minimal brain dysfunction); suppression of appetite in management of weight reduction	Dexedrine Bamadex (CD) Biphetamine (CD) Dexamyl (CD)
DIAZEPAM	Believed to reduce activity of some parts of limbic system (tranquilizer)	Relief of mild to moderate anxiety and tension without significant sedation	Valium
DICYCLOMINE	Believed to produce a local anesthetic action that blocks reflex activity responsible for spasm (antispasmodic)	Relief of discomfort from muscle spasm of the gastrointestinal tract	Bentyl Dispas Triactin (CD)

Name	Action	Prescribed for	Trade Names (CD = comb. drug)
DIGITOXIN	Increases availability of calcium within the heart muscle, thus improving conversion of chemical energy to mechanical energy; slows pacemaker and delays transmission of electrical impulses (digitalis preparations [cardiotonic])	Improvement of heart muscle contraction force (as in congestive heart failure); correction of certain heart rhythm disorders	Crystodigin Digitaline Purodigin
DIGOXIN	Same as above	Same as above	Davoxin Lanoxin Thegitoxin
DIPHENHYDRAMINE	Blocks action of histamine after release from sensitized tissue cells, thus reducing intensity of allergic response (antihistamine)	Relief of symptoms of hayfever (allergic rhinitis) and of allergic reactions of skin (itching, swelling, hives, rash)	Benadryl Ambenyl (CD) Benylin (CD)
DOXYLAMINE	Same as above	Same as above	Decapryn Bendectin (CD) Nyquil (CD)
EPHEDRINE	Blocks release of certain chemicals from sensitized tissue cells undergoing allergic reaction; relaxes bronchial muscles; shrinks tissue mass (decongestion) by contracting arteriole walls in lining of respiratory passages (adrenergic [bronchodilator])	Prevention and symptomatic relief of bronchial asthma; relief of congestion of respiratory passages	Bronkaid (CD) Bronkotabs (CD) Marax (CD) Nyquil (CD) Quelidrine (CD) Quibron Plus (CD) Tedral (CD)
ERGOTAMINE	Constricts blood vessel walls, thus relieving excessive dilation that causes pain of vascular headaches (migraine analgesic [vasoconstrictor])	Prevention and early relief of vascular headaches such as migraine or histamine headaches	Ergomar Bellergal (CD) Cafergot (CD) Migral (CD)

Name	Action	Prescribed for	Trade Names (CD = comb. drug)
ERYTHRITYL TETRANITRATE	Acts directly on muscle cells to produce relaxation which permits expansion of blood vessels, thus increasing supply of blood and oxygen to heart	Management of pain associated with angina pectoris (coronary insufficiency)	Anginar Cardilate
ERYTHROMYCIN	Prevents growth and multiplication of susceptible bacteria by interfering with formation of their essential proteins (antibiotic)	Elimination of infections responsive to action of this drug	Bristamycin E-Mycin Erythrocin Ethril Pfizer-E
ESTROGEN (Estrogenic Substances) Conjugated Estrogens, Esterified Estrogens (Estrone and Equilin)	Prepares uterus for pregnancy or induces menstruation by cyclic increase and decrease in tissue stimulation; when taken regularly, blood and tissue levels increase to resemble those during pregnancy, thus preventing pituitary gland from producing hormones that induce ovulation; reduces frequency and intensity of menopausal symptoms (female sex hormone)	Regulation of menstrual cycle; prevention of pregnancy; relief of symptoms of menopause	Amnestrogen Femogen Menotabs Menrium (CD) Milprem (CD)
GRISEOFULVIN	Believed to prevent growth and multiplication of susceptible fungus strains by interfering with their metabolic activities (antibiotic; antifungal)	Elimination of fungus infections responsive to action of this drug	Fulvicin-U/F Grifulvin V
HYDRALAZINE	Lowers pressure of blood in vessels by causing direct relaxation and expansion of vessel walls—mechanism unknown (antihypertensive)	Reduction of high blood pressure	Apresoline Dralserp (CD) Ser-Ap-Es (CD)
HYDROCHLOROTHIAZIDE	Increases elimination of salt and water (diuretic); relaxes walls of smaller arteries, allowing them to expand; combined effect lowers blood pressure (antihypertensive)	Elimination of excessive fluid retention (edema); reduction of high blood pressure	Esidrix HydroDiuril Oretic Thiuretic

Name	Action	Prescribed for	Trade Names (CD = comb. drug)
HYDROCORTISONE (CORTISOL)	Believed to inhibit several tissue mechanisms that induce inflammation (adrenocortical steroid [anti-inflammatory])	Symptomatic relief of inflammation (swelling, redness, heat, pain)	Cortef Cortril Hydrocortone
HYDROXYZINE	Believed to reduce excessive activity in areas of brain that influence emotional health (antihistamine; tranquilizer)	Relief of anxiety, tension, apprehension, and agitation	Atarax Vistaril Marax (CD)
INSULIN	Facilitates passage of sugar through cell wall to interior of cell (hypoglycemic)	Control of diabetes	Iletin Preparations Insulin Preparations: Lente Insulin NPH Insulin Regular Insulin Semilente Insulin Ultralente Insulin
ISONIAZID	Believed to interfere with several metabolic activities of susceptible tuberculosis organisms (antibacterial; tuberculostatic)	Prevention and treatment of tuberculosis	Laniazid Niconyl Nydrazid
ISOPROPAMIDE	Prevents stimulation of muscular contraction and glandular secretion in organ involved (antispasmodic [anticholinergic]	Relief of discomfort from excessive activity and spasm of digestive tract	Darbid Combid (CD) Ornade (CD)
ISOPROTERENOL/ ISOPRENALINE	Dilates bronchial tubes by stimulating sympathetic nerve terminals (Isoproterenol: adrenergic [bronchodilator]; Isoprenaline: sympathomimetic	Management of acute bronchial asthma, bronchitis, and emphysema	Isuprel Norisodrine Brondilate (CD) Isuprel Compound (CD)
ISOSORBIDE DINITRATE	Acts directly on muscle cells to produce relaxation which permits expansion of blood vessels, thus increasing supply of blood and oxygen to heart (coronary vasodilator)	Management of pain associated with angina pectoris (coronary insufficiency)	Isordil Sorbitrate Sorquad

Name	Action	Prescribed for	Trade Names (CD = comb. drug)
LEVODOPA	Believed to be converted to dopamine in brain tissue, thus correcting a dopamine deficiency and restoring more normal balance of chemicals responsible for transmission of nerve impulses (anti Parkinsonism)	Management of Parkinson's disease	Larodopa Parda Sinemet
LIOTHYRONINE (T-3)	Increases rate of cellular metabolism and makes more energy available for biochemical activity (thyroid hormone)	Correction of thyroid hormone deficiency (hypothyroidism)	Cytomel Euthroid (CD) Thyrolar (CD)
LITHIUM	Believed to correct chemical imbalance in certain nerve impulse transmitters that influence emotional behavior (antidepressant)	Improvement of mood and behavior in chronic manic-depression	Eskalith Lithane Lithotabs
MECLIZINE	Blocks transmission of excessive nerve impulses to vomiting center (antiemetic)	Management of nausea, vomiting, and dizziness associated with motion sickness	Antivert Bonine Vertrol
MEPERIDINE/PETHIDINE	Believed to increase chemicals that transmit nerve impulses (narcotic analgesic)	Relief of moderate to severe pain	Demerol
MEPROBAMATE	Not known (tranquilizer)	Relief of mild to moderate anxiety and tension (sedative effect); relief of insomnia due to anxiety and tension (hypnotic effect)	Equanil Kalmm Miltown SK-Bamate Tranmep
METHACYCLINE	Prevents growth and multiplication of susceptible bacteria by interfering with formation of their essential proteins (antibiotic)	Elimination of infections responsive to action of this drug	Rondomycin
METHADONE	Believed to increase chemicals that transmit nerve impulses (narcotic analgesic)	Relief of moderate to severe pain	Dolophine

Name	Action	Prescribed for	Trade Names (CD = comb. drug)
METHAQUALONE	Not known (hypnotic)	Low dosage: relief of mild to moderate anxiety or tension (sedative effect; higher dosage: at bedtime to relieve insomnia (hypnotic effect)	Quaalude Sopor Somnafac
METHYCLOTHIAZIDE	Increases elimination of: salt and water (diuretic); relaxes walls of smaller arteries, allowing them to expand; combined effect lowers blood pressure (antihypertensive)	Elimination of excess fluid retention (edema); reduction of high blood pressure	Enduron Diutensen (CD) Enduronyl (CD)
METHYLPHENIDATE	Believed to increase release of nerve impulse transmitter, which may also improve concentration and attention span of hyperactive child (primary action unknown) (central stimulant)	Management of fatigue and depression; reduction of symptoms of abnormal hyperactivity (as in minimal brain dysfunction)	Ritalin
NICOTINIC ACID/NIACIN	Corrects a deficiency of nicotinic acid in tissues; dilation of blood vessels is believed limited to skin—increased blood flow within head has not been demonstrated; reduces initial production of cholesterol and prevents conversion of fatty tissue to cholesterol and triglycerides (vitamin B-complex component; cholesterol reducer)	Management of pellagra; treatment of vertigo, ringing in ears, premenstrual headache; reduction of blood levels of cholesterol and triglycerides	Niacin Nicobid Nicotinex Elixir
NITROFURANTOIN	Believed to prevent growth and multiplication of susceptible bacteria by interfering with function of their essential enzyme systems (antibacterial)	Elimination of infections responsive to action of this drug	Furadantin Macrodantin Parfuran Trantoin
NITROGLYCERIN	Acts directly on muscle cells to produce relaxation which permits expansion of blood vessels, thus increasing supply of blood and	Management of pain associated with angina pectoris (coronary insufficiency)	Nitrobid Nitroglyn Nitrostat

Name	Action	Prescribed for	Trade Names (CD = comb. drug)
NYSTATIN	Prevents growth and multiplication of susceptible fungus strains by attacking their walls and causing leakage of internal components (antibiotic; antifungal)	Elimination of fungus infections responsive to action of this drug	Mycostatin Nilstat Declostatin (CD) Mycolog (CD)
ORAL CONTRACEPTIVES	Suppresses the two pituitary gland hormones that produce ovulation (oral contraceptives)	Prevention of pregnancy	Combination type: Enovid-E Ortho-Novum 2mg. Ovulen Zorane "Mini-Pill" type: Micronor 0.35mg. Ovrette
OXYCODONE	Believed to affect tissue sites that react specifically with opium and its derivatives (narcotic analgesic)	Relief of moderate pain; control of coughing	Percobarb (CD) Percodan (CD)
OXYTETRACYCLINE	Prevents growth and multiplication of susceptible bacteria by interfering with their formation of essential proteins (antibiotic)	Elimination of infections responsive to action of this drug	Oxlopar Terramycin Urobiotic (CD)
PAPAVERINE	Causes direct relaxation and expansion of blood vessel walls, thus increasing volume of blood which increases oxygen and nutrients (smooth muscle relaxant; vasodilator)	Relief of symptoms associated with impaired circulation in extremities and within brain	Cerespan Pavabid Vasopan

Name	Action	Prescribed for	Trade Names (CD = comb. drug)
PARA-AMINOSALICYLIC ACID (PAS)	Prevents growth and multiplication of susceptible tuberculosis organisms and makes them vulnerable to more potent drugs (antibacterial; tuberculostatic)	To increase effectiveness of other drugs used in management of tuberculosis	Pamisyl P.A.S. Rezipas
PAREGORIC (Camphorated Tincture of Opium)	Believed to affect tissue sites that react specifically with opium and its derivatives to relieve pain; its active ingredient, morphine, acts as a local anesthetic and blocks release of chemical that transmits nerve impulses to muscle walls of intestine (antiperistaltic)	Relief of mild to moderate pain; relief of intestinal cramping and diarrhea	Donnagel-PG (CD) Kaoparin (CD) Parepectolin (CD)
PENICILLIN G	Interferes with ability of susceptible bacteria to produce new protective cell walls as they grow and multiply (antibiotic)	Elimination of infections responsive to action of this drug	Pentids Pfizerpen G Sugracillin
PENICILLIN V	Same as above	Same as above	Ledercillin Pfizerpen VK Robicillin-VK V-Cillin Veetids
PENTAERYTHRITOL TETRANITRATE	Acts directly on muscle cells to produce relaxation which permits expansion of blood vessels, thus increasing supply of blood and oxygen to heart (coronary vasodilator)	Management of pain associated with angina pectoris (coronary insufficiency)	Peritrate SK-Petn. Miltrate (CD)
PENTOBARBITAL	Believed to block transmission of nerve impulses (hypnotic; sedative)	Low dosage: relief of mild to moderate anxiety or tension (sedative effect); higher dosage: at bedtime to induce sleep (hypnotic effect)	Nembutal Night-Caps Carbrital (CD)

Name	Action	Prescribed for	Trade Names (CD = comb. drug)
PHENACETIN (Acetophenetidin)	Believed to reduce concentration of chemicals involved in production of pain, fever, and inflammation (analgesic; antipyretic)	Relief of mild to moderate pain; reduction of fever	Bromo-Seltzer (CD) Empirin Compound (CD) Percodan (CD) Sinubid (CD)
PHENAZOPYRIDINE	Acts as local anesthetic on lining of lower urinary tract (urinary-analgesic)	Relief of pain and discomfort associated with acute irritation of lower urinary tract as in cystitis, urethritis, and prostatitis	Pyridium Azo Gantano (CD) Thiosulfil-A (CD) Urobiotic (CD)
PHENIRAMINE	Blocks action of histamine after release from sensitized tissue cells, thus reducing intensity of allergic response (antihistamine)	Relief of symptoms of hayfever (allergic rhinitis) and of allergic reactions of skin (itching, swelling, hives, and rash)	Inhiston Robitussin-AC (CD) Triaminicin (CD) Tussagesic (CD)
PHENOBARBITAL/ PHENOBARBITONE	Believed to block transmission of nerve impulses (anticonvulsant; hypnotic; sedative)	Low dosage: relief of mild to moderate anxiety or tension (sedative effect); higher dosage: at bedtime to induce sleep (hypnotic effect); continuous dosage: prevention of epileptic seizures (anticonvulsant effect)	Barbipil Bar-15, -25, -100 Eskabarb Stental
PHENTERMINE	Believed to alter chemical control of nerve impulse transmitter in appetite center of brain (appetite suppressant [anorexiant])	Suppression of appetite in management of weight reduction	Fastin Ionamin Tora Wilpo
PHENYLBUTAZONE	Believed to suppress formation of chemical involved in production of inflammation (analgesic; anti-inflammatory; antipyretic)	Symptomatic relief of inflammation, swelling, pain, and tenderness associated with arthritis, tendinitis, bursitis, superficial phlebitis	Azolid Butazolidin Azolid-A (CD) Sterazolidin (CD)

Name	Action	Prescribed for	Trade Names (CD = comb. drug)
PHENYLEPHRINE	Shrinks tissue mass (decongestion) by contracting arteriole walls in lining of nasal passages, sinuses, and throat, thus decreasing volume of blood (decongestant [sympathomimetic])	Relief of congestion of nose, sinuses, and throat associated with allergy	Neo-Synephrine Sinarest Nasal Spray Chlor-Trimeton Expectorant (CD) Co-Tylenol (CD) 4-Way Tablets, Nasal Spray (CD) Sinex (CD)
PHENYL PROPANOLAMINE	Same as above	Same as above	Allerest (CD) Contac (CD) Ornacol (CD) Sinutab (CD) Triaminicin (CD)
PHENYTOIN (formerly Diphenylhydantoin)	Believed to promote loss of sodium from nerve fibers, thus lowering their excitability and inhibiting spread of electrical impulse along nerve pathways (anticonvulsant)	Prevention of epileptic seizures	Dilantin Di-Phen Diphenylan Ekko
PILOCARPINE	Lowers internal eye pressure (antiglaucoma [miotic])	Management of glaucoma	Almocarpine Isopto-Carpine Pilocar
POTASSIUM	Maintains and replenishes potassium content of cells (potassium preparations)	Management of potassium deficiency	Kaon Kay Ciel Pfiklor Potassium Triplex
PREDNISOLONE	Believed to inhibit several mechanisms that induce inflammation (adrenocortical steroid [anti-inflammatory])	Symptomatic relief of inflammation (swelling, redness, heat, and pain)	Delta-Cortef Hydeltra Prednis Sterane

Name	Action	Prescribed for	Trade Names (CD = comb. drug)
PREDNISONE	Same as above	Same as above	Deltasone Delta Paracort Servisone
PROBENECID	Reduces level of uric acid in blood and tissues; prolongs presence of penicillin in blood (antigout [uricosuric])	Management of gout	Benemid Probalan Colbenemid (CD)
PROMETHAZINE	Blocks action of histamine after release from sensitized tissue cells, thus reducing intensity of allergic response (antihistamine); blocks transmission of excessive nerve impulses to vomiting center (antiemetic); action producing sedation and sleep is unknown (sedative)	Relief of symptoms of hayfever (allergic rhinitis) and of allergic reactions of skin (itching, swelling, hives, rash); prevention and management of nausea, vomiting, and dizziness associated with motion sickness; production of mild sedation and light sleep	Phenergan Prosedin Remsed Synalgos-DC (CD)
PROPANTHELINE	Prevents stimulation of muscular contraction and glandular secretion within organ involved (antispasmodic [anticholinergic])	Relief of discomfort associated with excessive activity and spasm of digestive tract	Norpanth Pro-Banthine Ropanth Probital (CD)
PROPOXYPHENE	Increases chemicals that transmit nerve impulses, somehow contributing to the analgesic effect (analgesic)	Relief of mild to moderate pain	Darvon Darvon-N Darvon Compound (CD) Proproxychel
PSEUDOEPHEDRINE (Isoephedrine)	Shrinks tissue mass (decongestion) by contracting arteriole walls in lining of nasal passages, sinuses, and throat, thus decreasing volume of blood (decongestant [sympathomimetic])	Relief of congestion of nose, sinuses, and throat associated with allergy	Sudafed Actifed (CD) Dimacol (CD) Emprazil (CD) Phenergan (CD)

Name	Action	Prescribed for	Trade Names (CD = comb. drug)
PYRILAMINE/ MEPYRAMINE	Blocks action of histamine after release from sensitized tissue cells, thus reducing intensity of allergic response (antihistamine)	Relief of symptoms of hayfever (allergic rhinitis) and of allergic reactions of skin (itching, swelling, hives, and rash)	Triaminic (CD) Triaminicin (CD) Triaminicol (CD)
QUINIDINE	Slows pacemaker and delays transmission of electrical impulses (cardiac depressant)	Correction of certain heart rhythm disorders	Cardioquin Cin-Quin Quinidex Quinidine M.B. (CD)
RESERPINE	Relaxes blood vessel walls by reducing availability of norepinephrine (antihypertensive; tranquilizer)	Reduction of high blood pressure	Rau-Sed Reserpoid Sandril Serp Serpasil
RAFAMPIN	Prevents growth and multiplication of susceptible tuberculosis organisms by interfering with enzyme systems involved in formation of essential proteins (antibiotic; tuberculostatic)	Treatment of tuberculosis	Rifadin Rifomycin Rimactane
SECOBARBITAL	Believed to block transmission of nerve impulses (hypnotic; sedative)	Low dosage: relief of mild to moderate anxiety or tension (sedative effect); higher dosage: at bedtime to induce sleep (hypnotic effect)	Seco-8 Seconal Tuinal (CD)
SULFAMETHOXAZOLE	Prevents growth and multiplication of susceptible bacteria by interfering with their formation of folic acid (antibacterial)	Elimination of infections responsive to action of this drug	Gantanol Azo Gantanol (CD) Bactrium (CD) Septra (CD)

Name	Action	Prescribed for	Trade Names (CD = comb. drug)
SULFISOXAZOLE	Same as above	Same as above	Gantrisin G-Sox SK-Soxazole Soxomide Sulfalar
TETRACYCLINE	Prevents growth and multiplication of susceptible bacteria by interfering with their formation of essential proteins (antibiotic)	Elimination of infections responsive to action of this drug	Achromycin V Cycline-250 Cyclopar Panmycin Robitet Sumycin Tetracyn Tetrex Achrostatin V (CD)
THEOPHYLLINE (Aminophylline, Oxtriphylline)	Reverses constriction by increasing activity of chemical system within muscle cell that causes relaxation of bronchial tube (bronchodilator)	Symptomatic relief of bronchial asthma	Amesec (CD) Brondecon (CD) Bronkotabs (CD) Elixophyllin (CD) Marax (CD) Quadrinal (CD) Quibron (CD)
THYROID (Thyroid Preparations)	Makes more energy available for biochemical activity and increases rate of cellular metabolism by altering processes of cellular chemicals that store energy (thyroid hormones)	Correction of thyroid hormone deficiency (hypothyroidism)	Armour Thyroid Proloid S-P-T Thyrobrom
THYROXINE (T-4)	Same as above	Same as above	Levothroid Synthroid Thyrolar (CD)

Name	Action	Prescribed for	Trade Names (CD = comb. drug)
TOLBUTAMIDE	Stimulates secretion of insulin by pancreas (hypoglycemic)	Correction of insulin deficiency in adult diabetes	Orinase
TRIDIHEXETHYL	Prevents stimulation of muscular contraction and glandular secretion in organ involved (antispasmodic [anticholinergic]	Relief of discomfort from excessive activity and spasm of digestive tract	Pathilon Milpath (CD) Pathibamate (CD)
TRIMETHOPRIM	Prevents growth and multiplication of susceptible organisms by interfering with formation of proteins (antibacterial)	Elimination of infections responsive to action of this drug	Syraprim Bactrim (CD) Septra (CD)
TRIPROLIDINE	Blocks action of histamine after release from sensitized tissue cells, thus reducing intensity of allergic response (antihistamine)	Relief of symptoms of hayfever (allergic rhinitis) and of allergic reactions of skin (itching, swelling, hives, and rash)	Actidil Actifed (CD) Actifed-C (CD)
VITAMIN C (Ascorbic Acid)	Believed to be essential to enzyme activity involved in formation of collagen; increases absorption of iron from intestine and helps formation of hemoglobin and red blood cells in bone marrow; inhibits growth of certain bacteria in urinary tract; enhances effects of some antibiotics (vitamin)	Prevention and treatment of scurvy; treatment of some types of anemia; maintenance of an acid urine	Ascorbicap Cetane Cevalin Synchro-C

CHAPTER 3

Thesaurus of Medical Terms

The *Thesaurus of Medical Terms* is designed to enable the reader to find the more technical terms that apply to a variety of health-related subjects. By locating the Key Word that applies to a particular subject and reading across the page, the pertinent adjective, study, specialist, and major disorders may be found. For example, if one wants to know the technical term for an eye doctor, one looks under the Key Word column for *eye,* and under Specialist, finds the words *ophthalmologist* and *oculist.* If one cannot recall the name of a common heart disease, one looks under *heart* in the Key Word column and finds, under Major Disorders, *angina* and other conditions listed. These disorders may in turn be looked up in the index for page references to the text.

KEY WORD	ADJECTIVE	STUDY
allergy	allergic	allergology
anesthesia	anesthetic	anesthesiology
blood	hemal	hematology
blood vessels	vascular	angiology
bone	osteal, osseous	orthopedics
brain *See* **nervous system.**		
cancer *See* **tumor.**		
causes of disease	etiologic, etiological	etiology
chest cavity	thoracic	thoracic surgery
children	pediatric	pediatrics
colon and rectum	proctologic, proctological	proctology
cosmetic surgery *See* **plastic surgery.**		
diet	nutritive	nutrition
digestive tract	gastroenteric	gastroenterology
disease	pathologic, pathological	pathology
ear	otologic, otological	otology
ear, nose, and throat	otolaryngological	otolaryngology
endocrine glands *See* **glands.**		
epidemics (geographical distribution of disease)	epidemic, epidemical	epidemiology
eye	ophthalmic	ophthalmology
foot	pedal	podiatry, chiropody
gastrointestinal tract (GI tract) *See* **digestive tract.**		
general medicine		
genital tract (female) *See* **reproductive system (female).**		
genital tract (male) *See* **urinogenital tract (male).**		
glands (endocrine)	glandular	endocrinology
hair *See* **skin and hair.**		
heart	cardiac, coronary, cardiologic, cardiological	cardiology
immunization	immunologic, immunological	immunology
internal medicine		
joints and muscles		rheumatology
kidney	renal, nephric	nephrology
law and medicine		forensic medicine, forensic pathology
liver	hepatic	hepaticology
lung	pulmonary	internal medicine

SPECIALIST	MAJOR DISORDERS
allergist, allergologist	respiratory and skin disorders, e.g. asthma and contact dermatitis
anesthesiologist	
hematologist	anemia, leukemia, hemophilia
vascular surgeon	varicose veins, phlebitis
orthopedist, orthopedic surgeon, orthopod	back disorders, fractures, trauma
etiologist	
thoracic surgeon	lung cancer, tuberculosis, emphysema
pediatrician	all diseases children are subject to
proctologist	hemorrhoids, cancer of the rectum or colon
nutritionist	malnutrition, obesity
gastroenterologist	digestive difficulties, ulcers, gallstones, inguinal hernia
pathologist	
otologist	hearing or equilibrium disorders
otolaryngologist, ENT specialist	hearing or equilibrium disorders, laryngitis, upper respiratory infections
epidemiologist	forms of cancer, cholera, influenza
ophthalmologist, oculist	glaucoma, cataract, detached retina
podiatrist, chiropodist	arch troubles, bunions, ingrown toenails
general practitioner (GP)	
endocrinologist	diabetes, hyperthyroidism, hypothyroidism
cardiologist, cardiovascular specialist	angina, coronary thrombosis (heart attack), atherosclerosis, hypertension
immunologist	poliomyelitis, measles, smallpox
internist	disorders of internal organs (heart, lungs, blood, GI tract)
rheumatologist	rheumatoid arthritis, osteoarthritis
nephrologist	nephritis, kidney failure
hepaticologist	hepatitis
internist	emphysema, lung cancer, tuberculosis

KEY WORD	ADJECTIVE	STUDY
medicine *See* general medicine, internal medicine, osteopathic medicine, rehabilitation.		
mental illness	psychiatric	psychiatry
muscles *See* joints and muscles.		
nervous system	neural, neurologic, neurological, neuro-pathological	neurology, neuropathology
nose *See* ear, nose, and throat.		
osteopathic medicine	osteopathic	osteopathy
plastic surgery		plastic surgery, cosmetic surgery
radiology	radiologic, radiological, X-ray	radiology, roentgenology
rectum *See* colon and rectum.		
rehabilitation		physical medicine
reproductive system (female)	obstetric, obstetrical, gynecologic, gynecological	obstetrics, gynecology
reproductive system (male) *See* urinogenital tract (male).		
skin and hair	dermal	dermatology
surgery	surgical	surgery
throat (*See also* ear, nose, and throat.)	laryngologic, laryngological	laryngology
tooth	dental, orthodontic, periodontal	dentistry, orthodontics, orthodontia, oral or dental surgery, periodontics, periodontia
tumor	oncologic	oncology
urinary tract (female)	urologic, urological	urology
urinogenital tract (male)	urologic, urological	urology
X ray *See* radiology.		

SPECIALIST	MAJOR DISORDERS
psychiatrist	neurosis, psychosis, psychosomatic disease
neurologist, neuropathologist, neurosurgeon	epilepsy, cerebral palsy, brain tumors, meningitis
osteopath	
plastic surgeon, cosmetic surgeon	scars, burns, cosmetic improvements
radiologist, roentgenologist	
physical therapist	
obstetrician, gynecologist, ob-gyn specialist	pregnancy and its complications, infertility, fibroid tumors, dysmenorrhea, birth control, ovarian cysts
dermatologist	dermatitis, acne, psoriasis
surgeon	
laryngologist	laryngitis, upper respiratory infections
dentist, oral or dental surgeon, orthodontist, periodontist, pediatric dentist	caries (tooth decay), periodontal disease, malocclusion, children's dental needs
oncologist	cancer, benign tumors
urologist	cystitis, nephritis
urologist	kidney stones, nephritis, prostate problems

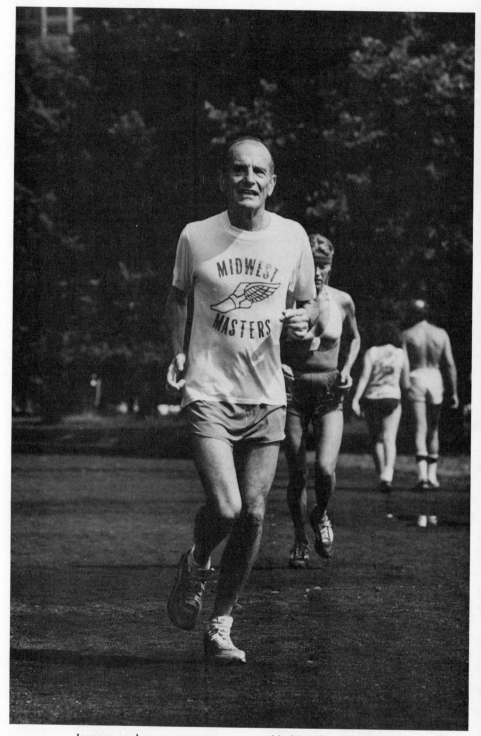

Joggers may be men or women, young or old, drawn from all groups in society—all trying to avoid the hazards of a sedentary lifestyle.

CHAPTER 4

Physical Fitness

One of the most important health studies of our time was started by the National Institutes of Health back in 1949. The population of an entire community was put under continuous scrutiny by a team of doctors who recorded the daily habits of thousands of men and women. For more than a quarter of a century, the citizens of Framingham, Massachusetts, have been observed at work, at play, and in the home. They have been measured and weighed repeatedly, their food analyzed, their cigarettes counted, blood pressure checked, and so on, without interfering with the normal life styles of the individuals.

The Framingham Study

Results of the Framingham Study of a generation of a typical American community reveal certain links between a way of life and the most common cause of death, which is cardiovascular disease. The links were found to be too many calories, mainly in the form of saturated fats and sugar, too many cigarettes, and too little exercise. Dr. William B. Kannel, Medical Director of the Framingham Study and a member of the Harvard Medical School faculty, reported that the most sedentary, or least active, men had about three times the heart attack risk as the most physically active. The rate of risk of cardiovascular disease seemed to be generally proportional to the degree of obesity, resulting from too many calories. The use of cigarettes was found to be associated with all manifestations of cardiovascular disease. One other link, which is still being explored, is high blood pressure.

The Framingham Study of the adult lives of some 5,000 subjects confirms what most doctors have suspected for many years—that

219

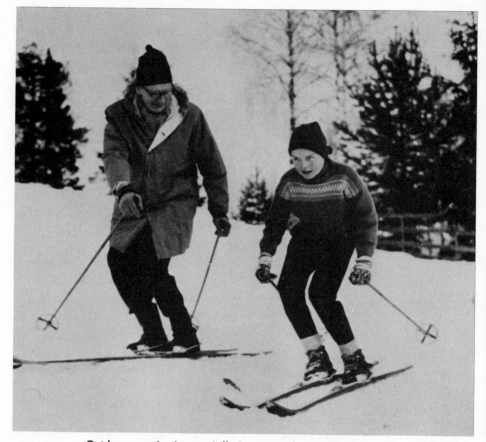

Outdoor exercise is especially important during the winter. This father and son have found an enjoyable winter recreation in skiing.

physical activity helps counteract the effects of overweight, diets rich in fats and sugar, blood pressure, and similar factors. Dr. Kannel's report added another explanation: physical exercise probably helps extend the life and health of even those people with cardiovascular disease by developing collateral circulation. In other words, a person who might otherwise develop heart trouble because of a diminished blood supply in his coronary arteries can forestall that threat to his life by physical exercise which promotes the increased flow of blood through alternate blood vessels.

There is a valuable lesson in the Framingham Study for every reader of this book: daily exercise, which requires no greater investment than a more efficient use of free time, can extend your life and retard certain organic diseases of the heart and blood vessels—diseases that account for more than half of the "natural" deaths in America each year.

Winter Exercise

If you are a typical American adult, the chances are that you are a "fair weather athlete." Although some men and women enjoy a hike through the freshly fallen snow to an outdoor ice skating rink, or an occasional visit to a ski run, too many individuals use the period between Indian summer and the return of spring as a time to take things easy, and indoors. That television producers save their best shows for the fall and winter months suggests that their careful surveys find most families indoors at that time. Sales of phonograph records and tape cassettes reach a peak as winter advances. And despite the letdown in physical activity, the long periods of relaxed entertainment seem to stimulate tremendous appetites for high-carbohydrate goodies like potato chips, pretzels, candy, beer, and soft drinks. This seasonal irony is compounded by the fact that autumn usually is marked by an increasingly heavy schedule of cocktail parties, business or club lunches, dinner parties, and holiday feasts that may stretch through several days.

The Value of Physical Fitness

The ancient Greek physician Hippocrates may have established the first rule of physical fitness some 2,400 years ago. He outlined what he called the Law of Use which governs the living organism: "That which is used develops; that which is not used wastes away." Modern medical practice still follows that Hippocratic concept in preventive medicine as well as in the rehabilitation of surgical patients. Dr. Harry J. Johnson, Chairman of the Medical Board of the Life Extension Institute, expresses the Hippocratic Law of Use this way: "Life itself is movement. Even the developing embryo moves

and stretches within the uterus by the fifth week of life—long before the mother becomes aware of it. And what does the mother say when she feels the first detectable stirring? She says she 'feels life.' "

After the birth of the baby, doctors have found that the mother recovers more quickly from the effects of childbirth if she gets out of bed and into action as soon as possible instead of lying in bed for a week or more to recuperate. The baby, during its hours of wakefulness, is in almost continuous motion—crawling, grasping, walking, running, jumping; the joy of activity continues in most normal children until adulthood.

There are exceptional people who almost literally keep moving throughout adult life. For example, Senator William Proxmire of Wisconsin is a strong advocate of jogging and regularly runs from his place of residence to his office on Capitol Hill. President Truman kept newsmen panting at his heels during his brisk morning walks. Individuals in all walks of life who spend a good deal of time in an office recognize the importance of daily exercise.

When Dr. Leonard Larson was president of the American Medical Association, he explained the importance of exercise in developing greater strength, stamina, endurance, and recuperative powers of the human body. "During exercise," said Dr. Larson, "the muscles need more oxygen and food. The blood circulates faster to meet the needs of the muscles and to carry off wastes. Body cells increase so that muscles gain strength and flexibility. There also is improved neuromuscular coordination."

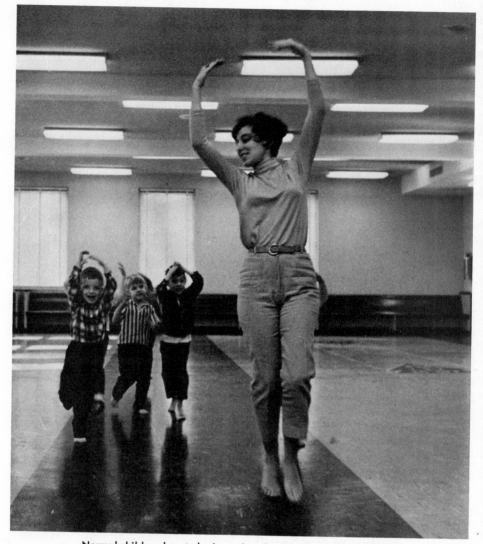

Normal children love to be in motion. Dancing is a natural form of exercise and a fine way to maintain muscle tone and good posture.

Everyday Emergencies

A frequently overlooked fringe benefit of physical fitness is an improved ability to survive everyday emergency situations that create a sudden demand for physical strength and endurance, which in turn require greater than normal performance by the heart and blood vessels, lungs, nerves, and muscles.

This was illustrated during a meeting of physicians to discuss the health hazards of flying. The medical director of one of the major airlines was asked if he had any records of passengers on his airline dying of a heart attack. "Yes," the medical director replied matter-of-factly. "Last year, seven of our passengers died of heart attacks. But not while they were flying. In each case, the passenger was running down a corridor to catch a flight when he collapsed and died." Each of the victims, it must be assumed, was "out of condition," perhaps a bit paunchy and flabby from lack of exercise, and unable to meet the ultimate test to fitness: the sudden demand on the body's organs to meet a brief modern emergency of running with suitcase in hand to reach the airline counter before the gates closed.

Running for a plane, running for a bus, running for a commuter train, pushing a stalled car, carrying an air conditioner up a flight of stairs— these are civilization's equivalents of the primitive human's battles with wild animals or hand-to-hand combat with tribal rivals. But the primitive man probably had a better chance for survival in an emergency because he maintained muscle, heart, and lung strength and endurance through the daily demands of his prehistoric life style.

Vigorous Recreational Activities

The alpine lakes of the mountains of Idaho were once stocked with

Racquetball not only provides vigorous physical exercise, but also—when played regularly—helps build endurance.

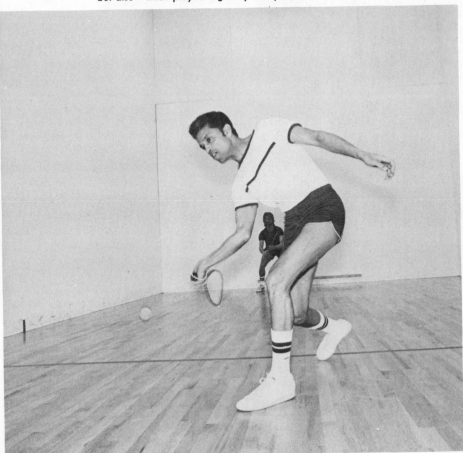

trout that were carried there in milk cans strapped to the backs of husky college boys. Some years out of college and softened by sedentary jobs, the same individuals, burdened only by sack lunches and fishing rods, had to stop several times for their "second wind" when they returned recently to the same lakes. There are still duck hunters who travel each autumn to a hilltop on the California-Oregon border; it is a favorite hunting ground for waterfowl that skim over the hill which separates two lakes on the Pacific Flyway. To reach the hilltop, the hunters have to scale a thousand feet of slippery lava rocks, and many drop out along the trail because of dizzy spells, painful leg cramps, and other discouraging symptoms. The peak bears the nickname of "Cardiac Ridge."

The point here is that true physical fitness involves more than a few easy or specialized exercises. A man can be a championship weight lifter with the physique of Mr. America, but he may not be able to compete in

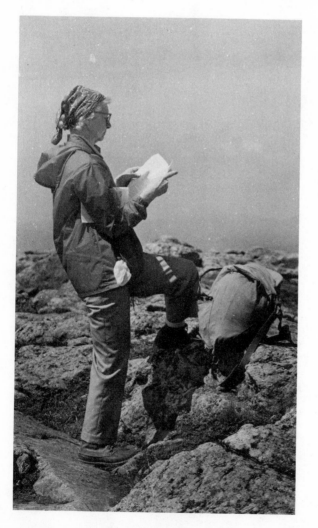

A senior citizen who has kept fit and is in good health enjoys a vigorous hike in the mountains.

running, swimming, or other sports activities unless he has developed and maintained strength and endurance in the heart, lungs, and muscles used for functions other than weight lifting. Conversely, an individual who considers himself in good physical condition because he has been jogging for the past two years might be unable to lift a portable TV set. The goal for anyone seeking an exercise program should be all-around physical fitness, with good heart and lung conditioning in addition to muscular strength.

Weight Control and Exercise

While no single set of exercises will guarantee physical fitness, neither will exercise alone control an overweight problem—although the Framingham Study has suggested a complementary relationship between exercise and weight control. The catch is that it takes a lot of exercise to get rid of a pound of fat. It would require, for example, about 90 minutes of swimming to burn up the calories you gain by eating a 450-calorie piece of chocolate layer cake; for most people, it would be easier to control weight by skipping the cake.

One pound of body fat is equivalent to about 3,600 calories of food. That amount of fat is about equal to a food intake of ten calories a day over a period of a year. In other words, you can add or lose a pound of fat by altering your diet by approximately ten calories a day. A three-inch cookie averages about 120 calories, slightly more than the amount of calories in ten medium potato chips. Translated into weight-control terms: if you eat one cookie a day beyond your body's normal food

requirements—or ten potato chips more—you should gain about 12 pounds in a year. Or if you regularly munch on such goodies, you should be able to reduce your weight by approximately 12 pounds a year simply by eliminating one cookie per day, or its equivalent.

Calorie Consumption During Normal Activities

An average human body needs about 1,500 calories a day just to survive; it burns about one calorie per minute in maintaining such simple body functions as breathing, keeping the body temperature at a normal level, and so on. A person who spends most of his time sleeping or watching TV doesn't need much more than a calorie per minute of food energy. A person who operates an electric typewriter for an hour requires only about 20 calories more for that period of work than a sleeping person. Driving a car for one hour might increase the body's need for calories by about 100 more than the amount needed for sleeping; one tablespoon of mayonnaise or a half-dozen saltine crackers will provide enough calories for one hour of driving.

By matching the calories in snack foods with the calorie needs of the human body for such low levels of inactivity as driving a car, watching TV, or operating an office machine, it is easy to see how pounds of body fat can accumulate within a short period of time.

Even walking, which is considered a mildly active way of utilizing calories, burns only three calories per minute above the basic needs of the body. So you would need to walk two hours to burn an extra 360

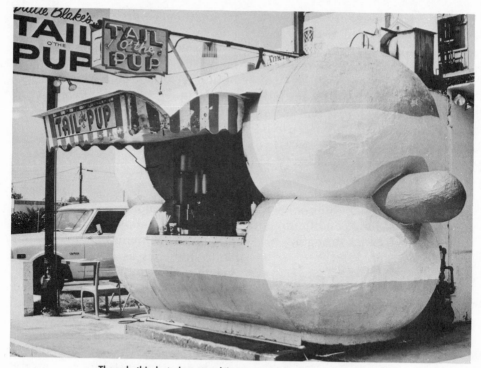

Though this hot dog stand is an amusing piece of Americana, snack foods such as hot dogs build unwanted fat in the body.

calories—the equivalent of a slice of cherry pie. The next time a friend assures you that you can burn up the calories in a piece of fruit pie by walking back to the office after lunch, make the friend promise to walk with you because it will require six miles of walking.

Lack of Exercise and Weight Gain

Nevertheless, it is better to walk for two hours after eating a piece of pie than to remain inactive after adding hundreds of excess calories to your body's fuel supply—if you can't resist the temptation to add the calories—because there *is* a relationship between weight control and exercise. Some people apparently gain weight even though they eat no more than their friends and relatives who remain slim. Careful studies made of obese people who ate only small or average amounts of food— in some cases as few as 1,800 calories a day—showed that they were simply less active than their slim friends and relatives who consumed the same amount of calories.

In one instance involving students, motion pictures were taken of the obese youngsters working out with their classmates in physical education classes. The investigators discovered by watching the movies that the overweight students were in effect faking the exercise routines; that is, they did not play enthusiastically, but merely went through the motions.

What about the need for fat deposits in the body as a source of energy? The answer is that while fat is indeed a rich source of energy for the body, the human body chemistry is geared to convert protein to energy, if needed. But the body is not equipped to build protein molecules from fat. As for sugar in the diet, the body gets all it needs from carbohydrates in fruits, vegetables, and other food sources.

Planning Your Own Physical Fitness Program

Any weight control program in connection with physical fitness improvement should be tailored to your individual needs and directed by a physician. Only your doctor knows for sure about your individual nutrition needs, and no two individuals are precisely alike. The same rule

applies to physical conditioning: you could have a hidden bodily deficiency that would not cause problems in a sedentary life style. But a sudden strenuous program of jogging, calisthenics, or other athletic activity could be enough to push you over the brink. After an examination, the doctor can recommend a program that will permit certain types of exercise but restrict or eliminate others. There are so many methods of exercise available today that an effective program can be built around any individual physical problems.

Exercises Keyed to Age

Age ordinarily is one factor in determining which exercises are most suitable for an individual, although

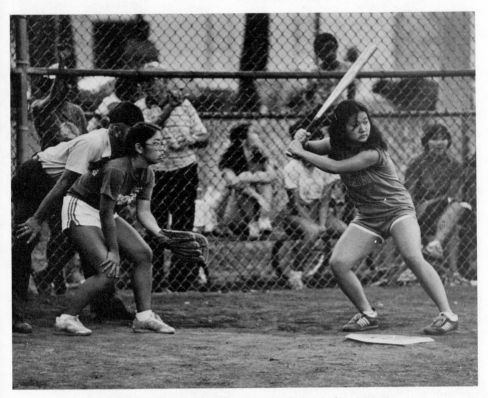

These girls had physical exams from their doctors before joining a baseball team, with all the physical effort that involves.

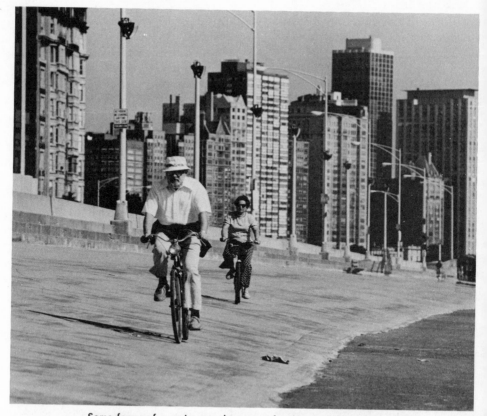

Some forms of exercise are dangerous for those over the age of 50, but bicycling is safe and beneficial for the fit older person.

everybody knows people who seem young at 60 and others who appear to be old at 30. The general rule for determining whether it is safe to begin an exercise program is this: if you are still in your 20s and have passed a standard physical examination within the past year, it should be safe to begin a progressive program of conditioning without further examination. But if you are over 30 years of age, you should have passed a complete physical examination that included an electrocardiogram within the past 90 days.

If you are over the age of 50, you can still begin a physical fitness program, but it should be a medically supervised program. For the over 50 group, the doctor may advise that certain activities, such as jogging and competitive sports, be restricted or eliminated. Jogging can be damaging to the spine in persons beyond the age of 40 and can aggravate signs of arthritis. But walking, golf, swimming, bicycling, and exercising on a stationary cycle are alternate types of exercising for the past-middle-age set.

Fitness and Mental Health

In addition to the physical benefits gained by exercise, Dr. Ernest Simonson of the University of Minnesota Medical School found in a study of 10,000 persons that physical activity can be a definite aid to mental health. Typical comments by his subjects reflect that they "feel more alive" when they exercise. Dr. Simonson reported after analyzing the improved mental health of his subjects: "It is common logic that if one feels better, his attitude toward others will be more congenial. When one is in a cordial, happy frame of mind, he will likely make wiser de-

cision, and his world in general will look better."

The late Dr. William Menninger, one of the world's foremost experts on mental health, explained that

Good mental health is directly related to the capacity and willingness of an individual to play. Regardless of his objections, resistances, or past practice, an individual will make a wise in-

Physicians now think that exercise helps contribute to a positive state of mental health—for all age groups.

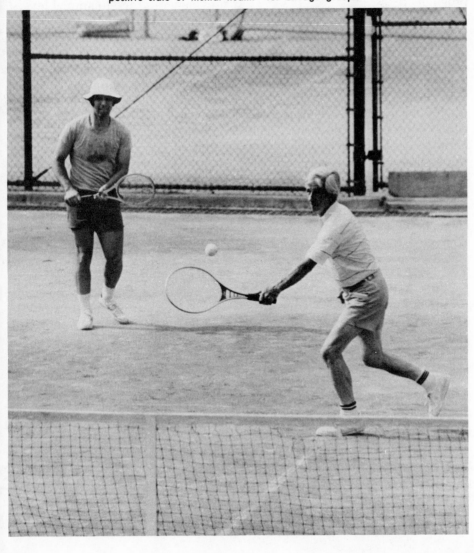

vestment for himself if he will budget some of his time each day for his play —and take it seriously.

Dr. Menninger added that play provides an outlet for instinctive aggressive drives that enable a person to "blow off steam." Physical activity, he said, is a necessary supplement to daily work.

At the Beginning

Two things to remember in planning your own physical conditioning program are:

• Tailor the exercises and sports to your own needs and interests. If you have wanted to ride a bicycle, or learn water skiing, or take regular fishing trips, this is your opportunity to begin.

• Follow a progressive program in which you start at the bottom and improve gradually over a period of weeks or months. Don't expect overnight miracles, and be willing to cut back on the pace of your workouts if you find the going tough; you may be pushing yourself too fast. Your goal is to improve your own physical condition to the highest level feasible for your age and other possible limiting factors. Don't expect to set any new world records; just try to do the best you can—for your own health.

WARM-UP EXERCISES: The easiest place to begin your exercise program is in your own home, with the kind of warm-up exercises that you performed each day in high school. The main difference is that you will be on your own, unless you can find a friend or family member to participate in the workouts. You can do your own counting.

The purpose of the warm-up exercise is to increase the blood flow to the muscles and gradually limber up the body. And a warm-up period of at least 20 minutes should be used before any strenuous exercise. Otherwise, you may experience strains and sprains, or worse. It is quite possible to rupture a tendon or injure a joint by starting with certain strenuous exercises without a preliminary warm-up period. Also, remember to taper off a workout period with mild muscular activity, such as walking, until breathing and body temperature have returned to normal levels.

The warm-up exercises include body benders, situps, pushups, bend and stretch, ankle stretch, knee lifts, straddle hops, walking, running-in-place, and rope-skipping workouts, among a wide assortment of calisthenics. You can select from the assortment of warm-up exercises illustrated on pp. 249–251 those that are best suited to your own situation. If you live in a house or apartment where you are likely to disturb your neighbors by running in place or skipping rope, you can find other exercises that stimulate the general body circulation. But if you have facilities, such as a basement or garage, or a ground-floor bedroom where there is room for straddle hops or rope skipping, the exercises that provide the better range of action should be followed. Most of the exercises can be done in a small area; airline personnel investigating a strange thumping in a jet aircraft at 30,000 feet altitude one morning discovered a passenger running in place in the rest room.

Although no special equipment is necessary, don't hesitate to invest in a few items of gym equipment—dumbbells, weights, a stationary cycle, or whatever you think you need to help you in your own fitness program. For the cost of one or two days in a hospital, you can buy enough exercising equipment to keep yourself out of the hospital for several years.

MUSCLE SORENESS: You can expect some muscular soreness for the first two or three weeks of the toughening stage of physical conditioning, particularly if you have shunned exercise for several years. Later on as you progressively increase the work load on your body you may experience some stiffness or soreness. Usually this is only a warning sign that you are moving up the fitness scale too quickly. On the other hand, if the muscle soreness is relatively mild and goes away overnight, you can assume that you are not overdoing the exercise routine.

If your muscles and joints appear to suffer from the exercise load, simply slow down to an easier pace and work back up the scale again at a more gradual rate. By working at your own pace, with only the goal of improving your muscular strength and endurance, you can build a lot of flexibility into your fitness program. You don't have to compete with others; if you need an extra day or week to advance from one stage to the next, take the extra time. It's your own conditioning routine, and the suggested benchmarks or guidelines for the accompanying exercises can be adapted to your own needs.

The Indoor Exercise Program

Based on the U.S. Army's 6–12 conditioning project, the Indoor Exercise Program on pp. 252–263 includes six sets of exercise routines. Each set requires 12 minutes a day to complete. Each of the sets, from I to VI, is in turn divided into three levels of activity. They are labeled A, B, C. The entire program, therefore, is designed to provide a progressive scale of physical conditioning for 12 minutes a day over a period of 18 weeks. You should begin at the C-level of set I and follow that routine for the first week. At the start of the second week, you progress to the B-level exercise routine of set I, and to the A-level routine at the beginning of the third week. Then, assuming that you follow the schedule according to its original design, you advance to the C-level routine of set II of the 6–12 exercises at the start of the fourth week, and so on.

The progression guides accompanying each table of 6–12 exercises represent suggested goals for healthy males. Women generally are not expected to match the suggested pace, although some may be able to do so. To follow the progression guide of Table I, read the first vertical column of numbers under the word *Exercises*. Under Exercise 1, in the age group of 17–29, are the numbers 15, 13, 11. These numbers show the repetitions of Exercise 1 to be completed within two minutes, the number indicated at the bottom of the column. The beginner in that age group should attempt to complete 11 side straddle exercises within two minutes, or at least he should work toward that primary goal. He also should try to complete 14 of the modified pushups in 1 minute, 12 situps in 1 minute, and so on. If he can accomplish the C level goals in the first week, he progresses to the B level goal of 13 side straddle exercises within two minutes, 16 modified pushups, 13 situps, and so on.

You will note that the total of the minutes suggested for the various exercises is 12 regardless of the age group or exercise level chosen. The greatest amount of time is allocated to running in place, and the number of steps ranges from a beginning level of 30, or six per minute, for men over 60 to a maximum of 250, or 50 per minute, for a young man in good condition.

Adapting the Program to Meet Your Needs

There is considerable flexibility in adapting this program to suit your own physical abilities, whether you are a man or woman. Each individual is as different in his physical strength and endurance as his fingerprints or other traits. The important thing about these sets of exercises is that most normal adults can perform most or all of them at one of the beginning levels, and with the beginning level as a benchmark the individual can gradually follow the progression guidelines to a higher level of fitness.

Some individuals may already be in such good condition that they can work up to the A-level of Table VI at the ninth week instead of the 18th week without any of the muscle stiffness or soreness that would indicate too fast a rate of advancement. Others may feel more comfortable if they spend two or three weeks at the C or B-level of Table I before moving to another level. There are no fixed rules to this program; the progression guides are merely suggestions that can be altered to fit your personal needs.

But don't go through the exercises half-heartedly. One purpose of exercising is to maintain a modest over-load on the muscles and the heart and lungs, which builds up a good reserve of strength and endurance. So you have to push a bit every day to make the plan work; if some of the exercises are less demanding of your muscles and circulatory system than your daily work responsibilities, you may be wasting your time. A man who moves pianos for a living would do little to improve his strength by lifting six-pound dumbbells for exercise.

On the other hand, there are people over the age of 45 who should be cautious about advancing beyond set IV of the Indoor Exercise Program. If they experience discomfort at the C-level of set V, they should drop back to the A-level of Table IV. This program is designed to fit all sorts of individual needs and abilities; some individuals probably should not advance beyond the Table III set of exercises. If there is any question about the level at which you should taper off your personal progressive program, discuss the matter with your doctor.

Maximum Performance Plateau

The rate of improvement in your physical condition will seem to be quite rapid at first, then increase slowly as you reach a plateau about halfway through the 18-week program. You can tell when you have reached your peak performance because you will begin to experience the huffing and puffing effects of an oxygen debt when you try to push yourself beyond that particular level—even though you have learned to overcome the need to pause for a "second wind" that you may have experienced earlier in the program.

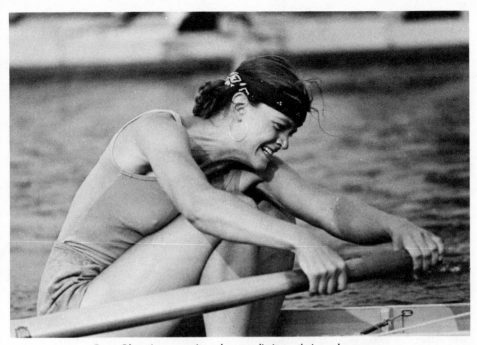

Even Olympic competitors have a limit to their endurance; a
woman training for Olympic crewing appears close to her limit.

There is a practical limit to the performance of anybody—even Olympic champions —when the heart and
lungs simply cannot supply oxygen
fast enough to sustain the activity of
the muscles. The muscle cells can
"borrow" oxygen that is dissolved in
the blood and other tissues in order
to function temporarily, but eventually that debt of oxygen has to be re-
paid. This is why you may occasionally see track stars collapse in a series
of agonizing gasps after they reach
the finish line: they have run their
oxygen debt to the point of bank-
ruptcy.

In your own conditioning program
based on the 6–12 exercise schedule,
you may reach a point where, for
example, you can do all of the exercises at the A level of Table V without experiencing an oxygen debt, but
you can't make it through the Table
VI routines without huffing and

puffing. Then you will know that you
are at your personal plateau of
maximum performance. But you
don't quit exercising at that point;
you simply continue working out at
the highest level that is comfortable
for you. If you drop out of the program after reaching the level of your
maximum performance your physical condition will deteriorate within
two or three weeks.

There are still goals ahead and
skills to be developed after you
reach your maximum performance
plateau—development of strength
and endurance for participation in
certain sports or improvement of the
function of special muscle groups
used in athletic activity. Rope skipping, a traditional conditioning exercise, always a favorite of professional
boxers in training, is an example of
an athletic activity that requires a
high level of coordination, muscular

function, and heart-lung performance to do well. Anyone who has
tried high-speed rope skipping for
more than three minutes without
missing a jump knows it is more than
a playground game; in fact, such a
test has been used by the army in
training soldiers for combat duty.

Weight Lifting

Another special method of developing strength and endurance is
weight lifting practice. See pp.
265–269. Weight lifting may be
one of the oldest known sports that
utilizes equipment; youths who
wanted to participate in the ancient
Greek Olympics in about 800 B.C.
were required to lift a heavy iron
weight to prove their strength before they were accepted into the
ritual. Weight lifting as a formal competitive sport was popular in Europe
for many generations, but it did not
attract much attention in North
America until the 1930s when the
United States organized its first
weight lifting team for Olympic competition.

Exercising With Barbells

Although competitive weight lifting generally is considered a masculine activity, there is no reason
why women could not work out with
barbells if they wanted to do so.
Body weight is not necessarily a factor; U.S. championship weight lifting has a minimum body weight
class of 114.5 pounds while A.A.U.
competition is held in a 123-pound
body weight class. However, most
women probably are not interested
in developing the muscle groups that
would benefit from lifting barbells.
The type of weight lifting that is
more compatible with female physi-

cal fitness goals, exercising with
dumbbells, is described later in this
chapter.

There are two approaches to
weight lifting as a part of physical
conditioning. One approach is to use
barbell weights in competitive lifting in which the participant lifts a
tremendous amount of weight off the
floor and holds it aloft for a brief
period of time. The other approach is
to use weights to develop the
strength and tone of major muscle
groups in the arms, legs, back, trunk,
and shoulder girdle. The effect is to
improve the blood flow to the muscles through more efficient pumping
volume of the heart and distribution
by the capillaries.

Muscle Overload

The principle of muscle overloading is particularly applicable in
weight lifting because of the added
demands made on the muscles
by lifting progressively heavier
weights. A person normally has no
more muscular strength than he
seems to need for daily work and
play routines. There is, therefore, little or no reserve for emergencies unless you create an artificial need by
overloading the muscles with heavy
weights three or four times a week.
The body responds to the extra demand by providing the extra muscle
fibers.

Each time you stimulate the body
to reach a certain plateau of muscle
overloading, you begin working toward the next higher level by adding
more weight to your barbell. You
may begin, for example, with 40 or
50 pounds of weight and add five
pounds when you are able. But do
not overload the muscles to the point
of a strain or a joint dislocation. Also,

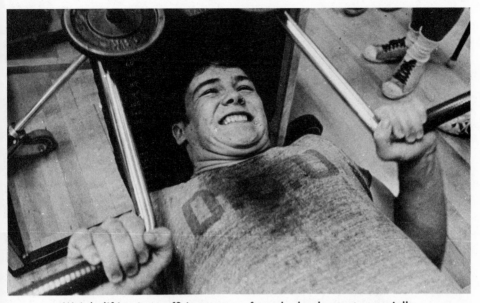

Weight lifting is an efficient means of muscle development, especially of the back and shoulders. Achievement depends on steady practice.

as you follow the basic barbell exercises described in this chapter, begin at the minimum number of repetitions. After you have learned to do six squats with 50 pounds of weight, continue at that rate for four or five days, then try seven squats with the same amount of weight. Do not advance to 55 pounds until you can handle 10 or 12 at the starting weight level.

WARM-UP EXERCISES: As mentioned above, you should go through a period of warm-up exercises before you begin a weight-lifting routine. Another factor to remember is that most weight-lifting exercises require postural control—which means you must hold the back straight during the lifting phase. Always squat to grasp the barbell from the floor; the bend-and-stretch technique could result in a serious back injury.

OTHER TIPS FOR WEIGHT LIFTING: Begin with the feet spread about 12 inches apart and the toes under the bar; otherwise the bar will tend to swing toward the feet when the lift movement begins. For most barbell exercises, grasp the bar overhand with the thumbs hooked under the bar; keep the arms spread apart by at least the width of the shoulders. For performing curls, reverse the hold with an underhand grip and the thumbs hooked above the bar. Breathe through the mouth and inhale as you lift; exhale on the return movement. Keep the weight evenly distributed between the hands.

Exercising With Other Weights

Another type of weight lifting is performed with dumbbells. There are at least ten different exercises that can be executed with these small, inexpensive weights to develop muscles from the waist to the shoulders and arms. Like the barbell exercises and the 6–12 program, they should be followed in a progressive order. Start with the minimum number of repetitions and advance gradually by adding one or two repetitions per week.

Dumbbells are somewhat deceptive in that they appear easy to handle when first viewed on the counter of a sporting goods store. And a pair is no heavier than a bag of groceries. But when the exercise routines with dumbbells are followed according to directions, you will discover muscles you didn't know you had.

Still other weight-lifting exercises designed to develop specific muscles are the war club swings and the twist grip. See the illustrations on p. 269. The war club weighs about 20 pounds with a handle 14 inches long attached to the weight. It is swung in circles with one or two hands or swung as a hatchet or a baseball bat. It is intended to improve the function of muscle groups in the trunk, back, and shoulders, but provides fringe benefits for the arms and waist also.

The twist-grip exerciser, which is used to develop muscles of the arms and hands, can be made at home from such simple objects as a foot-long piece of pipe, a length of rope, an empty container, and about 20 pounds of cement. The rope is attached to the pipe at one end and the other end is attached to the weighted container. By holding the pipe at arm's length and turning the pipe in the hands, the weight is raised and lowered, using alternately an underhand and overhand grip on the pipe.

Isometrics

Still another method of developing specific muscle groups is known as isometrics. Although isometrics was once popularized as an easy way to exercise, most physical fitness experts agree that there is no such thing as an easy exercise. This opinion applies especially to isometrics; if isometric exercises are performed according to the rules, they can be as difficult as any other kind of exercise. In fact, most isometric exercises should not be performed by an individual who has not been examined by a physician first. The effects of straining some muscle groups while holding the breath can prove dangerous for a person whose heart is not in good condition.

The term isometrics is used to describe a technique in which the muscle is contracted without moving the body part involved, and the muscle is held in contraction for about ten seconds before it is relaxed. Isometrics also are called static exercises, as contrasted with dynamic exercises or isotonic muscle activity in which the muscles not only contract but flex and extend extremities. Some exercise routines may include both isometrics and isotonics; in weight lifting, isometric muscle contractions are used to grasp the weight at the floor and to hold the weight in an overhead position but an isotonic contraction is involved in moving the weight through a curl or press between the isometric phases.

It should be understood that a specific isometric exercise generally is designed to develop only one specific group of muscles. To get the comparable benefits of a warm-up series of exercises and a 6–12 program you would have to perform a very large number of different isometric exercises to involve all of the body's muscles that need daily exercising. Also, they do not provide the aerobic effect of the more active exercise routines. *Aerobics* refers to the kind of physical activity that requires maximum or nearly maximum effort for at least four minutes in order to get the heart and lungs, as well as the muscles, involved in the conditioning effects. In other words, a ten-second isometric muscle contraction is not likely to require the kind of bodily effort that creates an oxygen debt.

Yet isometrics do have a place in physical conditioning, as one unit of an overall exercise effort that also includes warm-up routines and calisthenics, with perhaps a little running or jogging as well. Briefly, the best way to perform isometric exercises is to inhale deeply just before you start the muscle contraction. Hold your breath while you exert the greatest possible effort in muscle contraction. At that point the muscle should begin to quiver from the strain of the contraction. Hold the contraction for

at least five seconds, longer if the exercise requires; use a watch with a sweep second hand for timing. Then relax the muscle and exhale.

Most isometric exercises can be performed with little or no equipment; although special equipment is available for some exercises, many can be performed by using a desk, wall, or door jamb as an immovable object against which you can exert the force of your muscle contractions.

Jogging

Jogging has been viewed as a possible addition to an overall exercise program. But jogging or running may also be regarded as appropriate activities for men and women who take part in no other athletic activities (see *"Physical Fitness and Exercise,"* ["Jogging,"] pp. 623–624).

Jogging as a form of exercise for

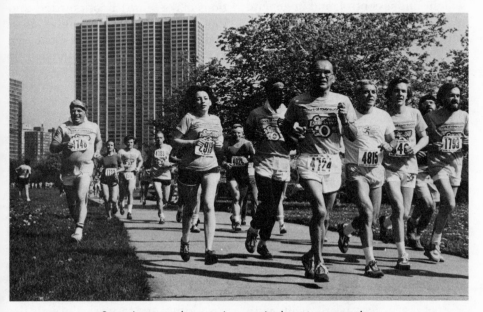

Some joggers take part in organized runs, or marathons, which often require an entry fee that is donated to a charity.

people of all ages and both sexes has acquired a kind of "mystique," or reputation. Jogging has been approached as the first step toward expert, skilled *running* or even competitive *foot racing*. But even if he or she does not go into running or racing the jogger reaps other benefits. For example, staying consistently with his jogging program, the jogger usually feels better. Experts on jogging, in fact, say that the exercise helps participants to feel better both mentally and physically.

Jogging enthusiasts make other claims. They say, for example, that jogging is the "best" exercise from all points of view. The jogger can go out alone to exercise—or can go in company. You can jog as long or as briefly as desired, setting your own pace; and in doing all these things you will be taking part in a form of exercise that ranks high among those that help strengthen the heart, keep weight under control, and in general contribute to fitness. In the average case the jogger is adding to his or her own life expectancy.

Giving testimony to the popularity of jogging, some 15 million Americans were reportedly jogging for better health and fitness in the early 1980s. Of those persons, one-third were women or girls and the rest men and boys. Many of them read books or magazines on the art of jogging. Most of them learned early that two factors, foot care and proper shoes, were important if the jogger was to gain the greatest benefit from the exercise.

Foot Care

Foot care has been dealt with from the podiatrist's point of view (see "The All Important Foot," p. 857). From the point of view of the jogger working toward physical fitness, foot care adds an element, and a very important one, to overall body care. But the feet require special attention.

Hygiene may rank at the top of the list of requirements for good foot care. The feet have to be kept clean; toe-nails should be closely trimmed. just as in running, a more strenuous exercise, in jogging the foot moves around inside the shoe during exercise. It moves particularly when the foot lands. As the toes move, they come into contact with the front of the shoe. Unless the toenails are carefully trimmed, they may become painful. They may even turn black in extreme cases; at that point they require medical attention.

For those joggers who tend toward athlete's foot, sprains, or other problems, some other precautions make sense. Foot powders and lotions may be recommended by a podiatrist. But the individual can avoid such potentially troublesome practices as walking or running barefoot on hard surfaces, unnecessary standing in one place or position for long periods of time, wearing high-heeled or platform shoes, and long continued squatting, crouching, kneeling, or sitting with crossed legs.

Foot injuries, even minor ones, send pain signals to the brain. A rule of thumb holds that if the pain becomes less, you can "run it out"; if the pain increases, or stays the same, you should stop. Where doubt exists . . .

• do not try to work through the pain, strain, or sprain; and

• do not change your jogging or running gait to accommodate the problem.

The warnings have a solid basis in logic. The jogger who ignores the signals from his foot may be making a minor condition worse. At the same time the jogger may not be taking the proper measures to deal with the problem.

The jogger cannot change some physical facts. He may have had childhood illnesses or diseases that predispose him to foot problems. He may be bringing to a fitness program such physical deficiencies as muscle imbalance, lateral pelvic tilt—a tilt toward the side—or other problems such as short leg, leg rotation, faulty leg alignment, outward foot rotation in jogging or running, and architectural defects of the lower leg or foot. While he may not be able to change many of these physical faults, he can nonetheless compensate for them in many cases. He may account for them by exercising in moderation.

Proper Shoes

There can be little wonder that jogging shoes should—must—be carefully selected. In running a mile, each of your feet strikes the ground about 800 times. Jogging 10 miles a week, you would put each foot down and pick it up an estimated 400,000 times a year.

Both socks and shoes should be chosen with those statistics in mind. Shoes in particular should be soft and well padded, with firm arch supports, to cushion the foot as it hits the jogging surface. The jogger has plenty of shoe makes and types to choose from: hundreds of quality running and jogging shoes have

appeared on the market. Many of them have been manufactured to fit the specific needs of different individuals of both sexes.

The needs can cover a broad range. Have you an overweight problem or a large frame? You may need extra cushioning between your feet and the ground. Have you been troubled by Achilles tendinitis? You may need cushioning at the bottom of the heel as well as good elevation. Have you had ankle sprains, or foot instability? You may also need a specially adapted arch support. Calluses on the soles of the feet may suggest a need for a deep toe area.

Have you had shin splints or heel problems? You may need heavier cushioning under the ball of the foot or cupping at the heel plus more flexible cushioning. Shin splints, a swelling of the muscles and tendons along the front of the lower leg, may be especially painful.

Knowing your own needs, you can usually buy the shoe that fits and does the job required. Some other guidelines have been suggested for those buying jogging—or running—shoes:

1. Don't buy shoes by look but by feel. Try them on—as many pairs as necessary. Run in them a little if you can.

2. Make up your own mind. The salesman who tells you a shoe is a perfect fit will not have to wear it—you will.

3. If you find a *brand* of shoe you like, you should in all probability stay with it when buying a new pair.

4. Break your shoes in gradually. In other words, give them some time to "wear in." Don't throw them away after one jog.

5. On the other hand, don't go

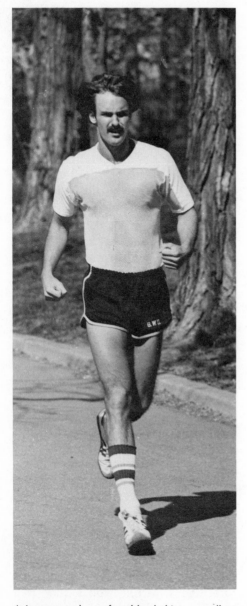

A jogger needs comfortable clothing as well as shoes that fit properly and provide the necessary support for his feet.

too long with a poorly fitting pair, a pair that irritates your foot seriously, or one that binds or pinches.

One other fact may help the jogger looking for shoes that will carry him or her to top fitness form. No person has two exactly identical feet. One foot is always larger than the other; one foot or the other may take somewhat longer to get used to the new shoes.

SHOE CHARACTERISTICS: The "anatomy of a shoe" has a number of key aspects. All of them should be given some attention at the time of purchase. One part can be of high quality while another may be faulty. The key parts:

TOE BOX: the part of the shoe that houses the toes should be large enough to make possible free movement of the toes. The box should exert no pressure.

SOLE: aside from providing the all-important running surface on the bottom of the shoe, the sole should be layered, with a soft cusion from heel to toe. The cushion under the ball of the foot should be at least a half-inch thick. The surface can be "waffle," "ripple," "suction cup," or some other style that gives good traction.

SHANK SUPPORT: for best support, the shoe should not have a "cutaway" arch that could break down under continuous pounding. The bottom of the shoe should, in short, be flat.

INSIDE SUPPORT: inside supports under the arch of the foot should be firm and durable. If necessary, custom-made arch supports should be used.

HEEL LIFT: the difference between the thickness of the sole under the ball of the foot and the maximum thickness of the heel represents the heel lift. The heel should usually ride half an inch higher than the ball.

UPPERS: selection of leather, nylon, mesh-nylon, suede, or other

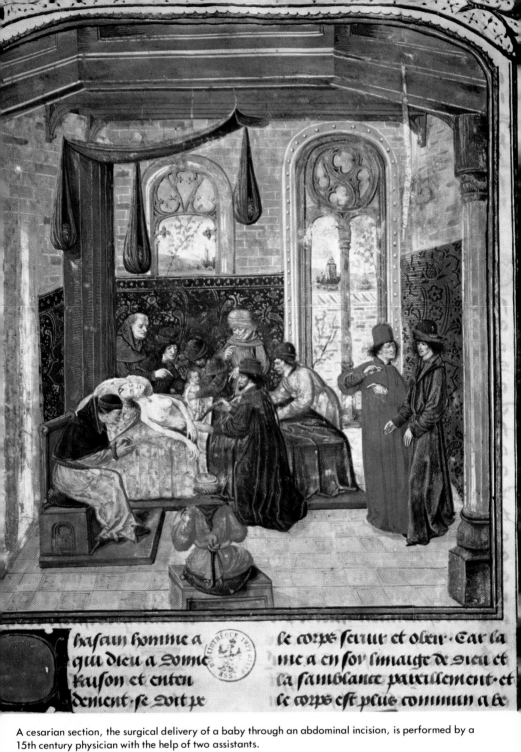

A cesarian section, the surgical delivery of a baby through an abdominal incision, is performed by a
15th century physician with the help of two assistants.
Credit: Bibliothèque Nationale, Paris

hec y est vn dea
ma figura ano
tomie in qua a
mouetur os ca
pitis causa facie
di amotum in p
ipius ossis 7 du
ax pclhcaulax · f · de
matset pie ma
ts et cerebu

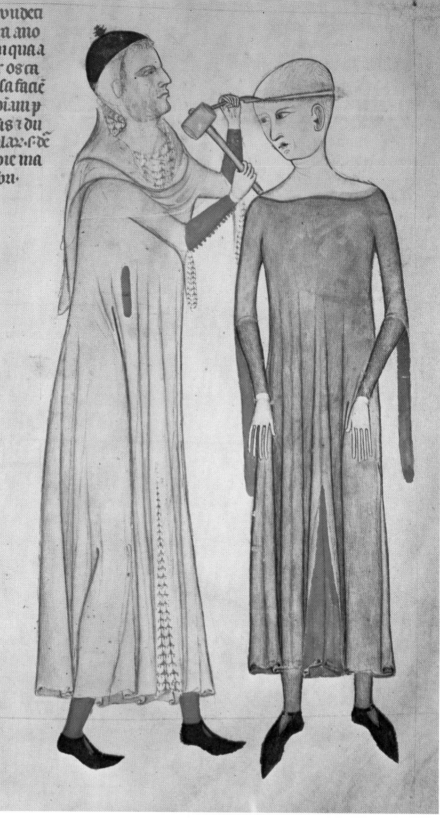

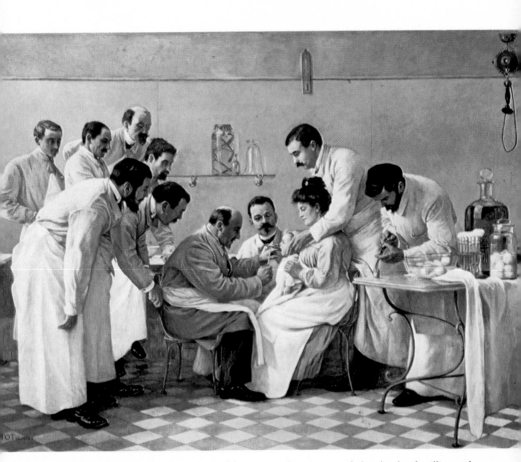

Diphtheria, a bacterial disease characterized by a sore throat, caused the death of millions of children by suffocation. Prior to the development of a diphtheria vaccine, doctors did what they could to alleviate the breathing problems associated with the disease. In "Le tubage par le Docteur Josis à Paris" by Georges Chicotot, a physician attempts to open a passage by inserting a tube down his young patient's throat.
Credit: Jean-Loup Charmet

In a 14th century French manuscript illustration (opposite), a patient's head is shaved and a chisel is used to perforate his skull. The operation, known as trephination, was used to treat various physical and mental disorders of the brain.
Credit: Jean-Loup Charmet

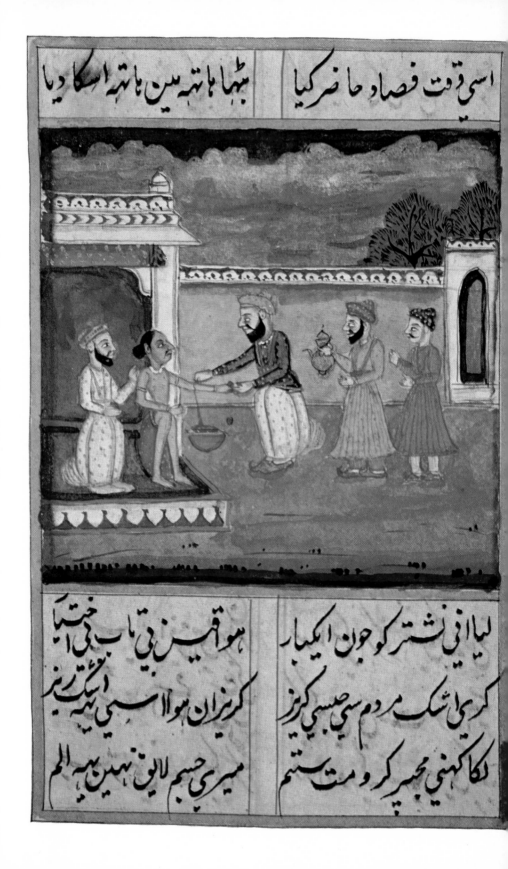

لیا اپنی نشتر کو جون ایکبار ہوا قین منی تاب نی اختیا
کری ائک مردم سی حبی کرو کہریزان ہوا اسپی یہ ایک رہز
لکا کہنی محبر پر کرو مت ستم میری حبسم لایو نہیں یہہ الم

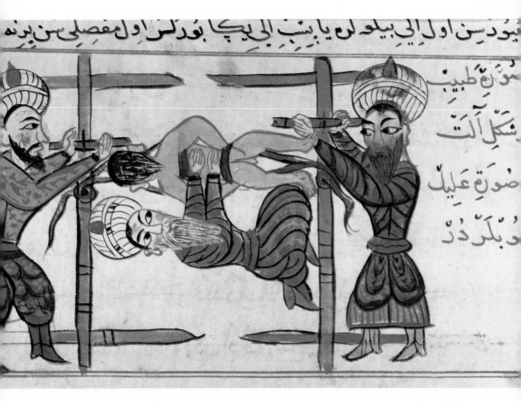

In many cultures useless or painful medical procedures were often performed by laymen. Bloodletting (opposite) was a common practice as a cure for most illnesses in many western and eastern societies. (above) A patient in the medieval Islamic world is treated for a bone fracture in a complicated splint device.

Credit, page 4: Putti Collection, Rizzoli Institute, Bologna

Credit, page 5: Bibliothèque Nationale, Paris

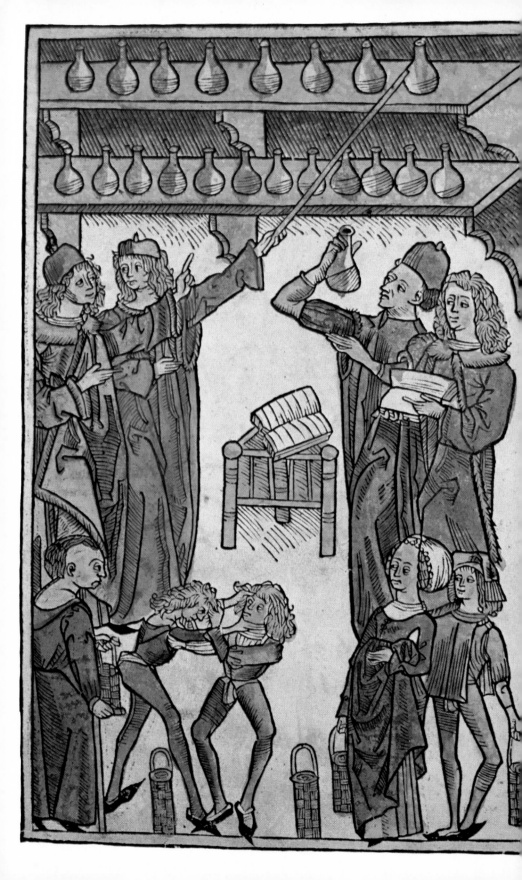

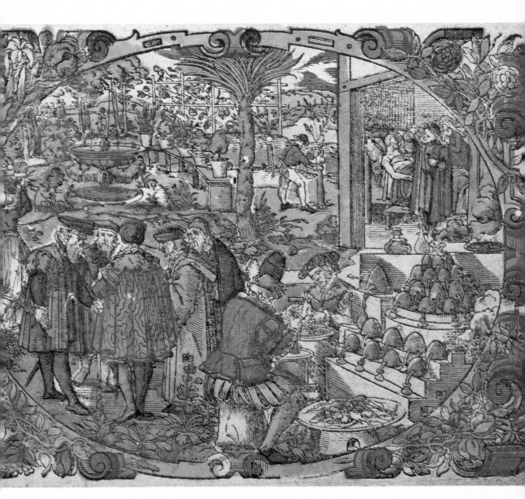

During the Renaissance herbs were one of the primary sources for medications. In a vignette from the title page of a sixteenth century herbal, physicians confer at an outdoor pharmacy while plants are collected and compounded into herbal concoctions.
Credit: National Library of Medicine, Bethesda, Maryland

For many centuries uroscopy (opposite) was such an important diagnostic technique that the urine flask became the symbol of the physician. Physicians carefully examined the color, texture, odor, and sometimes the taste of urine samples to determine the nature of a patient's ailment.
Credit: Francis A. Countway Library of Medicine, Boston; photograph, Eduardo Di Ramio

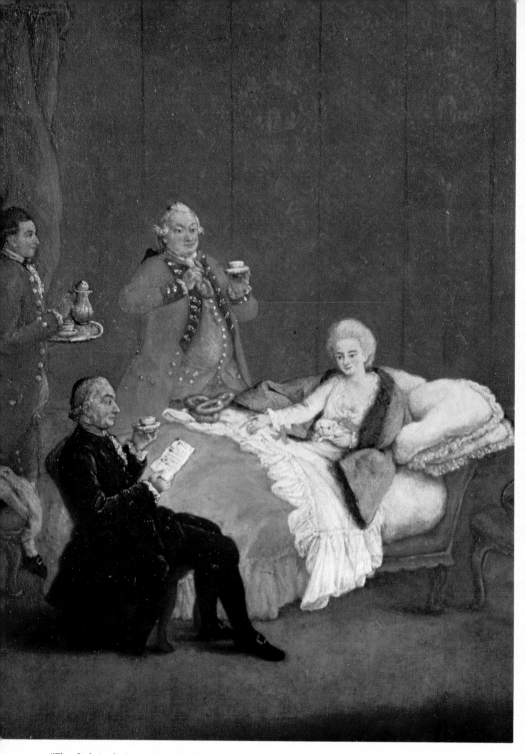

"The Sick Lady," painting by Pietro Longhi, consults with her physician at home. Before modern medical facilities were available, wealthy patients often summoned physicians to their bedsides for treatment.

Credit: Ca' Rezzonico, Venice; photograph, Scala/Editorial Photocolor Archives

type of upper portion of the shoe depends on taste and preference. Leather or nylon is usually preferred for durability, ease of care, and comfort.

SHOE WEIGHT: weight is again a matter of taste. A jogging shoe usually weighs between 10 and 12 ounces.

HEEL COUNTER: the counter, the wrapping around the back of the shoe, should cover the entire heel area for the greatest possible stability.

How all those parts move together—how the shoe bends —gives it its *flexibility*. Even when new a good shoe should flex 30 to 35 degrees without difficulty. The wise jogger tests the flexibility of the sole under the ball of the foot when buying.

SHOE ADD-ONS: Because the jogging shoe adds a critical component to every jogger's fitness program, the add-ons typically available should be noted. The custom-made arch support has been mentioned. A podiatrist will design such a support if needed.

Other add-ons range from heel lifts to insoles. Heel lifts raise the height of the heel, in that process easing the leg strain and pressures that can produce shin splints. Lifts may be one-quarter to one-half an inch or more in thickness; they differ from the heel cups that may be inserted into the shoe to cushion and stabilize the heel. Heel cups help many joggers and runners to avoid heel spurs, bruises, and even ankle sprains. Insoles fit inside the forward part of the shoe. They should be chosen carefully because they may disintegrate or bunch up when in extended use, when soaked by

rain, or when they are too large or too small for the shoe. They should be changed from time to time depending on their condition.

Arch supports present many serious joggers and runners with difficult problems. The supports that come with jogging shoes are often inefficient and inadequate. The solution, probably, is to experiment with supports purchased separately from reputable firms.

Exercises for Women

Physical conditioning programs for women are essentially the same as for men, although women are more likely to be conscious of bulging muscles that seem to produce bodily proportions they may regard as unattractive. However, there are exercise routines that can have the effect of balancing proportions. Running and cycling, for example, tend to favor development of the muscles from the hips downward. Weight lifting or other exercises designed to develop the muscles from the waist up can be used to advantage by women who want to reshape that part of the body. On the other hand, exercises that tend to develop musculature where it is unwanted can be avoided. Particularly recommended for women who plan to be mothers are exercises that strengthen the abdominal and back muscles. See the illustrations on pp. 270–272.

Basic exercises for women include running or jogging, bending and twisting at the waist, situps, and modified pushups, as well as standing on the toes while stretching the arms upward. Special exercises for enhancing the female figure can begin with a series of bustline exer-

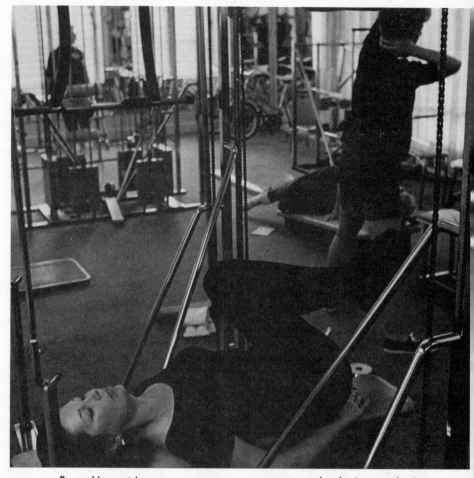

By working out in a gym, women can concentrate on developing muscles in some areas of the body while avoiding unwanted development in others.

cises. One is an isometric press that starts with the palms of the hands facing together, fingers clasped and pointed upward, and arms close to the chest. Inhale deeply and push the hands against each other with maximum effort. Hold the breath while pressing and continue for seven seconds. Then relax, exhale, and repeat the exercise. Two other exercises are performed while lying flat on the floor with a weight in each hand; dumbbells, bricks, or books can serve as weights. Start with weights in hands, arms stretched back over the head with backs of the hands on the floor. Next raise both arms without bending the elbows and move the weights overhead and down to the floor at the hips. While counting to yourself for rhythm, return to the original position and repeat the exercise. The second is a variation of the previous exercise, with the weights lifted straight overhead from a starting position of the arms extended sideward at shoulder level. Don't bend the elbows.

Cycle-type exercises and ballet stretches are recommended for hips and thighs. Ballet stretches can be performed from a standing position, with one hand on the hip and the other holding onto a steady object such as a chair. Another exercise for the hips and thighs is patterned after the "cheerleader" position. While kneeling on the floor, hands on hips and back straight, bend backward as far as is comfortable without bending the back or moving the knees. Return to the starting position and begin again.

Among the suggested exercises for calves and ankles is the rocker. With feet together and hands on hips, legs straight, rock back on your heels with toes off the floor. Then rock back with your weight on the toes and the heels off the floor.

Exercises for Special Situations

Persons recovering from an illness or surgery can help themselves by undertaking particular types of exercises. So can mothers who have just given birth, the elderly, and many others with special needs and, in some cases, special limitations.

Exercise after Illness or Surgery

Exercises designed to restore mobility and fitness after serious illness or surgery actually begin when the patient first sits up. When he or she starts to walk, an even more important step has been taken. But long hours of bed confinement can still, at that point, keep the patient weak. Bed exercises approved by a doctor can both help the time to pass and move the patient toward physical improvement.

Necessarily, the exercises must be kept simple. They have also to be prescribed with an eye to the patient's condition and the type of surgery or sickness. Exercises can begin with deep-breathing routines that will drive waste carbon monoxide out of the lungs and blood. Shifts of body position will be important because they relieve muscle tension. Even while largely bedridden, the patient can start a program including the following exercises suggested by Dr. James Graham and Donald G. Cooley in their book, *So You're Going to Have Surgery:*

• Rotation of the arms, forearms, and hands while the arms are stretched out straight from the shoulders

• Raising the arms from the stretched-out position until the hands touch over the body

• Stretching the arms upward, then back down, while palms are rotated

• With arms outstretched from the supine body, clenching fists and pressing elbows into the bed, then flex forearms until they touch chest

• Extending right arm at right angle from body, then reaching left arm across to the right until hand covers the right ear; repeat with left arm stretched away from body

• Lying supine, stretching feet and toes downward as far as they will go

• On back, with both legs straight, bending the toes up toward the head as far as they will go

• Lying on back, lifting first the right, then the left leg perhaps half an inch off the bed; repeat with the other leg

Other exercises for the recuperating patient cover a broad range.

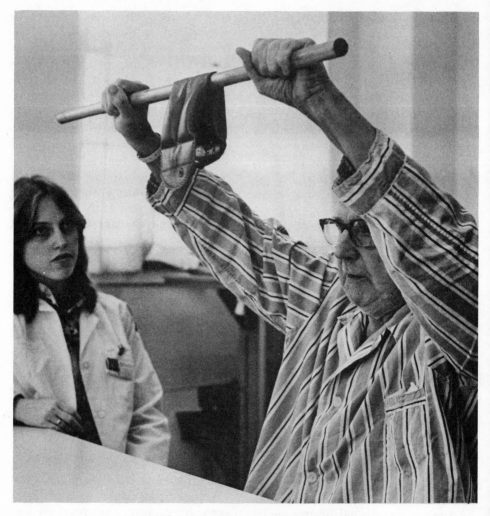

A special exercise program has been devised to
help this patient recover gradually from a stroke.

Their usefulness may depend on
what the patient was used to before
surgery. For example, a person
accustomed to lifting weights may
start working with a dumbbell very
soon after beginning to mend. Persons used to extensive exercise
programs may be able to start
bicycle movements, deep bends, or
even pushups within days after
beginning a rehabilitation program.

Many other exercises are adapted
to the patient's situation. Patients
with broken hips may need
extended therapy before they can
regain mobility. Amputees usually
require a supervised program of
therapy and rehabilitation. But in
nearly all cases recovery can proceed
at a steady rate if the exercises have
been properly selected.

Exercise after Breast Surgery

Breast surgery makes some special
physical demands (see "Mas-

tectomy," section, pp. 1034-1035). During the operation the surgeon may have removed important muscles at the front of the shoulder, the *pectoralis major* and *minor*. Exercises designed to restore movement and strength to the shoulders and arms may be quite extensive. They may, for instance, include:

• Hair brushing

• The "wall walk," in which the hands are "walked" up a wall as the patient stands facing it

• The rope swing, in which a rope is swung, lariat-fashion, in an ever-widening circle

• The rope pull, in which a rope is hung over a rod or hook so that the patient can pull the dangling ends first with one hand, then the other

• The arm swing, with the patient bending far over and swinging her arms

Exercise after Delivery

Expectant mothers today receive careful instructions on the types of exercises that will help them. The exercises are designed to maintain overall fitness and muscle tone, and to strengthen parts of the body that will be important during delivery. To a large extent, the same types of exercises also serve to bring the mother's body back to normal after her baby is born.

All such exercises require careful attention and a degree of concentration. Some of them are recommended for the ways in which they will improve special post-delivery conditions; but most contribute to overall physical fitness. All of them complement and extend such basic activities as walking, lifting normal weights, and performing various home and office tasks requiring physical movements.

At least nine basic categories of exercises have been recommended for the new mother. In any given case they should be integrated into the post-natal exercise program with a doctor's approval. The nine categories include:

1. *The leg strengthener:* From a supine position—lying on your back—slide first one leg and then the other along the floor until the leg is straight. The other leg remains bent; the back should be kept flat.

2. *The stomach reducer:* From the same position, one leg and then the other is drawn straight up, as close to the chest as possible, and then lowered at a steady rate. Repeat several times, then draw both legs up as high as possible. Repeat several times.

3. *The spine loosener:* To relax a tense spine, while kneeling and with the elbows on the floor raise your back upward. Lower the back while shifting the weight toward the heels. Repeat four or five times.

4. *The hip toner:* Lying supine with the knees bent and feet flat, lift the lower back and buttocks off the floor, then lower. Repeat several times, keeping the shoulders on the floor.

5. *The back relaxer:* Starting from the supine position with knees raised, sit up, clasp hands around the knees, and rock back and forth several times. Try the same exercise with first the left leg, then the right, stretched out straight on the floor.

6. *The arm stretcher:* From the supine position again, reach the arms over the head, on the floor, with the elbows slightly bent. With the head and arms leading the way,

move progressively into a sitting position. The hands should be brought all the way forward to touch the floor next to the ankles while the head rests on the knees.

7. *The thigh stretch:* Lying supine, with knees raised and turned out, place the soles of the feet together. Keep ing the soles together, extend both legs forward as far as possible, then straighten legs until the feet are pointing straight up. Repeat.

8. *The leg builder:* Start from kneeling position with hands flat on the floor. Draw right knee forward and up and place right foot flat on the floor between your hands. Return to starting position and repeat several times, alternating legs. With the last exercise, rise with your weight on the right leg and stride forward as if walking.

9. *The chest strengthener:* Standing at arm's length from a wall, place both hands flat on the surface. Keeping the hands stationary, turn your arms. The elbows should turn out. From the original position, turn your hands until the fingers point at one another.

With each exercise, rhythmic breathing should be practiced. Breathing in and breathing out should generally coincide with movements of parts of the body so that the movements are, in a sense, paced. When walking, sitting, or standing, good posture should be the rule. Posture then becomes an aid to fitness. Looking fit helps you to feel fit.

Exercise for the Elderly

Older persons trying to maintain a high level of physical fitness have other special challenges. For one thing, age has taken from them some of the vitality and spring of youth. For another thing, their muscles may have grown abnormally flabby and soft during the years they spent at work in office or home. Still a third factor may be noted: few exercise or fitness facilities exist for the elderly. Thus these "golden years" members of society often have to find or invent their own facilities.

Many elderly persons overcome the difficulties and lead healthy, active, exercise-or activity-filled lives. They pursue exercise or conditioning programs alone or in groups—at the local health club, at the YMCA, or elsewhere. When serious, they exercise daily, under all kinds of circumstances. In the process they acquire a sense of well-being as well as a reserve of strength for whatever life may bring.

A program of movement, of controlled exercise, for the elderly has some basic characteristics that other programs may lack. The program for the older person, for example, will usually encompass a number of simple, noncompetitive exercises. That program may include more strenuous exercises, but those should start only after the individual has "built up" to them. Many exercises for the elderly may also teach them basic physical skills that can prevent injuries and prolong life—such things as standing, sitting, and walking properly, making beds, improving posture, and so on. They may learn rocking-chair, bathtub, and bed exercises, and entire series of movements for the hands, feet, and other parts of the body.

A physical examination should always precede the start of any program. From that point on, with a doctor's approval, the elderly fitness fan usually tries to reach his or her level of participation, staying with certain exercises or moving on from one level to another. A typical progression would take the older person through finger, hand, and arm exercises to shoulder, chest, and neck hips, and back exercises. Competitive sports may follow: tennis, for example, or court games such as racquetball. These can be played as strenuously or noncompetitively as the player wishes. Normally, the wise course is to choose as a partner a person whose skills match one's own.

Most experts on exercise for the elderly stress the importance of proper breathing. Deep breathing constitutes a warmup or basic exercise in itself. Facial exercises may be included in many programs to minimize the wrinkling effects of age. Very often, group programs are conducted to the strains of enjoyable music.

Strengthening Particular Muscles

Exercises that serve the purpose of strengthening specific muscles can prove valuable whether or not a person has had an operation, disease, or illness. Hundreds of such exercises have been devised. Some involve the use of weights or other equipment; some are "free-form" exercises that require no equipment at all. The latter can be done at home, in a gym or workout room, or even in the office.

Usually, men and women pursue different exercise programs. But they have basically the same muscle structures. Their exercises differ because they want to *look different:*

in American society the ideal figures for men and women are different. Where men may work deliberately to develop heavier muscles, broad shoulders, and small hips, women more often choose exercises that ensure slimness, good muscle tone, and a slender waist.

For both sexes, symmetry and proportion constitute widely accepted targets of muscle-strengthening programs. But the task of building specific muscles takes consistent work. Aside from the need for consistency— performing exercise routines at particular times on specified days— fitness experts agree generally that . . .

1. as in jogging and other activities, every exercise session should include a warmup, basic participation, and cooling-down periods;

2. beginners at a muscle-building program should work up gradually to more advanced exercises. Where they are trying to develop muscles weakened by illness, an operation, or injury, or are real beginners, they should exercise under the supervision of a doctor;

3. exercises should be practiced at least two hours after eating—but there could be exceptions;

4. the proper exercise clothing should be worn for all sessions. Such clothing is loose and comfortable;

5. if your diet is already well balanced, don't change it simply because you are starting a muscle-building program;

6. when nearing completion of an exercise session, activity should be gradually reduced over a short period of time. The tension that accompanies exercise can then drop away.

Exercises can be found for

strengthening any part of the body. The table on the next page shows the names of major body muscles, their locations, and the types of exercises that will strengthen them. The table comes from the book, *The Zane Way to a Beautiful Body*, by Frank and Christine Zane.

The body regions in which the strengthening exercises. The five main regions are the neck and shoulders, the arms and chest or bosom, the waist and abdominal area, the hips and buttocks, and the legs and feet. In some cases the exercise variations will be prescribed by a doctor for specific conditions in one or more regions.

MUSCLES, THEIR LOCATIONS, AND EXERCISES
THAT STRENGTHEN THEM

Muscle	Location	Movement
Trapezius	Upper back and each side of neck	Shoulder-shrugging and upward-pulling movements
Deltoids	Shoulders	Arm raising and overhead pressing
Pectorals	Chest	Horizontal pressing and drawing arms across body
Latissimus Dorsi	Wide back muscle stretching over back up to rear Deltoids	Pulling and rowing movements
Serratus	Jagged sawtooth muscles between Pectorals and lattissimus Dorsi	Pullover and Serratus leverage movements
Spinal Erectors	Lower length of spinal column	Raising upper body from a bent-over position
Biceps	Front portion of upper arm	Arm bending and twisting
Forearms	Between wrist and elbow	Reverse-grip arm bending
Triceps	Back of upper arm	Pushing and straightening movements of upper arms
Rectus Abdominals	Muscular area between sternum and pelvis	Sit-up, leg-raising, knee-in movements
Intercostals	Sides of waist, running diagonally to Serratus	Waist twisting
External Oblique Abdominals	Lower sides of waist	Waist twisting and bending
Buttocks	Muscular area covering seat	Lunging, stooping, leg raising
Leg Biceps	Back of thighs	Raising lower leg to buttocks, bending forward and stretching
Frontal Thighs	Front of thighs	Extending lower leg and knee bending
Calves	Lower leg between ankle and knee	Raising and lowering on toes

WARM-UP EXERCISES

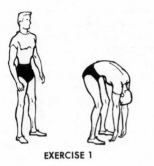

EXERCISE 1

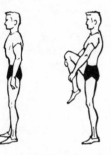

EXERCISE 2

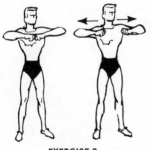

EXERCISE 3

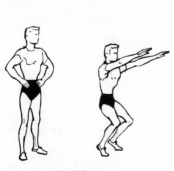

EXERCISE 4

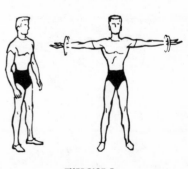

EXERCISE 5

Exercise 1: Bend and Stretch. Stand erect, feet shoulder-width apart. *Count 1.* Bend trunk forward and down, flexing knees. Stretch gently in attempt to touch fingers to toes or floor. *Count 2.* Return to starting position. *Note:* Do slowly, stretch and relax at intervals rather than in rhythm.

Exercise 2: Knee Lift. Stand erect, feet together, arms at sides. *Count 1.* Raise left knee as high as possible, grasping leg with hands and pulling knee against body while keeping back straight. *Count 2.* Lower to starting position. *Counts 3 and 4.* Repeat with right knee.

Exercise 3: Wing Stretcher. Stand erect, elbows at shoulder height, fists clenched in front of chest. *Count 1.* Thrust elbows backward vigorously without arching back. Keep head erect, elbows at shoulder height. *Count 2.* Return to starting position.

Exercise 4: Half Knee Bend. Stand erect, hands on hips. *Count 1.* Bend knees halfway while extending arms forward, palms down. *Count 2.* Return to starting position.

Exercise 5: Arm Circles. Stand erect, arms extended sideward at shoulder height, palms up. Describe small circles backward with hands. Keep head erect. Do 15 backward circles. Reverse, turn palms down and do 15 small circles forward.

WARM-UP EXERCISES

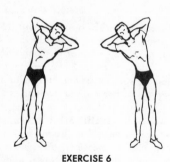

EXERCISE 6

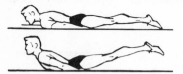

EXERCISE 7

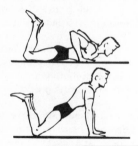

EXERCISE 8

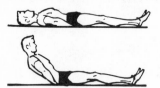

EXERCISE 9

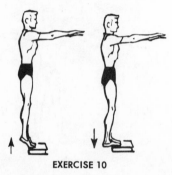

EXERCISE 10

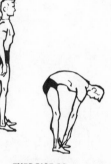

EXERCISE 11

Exercise 6: Body Bender. Stand, feet shoulder-width apart, hands behind neck, fingers interlaced. *Count 1.* Bend trunk sideward to left as far as possible, keeping hands behind neck. *Count 2.* Return to starting position. *Counts 3 and 4.* Repeat to the right.

Exercise 7: Prone Arch. Lie face down, hands tucked under thighs. *Count 1.* Raise head, shoulders, and legs from floor. *Count 2.* Return to starting position.

Exercise 8: Knee Pushup. Lie on floor, face down, legs together, knees bent with feet raised off floor, hands on floor under shoulders, palms down. *Count 1.* Push upper body off floor until arms are fully extended and body is in straight line from head to knees. *Count 2.* Return to starting position.

Exercise 9: Head and Shoulder Curl. Lie on back, hands tucked under small of back, palms down. *Count 1.* Tighten abdominal muscles, lift head and pull shoulders and elbows up off floor. Hold for four seconds. *Count 2.* Return to starting position.

Exercise 10: Ankle Stretch. Stand on a stair, large book or block of wood, with weight on balls of feet and heels raised. *Count 1.* Lower heels. *Count 2.* Raise heels.

Exercise 11: Toe Touch. Stand at attention. *Count 1.* Bend trunk forward and down keeping knees straight, touching fingers to ankles. *Count 2.* Bounce and touch fingers to top of feet. *Count 3.* Bounce and touch fingers to toes. *Count 4.* Return to starting position.

WARM-UP EXERCISES

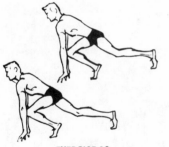

EXERCISE 12

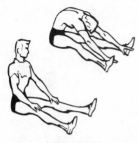

EXERCISE 13

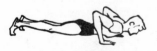

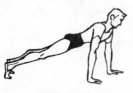

EXERCISE 14

Exercise 12: Sprinter. Squat, hands on floor, fingers pointed forward, left leg fully extended to rear. *Count 1.* Reverse position of feet in bouncing movement, bringing left foot to hands and extending right leg backward—all in one motion. *Count 2.* Reverse feet again, returning to starting position.

Exercise 13: Sitting Stretch. Sit, legs spread apart, hands on knees. *Count 1.* Bend forward at waist, extending arms as far forward as possible. *Count 2.* Return to starting position.

Exercise 14: Pushup. Lie on floor, face down, legs together, hands on floor under shoulders with fingers pointed straight ahead. *Count 1.* Push body off floor by extending arms, so that weight rests on hands and toes. *Count 2.* Lower the body until chest touches floor. *Note:* Body should be kept straight, buttocks should not be raised, abdomen should not sag.

Exercise 15: Situp (Arms Extended). Lie on back, legs straight and together, arms extended beyond head. *Count 1.* Bring arms forward over head, roll up to sitting position, sliding hands along legs, grasping ankles. *Count 2.* Roll back to starting position.

Exercise 16: Leg Raiser. Right side of body on floor, head resting on left arm. Lift left leg about 24" off floor, then lower it. Do required number of repetitions. Repeat on other side.

EXERCISE 15

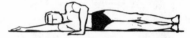

EXERCISE 16

INDOOR EXERCISE PROGRAM

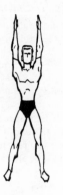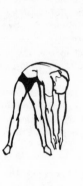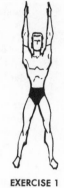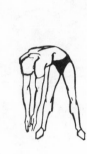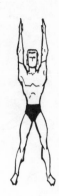

EXERCISE 1

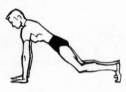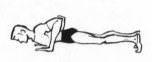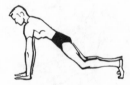

EXERCISE 2

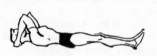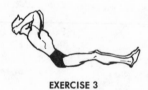

EXERCISE 3

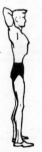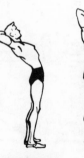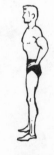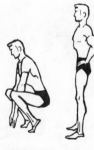

EXERCISE 4   EXERCISE 5

INDOOR EXERCISE PROGRAM

TABLE I: PROGRESSION GUIDE

AGE GROUP	LEVEL	1	2	3	4	5	6
		EXERCISES					
17	A	15	18	14	15	15	250
to	B	13	16	13	13	13	235
29	C	11	14	12	11	11	215
30	A	13	14	12	13	13	200
to	B	11	13	11	11	11	185
39	C	9	12	10	9	9	165
40	A	11	11	10	11	11	150
to	B	9	10	9	9	9	135
44	C	7	9	8	7	7	120
45	A	9	8	8	9	9	100
to	B	7	7	7	7	7	90
49	C	5	6	6	5	5	80
50	A	7	6	6	7	7	75
to	B	5	5	5	5	5	70
59	C	3	4	4	3	3	60
60	A	4	5	4	4	4	50
and	B	3	4	3	3	3	40
over	C	2	3	2	2	2	30
Minutes for each exercise		2	1	1	1	2	5

Exercise 1: Side straddle, arms overhead and straight, palms facing. Turn trunk to the left and bend forward over the left thigh, attempt to touch the fingertips to the floor outside the left foot, keep the knees straight. Alternate the movement to the opposite side. • Down and up to one side is one repetition.

Exercise 2: Kneeling front rest, hands shoulder width apart. The weight is supported on the knees and by the arms. Bend elbows and lower body until chest touches the floor. Keeping knees on the floor, raise body by straightening the arms. • Down and up is one repetition.

Exercise 3: Supine position, fingers interlaced and placed behind the head. Maintaining the heels on the floor, raise the head and shoulders until the heels come into view. Lower the head and shoulders until fingers contact the floor and head rests on the hands. • Up and down is one repetition.

Exercise 4: Body erect, feet slightly spread, fingers interlaced and placed on rear of neck at base of the head. Bend the upper trunk backward, raise the chest high, pull the elbows back, and look upward. Keep the knees straight. Recover to the erect position, eyes to the front. • Bending backward and recovery is one repetition.

Exercise 5: Body erect, feet spread less than shoulder width, hands on hips, elbows back. Do a full knee bend, at the same time bend slightly forward at the waist. Touch the floor with the extended fingers, keeping the hands about six inches apart. Resume the starting position. • Down into the touch position and return to the starting position is one repetition.

Exercise 6: Run in place, lift feet 4 to 6 inches off floor. At the completion of every 50 steps do 10 Steam Engines. Repeat sequence until the required number of steps is completed. • Count a step each time left foot touches the floor.

Steam Engines. Lace the fingers behind the neck and while standing in place raise the left knee above waist height, at the same time twist the trunk and lower the right elbow to the left knee. Lower the left leg and raise the right leg touching the knee with the left elbow thus completing the movement to that side. Continue to alternate the movement until the sequence is completed.

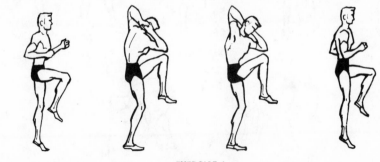

EXERCISE 6

INDOOR EXERCISE PROGRAM

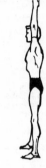
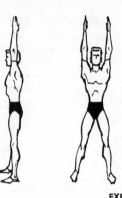
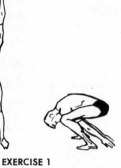

EXERCISE 1

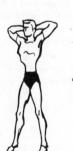
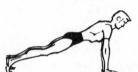

EXERCISE 2

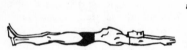

EXERCISE 3

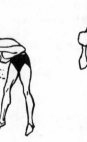
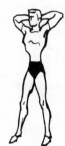

EXERCISE 4

EXERCISE 5

INDOOR EXERCISE PROGRAM

TABLE II: PROGRESSION GUIDE

AGE GROUP	LEVEL	EXERCISES					
		1	2	3	4	5	6
17 to 29	A	17	17	17	9	19	300
	B	15	15	15	8	17	270
	C	13	13	13	7	15	245
30 to 39	A	15	15	15	8	17	235
	B	13	13	13	7	15	210
	C	11	11	11	6	13	190
40 to 44	A	13	13	13	7	15	175
	B	11	11	11	6	13	155
	C	9	10	9	5	11	135
45 to 49	A	11	11	11	6	13	125
	B	9	9	9	5	11	110
	C	7	7	7	4	9	100
50 to 59	A	9	9	9	5	11	95
	B	7	7	7	4	9	85
	C	5	5	5	3	7	75
60 and over	A	6	7	7	4	9	70
	B	5	5	5	3	7	60
	C	4	4	4	2	5	50
Minutes for each exercise		1	1	1	1½	1½	6

Exercise 1: Wide side straddle, arms overhead and straight, palms facing. Bend at the knees and the waist, swing the arms down, and reach between the legs as far as possible. Look at the hands. The thighs are parallel to the floor during the bend. Recover to the starting position with a sharp movement. • Down and up is one repetition.

Exercise 2: Front leaning rest position with body straight from head to heels. Bending at the waist and keeping the knees locked, jump forward to a jack-knife position bringing the feet as close to the hands as possible. With the weight on the hands, thrust the legs to the rear resuming the front leaning rest position. • Up into the jack-knife position and return to the front leaning rest position is one repetition.

Exercise 3: Supine position with arms straight overhead, palms facing. With a sharp movement sit up, bringing the heels as close to the buttocks as possible and the knees to the chest. Swing the arms in an arc overhead to a position outside the knees and parallel to the floor. To recover swing the arms overhead keeping them straight. At the same time move the legs forward until they are straight. • Sitting up and returning to the supine position is one repetition.

Exercise 4: Feet spread more than shoulder width apart, fingers laced behind the neck and elbows are back. Bend forward at the waist vigorously, then twist the trunk to the left, then to the right and return to the erect position. Keep the knees locked and back straight. • Bend forward, twist left, twist right, and return to the erect position is one repetition.

Exercise 5: Bend forward at the waist, grasping the right toes with right hand, left toes with left hand, knees are slightly bent. Walk forward retaining this position. • Count a repetition each time a foot contacts the floor.

Figure 6: Run in place, lift feet 4 to 6 inches off floor. At the completion of every 50 steps do 10 Heel Clicks. Repeat sequence until the required number of steps is completed. • Count a step each time left foot touches the floor.

Heel Clicks. Jump upward about 12 inches and bring the heels together. Before landing on the floor, separate the feet 15 to 18 inches. Immediately upon contact with the floor repeat the jump and heel click.

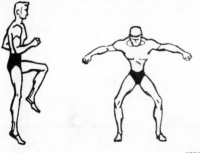
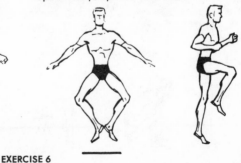

EXERCISE 6

INDOOR EXERCISE PROGRAM

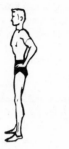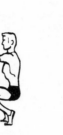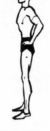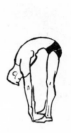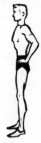

EXERCISE 1

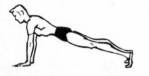

EXERCISE 2

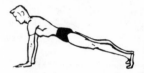

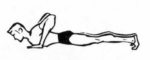

EXERCISE 3

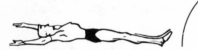

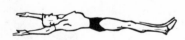

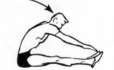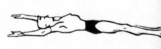

EXERCISE 4

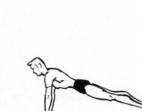

EXERCISE 5

INDOOR EXERCISE PROGRAM

TABLE III: PROGRESSION GUIDE

AGE GROUP	LEVEL	1	2	3	4	5	6
			EXERCISES				
17	A	10	19	19	16	10	350
to	B	9	17	17	15	9	315
29	C	8	15	15	14	8	280
30	A	9	17	17	14	9	270
to	B	8	15	15	13	8	240
39	C	7	13	13	12	7	210
40	A	8	15	15	12	8	200
to	B	7	13	13	11	7	180
44	C	6	11	11	10	6	160
45	A	7	13	13	10	7	150
to	B	6	11	11	9	6	135
49	C	5	9	9	8	5	120
50	A	6	11	11	8	6	115
to	B	5	9	9	7	5	105
59	C	4	7	7	6	4	95
60	A	5	9	9	7	5	90
and	B	4	7	7	6	4	80
over	C	3	5	5	4	3	70
Minutes for each exercise		1½	1	1	1½	1	6

Exercise 1: Feet spread less than shoulder width apart, hands on hips, elbows back. Do a full knee bend, trunk erect and thrust the arms forward. Recover to the erect position, and with knees locked, bend forward at the waist and touch the toes and recover to the erect position. • Down into the full knee bend, recover, touch toes and recover is one repetition.

Exercise 2: Front leaning rest position with body straight from head to heels. Lower the body until the chest touches the floor, keep body straight. Recover by straightening the arms and raising the body. • Down and touch the floor and recovery to the front leaning rest position is one repetition.

Exercise 3: Supine position, arms overhead, palms facing. With a sharp movement sit up, thrust the arms forward and touch the toes. Keep the legs straight and the heels in contact with the floor. • Sit up, touch toes, and resume the supine position is one repetition.

Exercise 4: Supine position, arms overhead, palms upward. Raise the legs and swing them backward over the head until toes touch the floor. Recover by returning legs to the starting position. • Touch toes overhead and recover to the supine position is one repetition.

Exercise 5: Erect position, feet together. Bend knees and place hands on floor, shoulder width apart. Thrust legs to the rear, body straight from head to heels. Move legs forward assuming squat position, elbows inside of knees. Assume erect position. • Down into full squat, legs to the rear, back to full squat and return to the erect position is one repetition.

Exercise 6: Run in place, lift feet 4 to 6 inches off floor. At the completion of every 50 steps do 10 Knee Touches. Repeat sequence until the required number of steps is completed. • Count a step each time the left foot touches the floor.

Knee Touches. From a stride position, bend the knees and touch the knee of the rear leg to the floor, straighten legs, jump upward and change position of the feet. Again bend knees and touch the opposite knee. Continue alternately touching each knee.

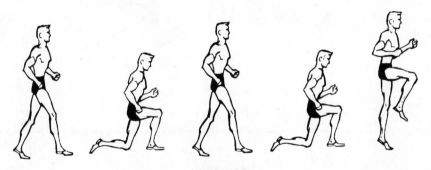

EXERCISE 6

INDOOR EXERCISE PROGRAM

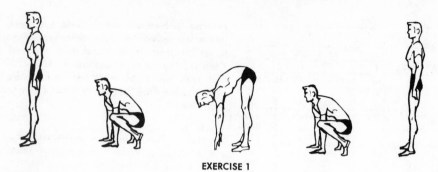

EXERCISE 1

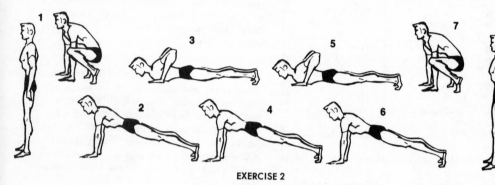

EXERCISE 2

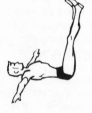

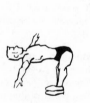
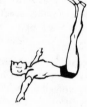
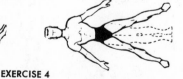
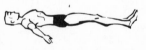

EXERCISE 3

EXERCISE 4

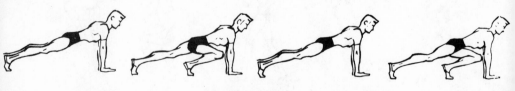

EXERCISE 5

INDOOR EXERCISE PROGRAM

TABLE IV: PROGRESSION GUIDE

AGE GROUP	LEVEL	EXERCISES					
		1	2	3	4	5	6
17 to 29	A	12	9	12	24	25	400
	B	11	8	11	22	23	380
	C	10	7	10	21	21	360
30 to 39	A	11	8	11	23	23	305
	B	10	7	10	21	21	290
	C	9	6	9	20	20	275
40 to 44	A	10	7	10	20	21	225
	B	9	6	9	18	18	215
	C	8	5	8	16	16	205
45 to 49	A	8	6	8	16	16	175
	B	7	5	7	14	14	165
	C	6	4	6	12	12	155
50 to 59	A	6	5	6	13	13	135
	B	5	4	5	11	11	130
	C	4	3	4	10	10	120
60 and over	A	5	4	5	10	10	100
	B	4	3	4	9	9	95
	C	3	2	3	8	8	90
Minutes for each exercise		1	2	1	1	1	6

Exercise 1: Erect position, hands at sides, feet spread slightly. Bend knees, incline trunk forward, and place hands on floor between legs. Straighten knees, keeping feet in place and fingers touching floor. Again bend knees and resume the first position. Recover to the erect position. • The above sequence is one repetition.

Exercise 2: Erect position, hands at sides, feet together. Bend knees, place hands on floor between legs. Thrust legs to the rear. Execute two complete pushups and then thrust the legs forward bending the knees with arms between the knees. Recover to the erect position. • The completion of all eight counts is one repetition.

Exercise 3: Back position with arms out to sides and legs raised to the vertical. Lower legs to the left, raise legs to the vertical, lower to the right, again raise to the vertical. Keep legs together and the head and hands in contact with the floor throughout the exercise. • The above sequence is one repetition.

Exercise 4: From back position, raise legs with heels 10 to 12 inches from the floor. Spread legs as far as possible, close them together. Continue to open and close legs until required repetitions have been completed. • Opening and closing legs is one repetition.

Exercise 5: Front leaning rest position, body straight from head to heels. Bend the left knee and bring the left foot as far forward as possible, return left leg to original position. Repeat movement with the right leg. Continue exercise alternating left and right legs. • A leg thrust forward and returned to the rear is one repetition.

Exercise 6: Run in place, lift feet 4 to 6 inches off floor. At the completion of every 50 steps do 10 Jumping Jacks. Repeat sequence until the required number of steps is completed. • Count a step each time left foot touches the floor.

Jumping Jacks. Feet spread shoulder width apart, arms extended overhead. Jump upward, bring heels together and at same time squat to a full knee bend position, bring the arms downward and place hands on the floor, elbows inside of knees, directly under the shoulders. Jump to the side straddle and swing the arms sideward overhead.

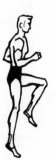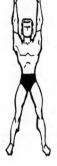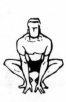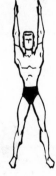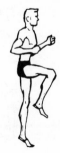

EXERCISE 6

INDOOR EXERCISE PROGRAM

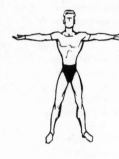
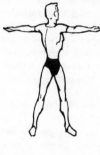
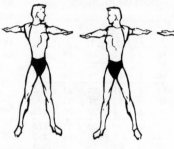

EXERCISE 1

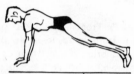
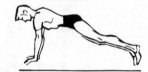

EXERCISE 2

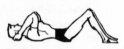

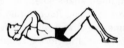

EXERCISE 3

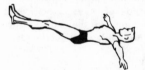

EXERCISE 4

EXERCISE 5

INDOOR EXERCISE PROGRAM

TABLE V: PROGRESSION GUIDE

AGE GROUP	LEVEL	EXERCISES					
		1	2	3	4	5	6
17	A	14	13	28	14	30	450
to	B	13	12	27	13	28	430
29	C	12	11	26	12	26	410
30	A	12	12	25	12	26	350
to	B	11	11	24	11	24	330
39	C	10	10	23	10	22	310
40	A	11	11	23	11	23	250
to	B	10	10	21	10	21	240
44	C	9	9	19	9	19	230
45	A	9	9	20	9	20	200
to	B	8	8	18	8	18	190
49	C	7	7	16	7	16	180
50	A	7	7	16	7	16	170
to	B	6	6	14	6	14	155
59	C	5	5	12	5	12	140
60	A	6	6	12	6	12	115
and	B	5	5	11	5	10	110
over	C	4	4	9	4	9	105
Minutes for each exercise		2	1	1	2	1	5

Exercise 1: Feet spread more than shoulder width, arms sideward at shoulder level, palms up. Turn trunk to the left as far as possible, recover slightly, repeat to the right and recover slightly. The head and hips remain to the front throughout the exercise. • The above sequence is one repetition.

Exercise 2: Front leaning rest position, body straight from head to heels. Bend the elbows slightly and push with the hands and toes, bouncing the body upward and completely off the floor. In contact with the floor resume the front leaning rest position. • Propelling the body upward and the return to the floor is one repetition.

Exercise 3: Back position, hands interlaced and placed under head, knees bent with feet flat on the floor. Sit up bending the trunk forward and attempting to touch the chest to the thighs. Recover to the back position without moving the feet. • Sit up and recovery to the back position is one repetition.

Exercise 4: On back, arms sideward, feet raised 12 inches from the floor, knees straight. Keeping the legs together, swing legs as far to the left as possible, swing legs overhead, then to the right as far as possible and recover by swinging legs to the front. Legs stop momentarily at each position and do not contact floor until all repetitions are complete. • One repetition is completed when legs make the complete circle.

Exercise 5: From a stride position do a deep knee bend and grasp the right ankle with the right hand, left ankle with the left hand, arms outside knees. Walk forward maintaining the grasp of the ankles. • One repetition is counted each time the left foot contacts the floor.

Exercise 6: Run in place, lift feet 4 to 6 inches off floor. At the completion of every 50 steps do 10 Hand Kicks. Repeat sequence until required number of steps is completed.

Hand Kicks. Stand in place and kick left leg upward, at the same time extend the right arm touching the toe and hand. Repeat with right leg, extending left arm.

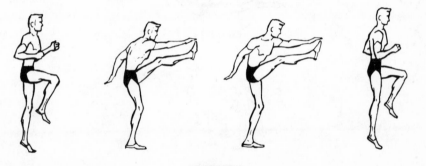

EXERCISE 6

INDOOR EXERCISE PROGRAM

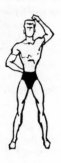
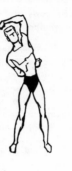
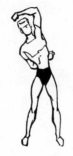
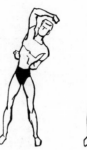
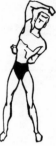

EXERCISE 1

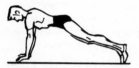
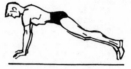
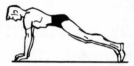

EXERCISE 2

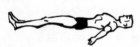

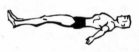

EXERCISE 3

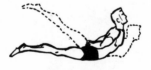

EXERCISE 4

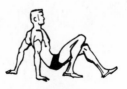

EXERCISE 5

INDOOR EXERCISE PROGRAM

TABLE VI: PROGRESSION GUIDE

AGE GROUP	LEVEL	EXERCISES 1	2	3	4	5	6
17	A	17	15	32	32	35	500
to	B	16	14	30	30	33	480
29	C	15	13	28	28	31	460
30	A	15	13	30	30	31	400
to	B	14	12	28	28	29	380
39	C	13	11	26	26	27	360
40	A	13	10	27	27	27	310
to	B	12	9	25	25	25	285
44	C	11	8	23	23	23	265
45	A	11	9	23	23	23	250
to	B	10	8	21	21	21	230
49	C	9	7	19	19	19	210
50	A	9	8	19	19	19	200
to	B	8	7	17	17	17	190
59	C	7	6	15	15	15	175
60	A	8	7	15	15	17	140
and	B	7	6	13	13	15	130
over	C	5	5	10	10	12	120
Minutes for each exercise		2	1	1	1	1	6

Exercise 1: Feet spread shoulder width apart, left fist clenched and overhead, right fist clenched at waistline in rear of body. Simultaneously thrust the left fist as far to the right as possible and the right fist as far to the left as possible. Recover and repeat. Reverse the hands with the right fist above the head and the left in rear at the waistline. Repeat the movement to the opposite side by thrusting the upper body to the left with the arm motion. • The above sequence is one repetition.

Exercise 2: Front leaning rest position. Bend elbows slightly and push with the hands and toes bouncing the body upward and completely off the floor. At the height of the bounce, clap the hands and quickly return them to a position directly under the shoulder to catch the body weight. • Push off the floor, clap hands, and return to the front leaning rest position is one repetition.

Exercise 3: Back position, arms extended to the side at 45 degrees. Raise the legs and the trunk into a V position bringing the trunk and legs as close as possible. Return to back position. • Raising the legs and trunk and recovery to the back position is one repetition.

Exercise 4: Prone position with hands clasped in small of the back. Arch the body, holding the head back and rock forward, relax and repeat the movement. • Arch the body, rock forward, and relax is one repetition.

Exercise 5: From a sitting position lift the hips, supporting the body on the hands and feet. By moving the arms and legs walk on all fours either forward or backward. • A repetition occurs each time the left hand contacts the floor.

Exercise 6: Run in place, lift feet 4 to 6 inches off floor. At the completion of every 50 steps do 10 Pike Jumps. Repeat sequence until required number of steps is completed.

Pike Jumps. Jump forward and upward from both feet, keeping the knees straight. Swing the legs forward and touch the toes with the hands at the top of each jump.

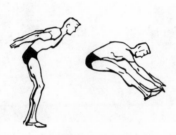
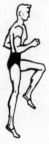

EXERCISE 6

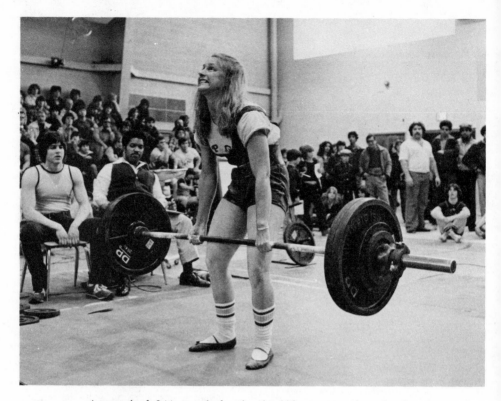

A record of 344 pounds for the dead-lift category is set by this contestant in the New England Regional Powerlifting Championships.

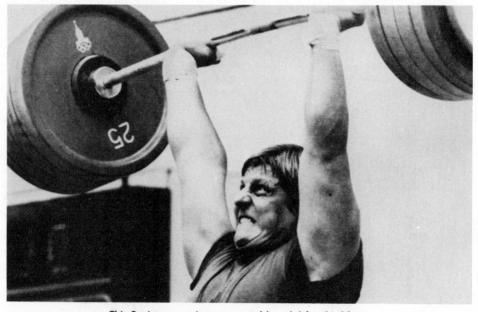

This Soviet competitor won a gold medal for this lift at the 1980 Summer Olympic Games in Moscow, U.S.S.R.

WEIGHT LIFTING

Basic Barbell Exercises

Exercise 1: Squat. 6 repetitions, 50 pounds (commonly called the *flatfoot deep knee bend*). Place the bar upon the shoulders. Stand with feet about 18 inches apart. Keeping the feet flat, lower the body into the low squat position. Come erect and repeat. Exhale as you lower into the squat position and inhale as you come up.

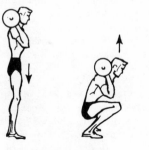

EXERCISE 1

Exercise 2: Waist Bender. 6 repetitions, 40 pounds. Assume the standing position with the bar across the shoulders, feet shoulder-width apart. Bend forward at the waist until the upper body is parallel to the ground; return to the starting position. • Each time you return to the upright position will constitute one repetition.

Exercise 3: Curl. 6 repetitions, 40 pounds. Grasp the barbell with the palms facing to the rear and assume the standing position, feet shoulder width apart. With the barbell held in front of the hips, flex the elbows and lift the weight until the bar touches the upper chest. Lower the barbell back to the hip level position. Inhale deeply with the upward movement and exhale on the downward movement. • Each time the bar touches the chest will constitute one repetition.

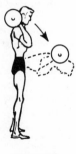

EXERCISE 2

Exercise 4: Side Bender. 6 repetitions per side, 40 pounds. Assume the standing position, feet shoulder width apart, with the bar across the shoulders. Bend to the left as far as possible and return to the starting position. Repeat six times and then execute the same procedure to the right for six repetitions.

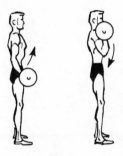

EXERCISE 3

EXERCISE 4

WEIGHT LIFTING

Exercise 5: Standing Press. 6 repetitions, 45 pounds. Grasp the bar with the palms facing forward and assume the starting position. Curl the weight to the upper chest position. Inhale deeply and press the bar upward to an overhead position. Exhale as you lower the bar to the chest position. • Each time the bar is pressed upward constitutes one repetition.

Exercise 6: Upward Row. 6 repetitions, 40 pounds. Grasp the bar, hands close together, palms to the rear, and assume the standing position. Starting with the bar held in front of the hips, flexing the elbows and the shoulder girdle muscles, lift the bar straight up to an overhead position. Inhale deeply as you lift the bar. Exhale as you lower the bar to the hip position. • Each time the bar returns to the hips will constitute one repetition.

Exercise 7: Shoulder Curl. 6 repetitions, 25 pounds. Grasp the bar palms down, and assume the standing position. Keeping the elbows locked, curl the bar, pivoting the arms at the shoulders until the bar is in an overhead position and as far to the rear as possible. Return the bar in the same manner to the hip position. • Each time the bar returns to hip position constitutes one repetition.

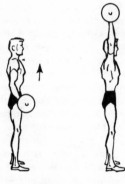

EXERCISE 5

EXERCISE 6

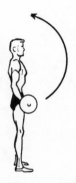
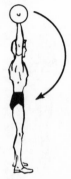

EXERCISE 7

WEIGHT LIFTING

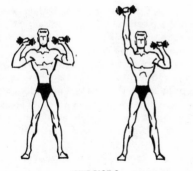

EXERCISE 1

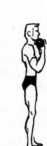

EXERCISE 2

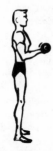

EXERCISE 3

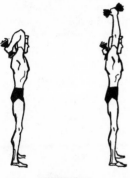

EXERCISE 4

Basic Dumbbell Exercises

Exercise 1: To develop shoulders and the back of the arm. Hold dumbbells at shoulder height. Push bells overhead to a full extension with the palms forward. Lower the bell back to the shoulder. Alternate right and left arm. Inhale as you push weight to full extension. Exhale as you lower the weight to the shoulder. • Repetitions: first week, 8; second week, 10; third week, 12.

Exercise 2: To develop the front of the upper arm. Hold dumbbells at arm's length parallel to the feet. Curl the weight to the shoulder, rotating the bell as the biceps contract. Lower the bell back to the starting position, reversing the rotation. Contract the triceps (back of the arm) to insure a full extension. This is done only after the bell has reached the starting position. Keep the bell under control as you lower it. Alternate right and left arms. Inhale as you curl the weight. Exhale as you lower the weight. • Repetitions: first week, 8; second week, 10; third week, 12.

Exercise 3: Curl weight until forearm is parallel to the floor. Return to the starting position. Repeat required number of repetitions. Curl bells to the shoulders. Lower weight until forearm is parallel to the floor. Return to the shoulder position. Repeat required number of repetitions. Lower bells to the starting position and curl required number of repetitions through full range of movement. Curl both bells at same time. • Repetitions: first week, 4 each movement; second week, 5 each movement; third week, 6 each movement.

Exercise 4: To develop the back of the upper arm. Hold dumbbells above and back of each shoulder by pointing the elbows up and holding them close to the head. Hold the elbows in place and extend the weight overhead by contracting the triceps. Lower the weight to the starting position. Alternate right and left arm. Inhale as you push weight to full extension. Exhale as you lower the weight to the shoulder. • Repetitions: first week, 8; second week, 10; third week, 12.

WEIGHT LIFTING

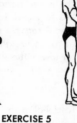

EXERCISE 5

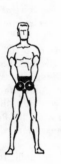

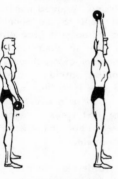

EXERCISE 6

EXERCISE 7

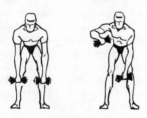

EXERCISE 8

Exercise 5: To develop the shoulders. Use the standing position, holding the bells at arm's length in front of the thighs with the palms to the rear. Raise the bells to the shoulder, keeping the weight close to the body as the elbows go up and out. Lower the weight to the starting position, keeping the weight under control. Inhale as the weight goes up. Exhale as the weight goes down. • Repetitions: first week, 12; second week, 14; third week, 16.

Exercise 6: To develop the shoulders. Use the standing position. Place the feet at shoulder's width apart, bending the knees a little more than usual. Roll the hips back slightly. Hold the bells at arm's length in front of you. Now, raise both bells laterally rotating the arms so the back of the hands come together on completion of the contraction. Keeping the bells under control, lower them to the starting position. Elbows should be slightly bent to avoid strain. • Repetitions: first week, 6; second week, 8; third week, 10.

Exercise 7: To develop the shoulders. Use the standing position holding the bells at arm's length with the palms to the rear. With the elbows slightly out of locked position, raise the bells overhead without rotating the arm. Return to the starting position. Inhale as you raise weight over head. Exhale as you lower weight to starting position. • Repetitions: first week, 6; second week, 8; third week, 10.

Exercise 8: To develop the upper back. Stand with feet at shoulders' width apart. Bend the knees and lean forward until the trunk is parallel to the floor. Hold the bells at arm's length directly below the shoulder. Raise the bells alternately to the shoulder by driving the elbow up and to the rear. Inhale as you pull weight up. Exhale as you lower the weight to the starting position. • Repetitions: first week, 12; second week, 14; third week, 16.

WEIGHT LIFTING

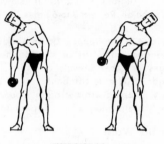

EXERCISE 9

Exercise 9: To develop the upper back. Stand with feet at shoulders' width apart. Bend the knees and lean forward until the trunk is parallel to the floor. Hold the bells at arm's length directly below the shoulders. Extend the arms laterally until they are parallel with the floor. Return to the starting position and repeat. Inhale as the bells are extended laterally. Exhale as the bells are lowered to the starting position. • Repetitions: first week, 6; second week, 8; third week, 10.

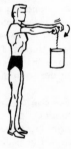

EXERCISE 10

Exercise 10: To exercise the waist. Stand with the feet shoulder width apart. Hold one bell in the right hand at arm's length by the right thigh. Do not bend forward or backward, but lean to the right, lowering the bell below the right knee. Now, lean to the left touching the left hand below the left knee. Repeat the desired number of repetitions. Change the bell to left hand to exercise the right side of the waist. Inhale as weight rises. Exhale as weight goes down. • Repetitions: first week, 15; second week, 20; third week, 25.

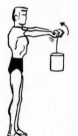

TWIST GRIP

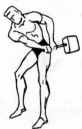
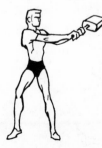
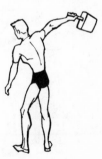

WAR CLUBS

EXERCISES FOR WOMEN

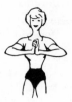

EXERCISE 1

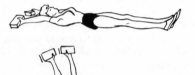

EXERCISE 2

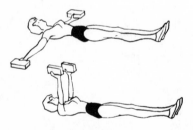

EXERCISE 3

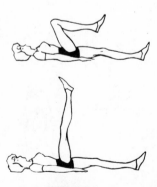

EXERCISE 4

For the Bustline

Exercise 1: The Press. Stand or sit erect. Clasp hands, palms together, close to chest. Press hands together hard and hold for 6 to 8 seconds. Repeat three times, resting briefly and breathing deeply between repetitions.

Exercise 2: Pullover. Lie on back with arms extended beyond head. Hold books or other objects of equal weight in hands. *Count 1.* Lift books overhead and down to thighs, keeping arms straight. *Count 2.* Return slowly to starting position. Repeat 3 to 6 times.

Exercise 3: Semaphore. Lie on back with arms extended sideward at shoulder level. Hold books or other objects of equal weight in hands. *Count 1.* Lift books to position over body, keeping arms straight. *Count 2.* Lower slowly to starting position. Repeat 3 to 6 times.

For the Waist

Exercise 4: Knee Lifts. Lie on back with knee slightly bent, feet on floor and arms at side. *Count 1.* Bring one knee as close as possible to the chest, keeping hands on floor. *Count 2.* Extend leg straight up. *Count 3.* Bend knee and return to chest. *Count 4.* Return to starting position. Repeat 5 to 10 times, alternating legs during exercise. The *double knee lift* is done in the same manner, raising both legs at the same time. Do 5 to 10 repetitions.

Exercise 5: Crossover. Lie on back, arms extended sideward, palms down. *Count 1.* Raise right leg to vertical position and move slowly to left until almost touching floor. Keep arms, head and shoulders on floor. *Count 2.* Return to starting position. *Counts 3 and 4.* Same action to other side. Do 5 to 10 repetitions.

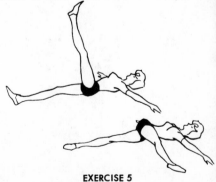

EXERCISE 5

EXERCISES FOR WOMEN

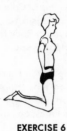

EXERCISE 6

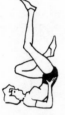

EXERCISE 7

For Hips and Thighs

Exercise 6: Cheerleader. Kneel on floor, back straight, hands on hips. *Count 1.* Bend backward as far as possible, keeping knees on floor and body straight. *Count 2.* Return to starting position. Repeat 10 to 15 times.

Exercise 7: Bicycle. Lie on back with hips and legs supported by hands. Simulate bicycle pumping action with legs. Pump 50-100 times.

Exercise 8: Ballet Stretch. Stand erect with left hand resting on back of chair for support. *Count 1.* Raise right leg sideward as high as possible. *Count 2.* Return to starting position. *Count 3.* Swing right leg forward as high as possible. *Count 4.* Return to starting position. *Count 5.* Swing right leg back as high as possible. *Count 6.* Return to starting position. Do 5 to 10 repetitions, then repeat exercise with left leg.

Exercise 9: Two-Way Stretch. Kneel with hands on floor, back straight. *Count 1.* Arch back, bend head down and bring left knee as close as possible to chin. *Count 2.* Lift head high and extend left leg as far backward and up as possible. Repeat 6 to 10 times with each leg.

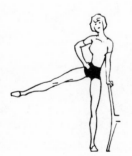
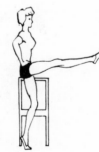
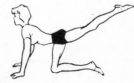

EXERCISE 8

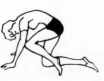

EXERCISE 9

EXERCISES FOR WOMEN

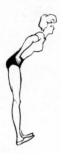

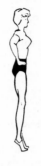

EXERCISE 10

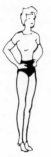

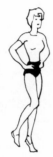

EXERCISE 11

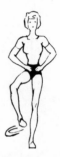

EXERCISE 12

For Calves and Ankles

Exercise 10: Rocker. Stand erect, feet together, hands on hips. *Count 1.* Rock back on heels, keeping legs straight and raising toes off floor. *Count 2.* Rock forward on toes, lifting heels off floor. Repeat 10 to 20 times.

Exercise 11: Hop. Stand erect, feet close together, hands on hips. Hop lightly on both feet 50 times, on the right foot 25 times, on the left foot 25 times, on both feet 50 times.

Exercise 12: Stemwinder. Stand erect, left foot lifted clear of floor. Rotate left foot in small circles 20 times. Repeat with right foot.

CHAPTER 5

Questions and Answers

Accidents

Q. Are falls a major cause of death among children?

A. No, less than five percent of falls that result in death involve children 14 or under. Fatal falls are a much more serious problem for old and middle-aged people.

Acetaminophen

See ASPIRIN.

Acne

See SKIN CARE.

Adams-Stokes disease

Q. Does the heart ever really skip a beat?

A. Although the expression is used figuratively about anyone who is excited, "skipping a beat" is something that normal, healthy hearts do not do. The skipping of a beat—the failure of the heart to contract and pump blood on schedule—is a symptom of *Adams-Stokes disease* and is marked by temporary loss of consciousness. Anyone suffering from this symptom should seek medical advice promptly.

Aging

Q. Why is the sense of taste lost in old age?

A. One reason is that taste buds diminish as one gets older until elderly persons have only 20 percent as many taste buds on the tongue as youngsters. Some brain cells also are involved, causing older persons to make more mistakes in identifying specific tastes.

Air travel

Q. Does flying in a jet airplane affect digestion or other body processes?

A. Modern jet aircraft cabins are pressurized to produce a simulated altitude of about 7,500 feet. While normal pressure is maintained, there is no health threat from a lack of oxygen or gaseous expansion in the digestive tract. See also EAR DISCOMFORT.

Albumin (in urine)
See TESTS AND DIAGNOSTIC PRO-
CEDURES/URINE.

Allergy

Q. What is an allergy?

A. An allergy is a sensitivity in an individual to a substance that is harmless to others. The sensitivity may be marked by sneezing, a skin rash, digestive disturbance, or some other reaction. Eczema, hives, and asthma may be allergic reactions.

Q. What is an antibody?

A. An antibody is a substance produced by the body to combat an allergen or foreign substance that has invaded the body tissues; the antibody may combine with the foreign substance, neutralize its toxin, or otherwise render it inactive.

Q. What causes allergic symptoms?

A. In a typical allergic reaction, an allergen such as pollen or dander combines with an antibody and triggers the release of histamines. This in turn results in itching, swelling, redness, nasal discharge, watery eyes, or other physical effects.

Q. What are histamines?

A. Histamines are chemicals naturally present in human body tissues; they dilate blood vessels and render them more permeable, stimulate certain muscles and glandular secretions, and are actively involved in allergic reactions.

Q. Why do allergic symptoms resemble cold symptoms?

A. The eyes, nose, and throat are "shock organs" for several diseases transmitted by the atmosphere, including the rhino-virus responsible for the common cold. As in some allergic reactions, histamines are released by antibody reaction to the invading virus, causing nasal congestion, nasal discharge, etc.

Q. How can you find out what you are allergic to?

A. Very dilute solutions of suspected allergens can be applied to eye or nose membranes or into the skin of the patient. A sensitive person will react with typical allergic symptoms; some allergic individuals may react to a number of possible allergens in skin tests.

Q. What is "hay fever"?

A. Hay fever is a common name for allergic rhinitis, an allergic reaction to wind-borne pollens or fungi marked by nasal discharge, swollen nasal membranes, coughing, sneezing, and conjunctivitis. It usually is seasonal and affects about ten percent of the population.

Q. Some people seem to develop asthma during the Christmas season. Could they be allergic to Christmas trees?

A. Allergic reaction to spruce, fir, or pine trees is not unusual. The cause may be sensitivity of the person to the odors of evergreen or to molds commonly found on the trees. A simple way of avoiding the problem is to use artificial trees instead of evergreens.

Q. Is it possible to develop a rash from using perfume or cologne on the skin?

A. Yes. Some individuals are sensitive to oil of bergamot, a plant product used in colognes and perfumes. The effect is intensified by exposure of the perfumed skin to sunlight.

Q. Some people develop a skin rash after drinking even a small amount of alcohol. Could this be due to an allergy?

A. Some individuals experience allergic reactions similar to asthma and eczema after ingesting alcohol. They may be sensitive to alcohol itself or the alcohol may increase sensitivity to other allergens, such as ragweed or certain foods.

Q. Can allergy-caused sinus trouble be cured by moving to an area with a dry climate, like the desert southwest?

A. Many people who have moved to other regions found that a change in climate did not help their sinusitis, possibly because their sinuses were irritated by the dust in the desert atmosphere.

Ambulation
See HOSPITALIZATION/AMBULATION.

Angina
See HEART DISEASE.

Apoplexy
Q. What is apoplexy?

A. Apoplexy is a rather old-fashioned term for stroke or brain-tissue damage caused by a hemorrhage in the region of the brain.

Arthritis
Q. How common is rheumatoid arthritis?

A. It has been estimated that between two to four percent of the population have this disorder.

Q. At what age do arthritis symptoms first become apparent?

A. In most cases, at about the age of 40.

Q. Is arthritis a disease of old people?

A. Although the disease usually occurs in people 40 or over, it can occur at any age. About five percent of arthritis sufferers are young children.

Q. Are women more often afflicted with this disease than men?

A. Yes, three times as many women have arthritis as men. A

common time for the onset of the disease in women is at or shortly after the menopause.

Q. Can arthritis cause a low-grade fever?

A. Some forms of arthritis are associated with a mild fever. But the cause may be an inflammation related to the pain of arthritis and should be checked by a physician.

Q. Are mud baths or mineral baths helpful in treating osteoarthritis?

A. Most of the benefit from so-called "spa" therapy probably is due to rest, relaxation, a change of environment, and diet rather than the baths themselves.

Aspirin
Q. Aspirin can irritate the stomach. Is there a nonprescription painkiller that can be used instead?

A. Acetaminophen drugs frequently are used to relieve pain in persons sensitive to aspirin. Special aspirin formulations designed to reduce stomach irritation also are available.

Q. Can a patient substitute acetaminophen for aspirin in treating rheumatoid arthritis?

A. No. Acetaminophen has not been found to relieve the inflammation symptoms of rheumatoid arthritis.

Q. Is it safe to pack aspirin around a tooth that aches?

A. The aspirin would do more good if you swallowed it with a glass of water, because aspirin must get into the bloodstream through the digestive tract to be effective.

Q. Is is true that aspirin prevents blood from clotting?

A. Experiments show that it takes several minutes longer for blood to clot in a wound of a person using aspirin. But the effect is not a serious problem except for hemophiliac patients or for those who take large quantities of aspirin over an extended period of time.

Q. Why is it necessary to drink a glass of water every time aspirin is taken?

A. Because aspirin must be dissolved in a watery solution to get into the bloodstream, and a generous amount of water is needed to dissolve the drug properly. Otherwise, the aspirin may irritate the stomach lining while slowly dissolving in whatever fluid is in the stomach.

Asthma
See ALLERGY.

Atherosclerosis
See HEART DISEASE.

Backache
Q. Are men or women more likely to have backache?

A. Backache is common among both men and women.

Q. Are tall, thin people more subject to backache than short people?

A. Generally speaking, taller people, especially if they have long backs, are more likely to develop back trouble than shorter people. Erect posture is more of a strain for them because they lack the stability of shorter people.

Bags under the eyes
See SKIN CARE.

Bilirubin
See TESTS AND DIAGNOSTIC PROCEDURES/BLOOD.

Biopsy
See TESTS AND DIAGNOSTIC PROCEDURES/BIOPSY.

Blood
See TESTS AND DIAGNOSTIC PROCEDURES/BLOOD.

Blood circulation
Q. Are there any exercises that help improve poor blood circulation in the legs?

A. One simple exercise is to lie on your back with your legs raised at a 45 degree angle for a few minutes, draining the blood from your feet. Then sit on the edge of a bed or chair until the blood returns to the feet. Repeat this several times a day.

Blood pressure
Q. Is low blood pressure dangerous?

A. Disorders due to low blood pressure are rare; your blood pressure must be very low before it can be considered a cause for concern.

Q. Sometimes a doctor will check the blood pressure of your right arm and then of your left arm. Isn't the blood pressure the same on both sides?

A. Not always. There are certain disorders in the body that can be detected by comparing the two blood pressure readings. See also TESTS AND DIAGNOSTIC PROCEDURES.

Blood sugar
See TESTS AND DIAGNOSTIC PROCEDURES/BLOOD.

Body odor
See PERSPIRATION.

Body temperature
Q. Is it possible for an otherwise normal person to have a "fever"?

A. Yes. Some people lack the ability to sweat properly and thus are unable to lower their body temperature in a hot, humid environment.

Q. Is a high body temperature serious?

A. Yes. It is a sign that body cells are working faster and breaking down, leading to dehydration. Each degree of fever also increases the work load of the heart and threatens the nervous system. A critical point is 103° F.

Q. Do body temperatures change during the day?

A. Yes, temperatures generally are slightly higher in the afternoon and evening, and lower in the morning. Also, the temperature in women varies with different stages of the menstrual cycle.

Boils
See SKIN CARE.

Brain/speech

Q. Is speech controlled by one hemisphere of the brain? If so, which one?

A. Among right-handed people, who probably make up about 93 percent of the population, speech is almost always controlled by the left hemisphere—the same one that controls their right-handedness. Among left-handed people, about 60 percent also have speech controlled by the left hemisphere in spite of having their dominant hand controlled by the other.

BUN
See TESTS AND DIAGNOSTIC PROCEDURES/BLOOD.

Cancer

Q. What is the leading cause of death from cancer among men?

A. Lung cancer.

Q. Does cigarette smoking increase the chances of getting lung cancer?

A. Men who smoke are ten times more likely to die of lung cancer then men who don't.

Carbuncles
See SKIN CARE

Cats
See TOXOPLASMOSIS.

Chest
See FUNNEL CHEST; PIGEON BREAST.

Children

Q. Some say that soap solutions sold for children's bubble blowing can be harmful to a child. Is this true?

A. Several of the special "soap" bubble preparations have been found to acquire disease organisms when exposed to the environment. Parents should supply freshly prepared solutions made from liquid laundry detergents or "no-tear" shampoos for use in blowing bubbles.

Cholesterol

Q. What level of cholesterol is dangerous?

A. In the U.S., the *average* blood cholesterol level is 245 milligrams (per 100 milliliters—the standard index). Heart disease linked to atherosclerosis (hardening of the arteries) is very high in the U.S. In some other countries, where the average blood cholesterol level is probably about 100–170 milligrams, this type of heart disease is rare. There is no one danger point for every individual, but statistically anyone with a blood cholesterol level over 250 milligrams has a much greater chance—perhaps as much as five times greater—of developing atherosclerotic heart disease than someone with a lower cholesterol level.

Q. Can blood cholesterol levels be reduced through a change in diet?

A. There is evidence that by cutting down on consumption of saturated fats (fatty meats and dairy products) and by increasing the consumption of polyunsaturated fats (vegetable oils, fish, etc.), serum cholesterol levels can be moderately reduced. In any case, it seems wise to take steps along the lines indicated simply to keep your cholesterol level from getting any higher. Adding polyunsaturated fats to the diet, without decreasing the intake of saturated fats, will not lower your serum cholesterol level. See also TESTS AND DIAGNOSTIC PROCEDURES/BLOOD.

Colds

Q. Are the symptoms of the common cold caused by a single virus?

A. No. About 150 different viruses have been identified as causing common cold symptoms. The fact that so many different viral strains cause the infection precludes the possibility of creating an effective immunizing vaccine.

Q. Is it all right to blow your nose when it's blocked by a cold?

A. If the nose is completely blocked by swollen membranes during a cold, blowing will not open it. Forceful blowing may only spread the infection into the sinuses and Eustachian tubes.

Q. Will nose drops help open a "stuffed" nose?

A. Nose drops should be used cautiously; they give temporary relief which may be followed by greater congestion. Continued congestion may lead to continuous use of nose drops in a vicious cycle.

Contagious diseases
See INFECTIOUS AND CONTAGIOUS DISEASES.

Corneal transplant
See EYE DISEASE.

Cough plate
See TESTS AND DIAGNOSTIC PROCEDURES.

Crohn's disease
Q. What is Crohn's disease?

A. Crohn's disease, another name for regional enteritis, is an inflammation of the part of the small intestine where the small and large intestines are joined. See also ENTERITIS, REGIONAL.

Dandruff
Q. What causes dandruff?

A. Unfortunately, the cause is so far unknown. Theories abound, but no one has been able to prove that bacteria, for example—represented as the cause in one theory—exist in scalps affected by dandruff.

Q. Do any dandruff shampoos or other treatments sold over the counter really help?

A. Yes, some are reasonably effective in controlling dandruff. Certainly, if you have a problem with dandruff, it would pay to experiment with various brands until you find one that works for you. If nothing seems to help, see your physician or ask him to recommend a more effective medication.

Delirium tremens
Q. Is it possible to develop delirium tremens from overuse of tranquilizers?

A. Convulsions, tremors, and other characteristic symptoms of delirium tremens can occur as side effects of certain tranquilizing drugs.

Q. What is the cause of delirium tremens?

A. This is a psychotic disorder marked by delirium, tremors, and vivid hallucinations. It occurs in people who have been chronic alcoholics for several years.

Devil's pinches

Q. What are "devil's pinches"?

A. "Devil's pinches" is a common term for a hereditary disorder marked by the mysterious appearance of bruises on the body. The bruises are essentially harmless and there is no permanent cure for them.

Diabetes

See EYE DISEASE/DIABETIC RETINOPATHY; TESTS AND DIAGNOSTIC PROCEDURES/BLOOD/URINE.

Diagnostic tests

Q. What can a doctor tell about your health by examining spinal fluid?

A. There are at least two dozen physical conditions that can be revealed by study of the spinal fluid, including meningitis, poliomyelitis, brain tumor, lead poisoning, and rabies.

Doctors and patients

The following series of questions and answers relating to doctors and patients is an edited transcription of an interview with Dr. Richard J. Wagman, editor of *The New Complete Medical and Health Encyclopedia*. The interviewer was Sidney I. Landau, managing editor of the Ferguson staff.

Q. Why don't doctors tell the patient more than they do? Why do they often seem so reluctant to tell him what underlies his condition?

A. I think this situation has changed significantly, especially as more and more people are becoming more sophisticated about illness and health. It is extremely foolish for a doctor not to discuss what is going on with his patients. It is far more frightening to the patient to be kept in the dark about his real condition.

Q. Do you think that younger doctors are prone to tell more than older doctors?

A. I think it depends on the individual. I have seen a lot of younger doctors who behave like they are 80, and a lot of older doctors who behave like young people.

Q. What about doctors who do not explain the full reason for performing an operation, for example delivering a baby by Caesarian section?

A. This is the kind of thing that would make me very upset with my doctor, because he would be talking down to me. I am speaking not only as a doctor but as a person who is involved with using doctors. I have a family of my own, after all. I don't like being talked down to. Speaking as a physician, I don't like talking down to people.

Q. Would you tell the truth to someone who was suffering from a terminal illness?

A. I like to tell the truth, and I like to tell the patient as much as I think he can tolerate, if I think the patient wants to know. This is not a yes or no sort of phenomenon; this is picked up by hints, by clues, by innuendos, by the whole approach of the patient to me in terms of the questions he or she asks about his or her illness. I prefer to answer the questions honestly.

If a patient with cancer asks me point-blank, "Do I have cancer?" I will answer yes. I won't necessarily say more. I answer the specific question. If the patient asks more I will go on and answer each specific question and no more.

If you lie to the patient you wind up isolating him, often from his own family, which has to know. At least some responsible member of the family has to know. They may find it difficult to talk to the patient since they are hiding the truth. All of a sudden the patient winds up in an untenable position: he or she has no one to talk to honestly.

This is also predicated on the belief that most patients who are seriously ill know what's going on. They sense the concern of their family and friends. Most people close to the patient are poor liars. I am against isolating the patient like this.

On the other hand, there are some patients who cannot tolerate the truth in this kind of situation, and again I think it is the role of the physician to be sensitive to the clues that the patient gives him.

Q. How should a layman act when visiting someone in the hospital who is gravely ill? Should he pretend he's going to get well? Can you make any blanket rule about this?

A. Two very simple rules. One, the visitor should be himself, and should be friendly and cheerful. Two, he should stay only a short period of time.

House Calls and Telephone Calls

Q. To what extent can the telephone replace office calls and house calls?

A. I am very accessible, and most of my patients do not abuse the privilege of calling. That is, they generally call—not always, but generally—during office hours. A high percentage of the calls can be screened by my nurse, and most of the calls involve problems of anxiety and fear rather than medical emergencies—concerns which are quite legitimate. They often make office visits unnecessary, if it's simply a matter of a patient asking a question about something that has been bothering him.

Q. Why don't doctors make house calls any more?

A. I speak for myself only. I make almost no house calls, and there are a variety of reasons. I say this as a big-city practitioner. There are simply not enough hours in the day. It becomes impossible in terms of getting around. Ninety-nine percent of the house calls are not really and truly necessary. If a patient is seriously ill—for example, someone is having chest pains—he should be seen by a physician, but he also needs to have an electrocardiogram done, for example, and the best place to do this is either in the office or in the hospital. I am very limited in terms of what I can do at a patient's home. I don't carry an electrocardiograph machine in my car. If someone really needs a house call, for instance, in a city like New York, I can arrange for someone to see one of my patients at home and call me and let me know what he has found.

Q. What if a person is too sick to come out?

A. This is nonsense. The question is, must you be seen? And if you have to be seen, then the best place for an X ray or a blood test is the hospital or the office. The trouble is, in order for me to do the greatest good for the greatest number under my care, I have to put the responsibility on the patient to come to the office or, in emergencies, to the hospital.

Q. What if a child has a fever of 105° or something like that?

A. There are emergency measures that can be dealt with on the phone, in terms of the *immediate* care that can be given. In general, pediatric emergencies present another spectrum of disease. The question is, if you have a child who has a high fever or has had a convulsion, must you come out? The answer is, something has to be done immediately—before you can either physically get dressed, get into the car, or what have you. Advice can be given on the phone. That sums up what to do until either you come or one of your delegates comes. I think the patient has to be seen.

Q. What about a bleeding ulcer in an older person?

A. Hospital.

Q. What about heart attacks?

A. The only thing you can do in the case of a heart-attack patient in terms of coming to the house is to give relief of pain. Again, in a big city so much time is lost getting from one end of the city to the other. It is much more sensible to make all the arrangements to get the patient to the hospital. This means that the person is going to be in discomfort or distress no matter what you do, but you are going to get the patient to a place where something can be done as quickly as possible.

Answering Services

Q. How should one deal with an answering service that won't give you your doctor's home phone number?

A. My own attitude with answering services—which leave a great deal to be desired as a general rule—is that you must explain to them that this is an emergency and what you hope for is that they will get either your doctor or whoever is covering for your doctor in his absence. You are not calling directly, but theoretically the answering service should relay the message to the doctor or his substitute who will then call you back.

I tell my patients that if there is something urgent and they have problems with the answering service, that it is their obligation to badger the answering service to impress upon them the urgency of the call. You have to call back if you do not hear from the doctor within a given period of time, depending upon the actual degree of urgency or your anxiety, or both.

Psychosomatic Complaints

Q. In a recent poll of doctors, over 90 percent said their patients suffered from hypochondria and psychosomatic ailments. Have you found this to be true?

A. I can't say 90 percent, but a high percentage of patients who call are troubled with problems in terms of anxiety about their health, including patients who have serious, real illnesses. Usually the reason for the call is something involving fear, fright, worry, or whatever word you want to use.

Q. What about those who come to see you?

A. Also a high percentage.

Q. More pronounced in women than in men? In old people than in young?

A. I can't quote statistics. But higher in women. Women come more freely to doctors than men do anyway.

Q. Older women?

A. Most patients who come to an internist are in the older age group.

Specialists and GPs

Q. How does an internist differ from a general practitioner?

A. The internist is someone who practices only adult medicine. He deals with medical diseases involving, for example, heart, lungs, GI tract, kidneys, blood, the entire gamut of illnesses in adults. He does not practice pediatrics, and he does not deal with surgery, does not deal with obstetrics or gynecology.

The internist as a specialist has really come of age only relatively recently. The internist is rather like the medical counterpart to the surgeon as a specialist.

Q. In what way is the internist a specialist?

A. Internal medicine is considered, at least in most Western countries, as a specific specialty—with special requirements in terms of training. For example, my own training involved a year of internship specifically in medicine. I didn't spend time going through a pediatric service, ob-gyn [obstetrics-gynecology], or surgery. Internists deal entirely with medical problems as an intern, then two or three years of residency, and generally a subspecialty—in my case, cardiology. A general practitioner usually has one to two years of training in postmedical school with a little bit of everything—a little pediatrics, a little bit of surgery, a little bit of ob-gyn, dermatology, etc.

Q. An internist does not have that?

A. That is right.

Q. Is there any need for a general practitioner today?

A. A good GP is worth his weight in gold. He is, in many communities, the family physician—the number one contact for the patient. He may take care of all the individual's health needs or be the one to refer him to the proper specialist. In the big cities, frequently the internist has taken over the role of the family physician.

Q. But isn't it true that often you go to your family doctor, who is an internist, and it seems that he is sort of an agent for leading you on to other doctors who are more specialized in various things? From the point of view of the patient, in purely practical terms, you are paying twice. The temptation is to think twice about going to the doctor at all.

A. There is a lot of truth to that, and I agree with you. This involves, in my opinion, a great deal of responsibility on the part of your—what I call your primary—physician, in this case, the internist. Before he refers you to someone else, he will have to sit back and say, can I handle this myself? Does it need handling by someone else? And this means also he has to realize that this is going to cost the patient money, and consider whether it's really necessary. Unfortunately, I am not sure that everybody does think this way. I think one should.

Q. If your regular doctor is an internist and you want medical advice about digestive troubles, should you go to him or to a GI specialist?

A. I think that is jumping the gun. I think that your internist should be able to handle this very easily. If you have an internist or a GP, one of the things you have to do is have enough faith in him. He is the one who is going to decide when you need a specialist in any field. But don't be afraid to ask him if he thinks a consultation is necessary.

Q. If a doctor you know and respect recommends surgery, is it still advisable to get a second opinion?

A. It depends on how much anxiety you have, how clearcut the situation is, and how much faith and trust you have in the doctor and the doctor's advice. For example, if you have a hernia the treatment is surgical. If you have gallstones, and you had an attack from your gallstones, the treatment is surgical. There are other areas, of course, where the treatment is less clear, such as duodenal ulcer. It all boils down to the old business of whether or not you trust the person who is taking care of you. If you don't, then I think you are in trouble to begin with. You must be able to say to your doctor: I am not sure; let's talk about it.

Q. What is an osteopath?

A. An osteopath is a physician who has graduated from a school of osteopathy. The training is similar to an MD's training but slightly different. There is a bit more orientation towards bones, joints, etc.

Q. Are MD's overqualified? Don't they spend a great deal of time learning more than they have to know in order to do the job they do?

A. If you are asking me is our training too long, yes, because so much of what we learn could probably be taught in shorter form. There are several experiments going on in medical education now—for example, taking people in their final year of medical school and making them interns. At least in my personal experience with people in this program, it is quite successful. So far as medical school goes, I do think it could probably be shortened.

Changing Doctors

Q. What is the best way of finding a doctor if you do not have one?

A. There are many ways: one is by referral from someone in the community who has a doctor he is satisfied with; by calling the county medical society; or by calling the local hospital, if it is a small town, and having them recommend one of several doctors who are near you. This is a very reasonable approach.

Q. How can a patient tell if his doctor is unsatisfactory?

A. I think this is better asked of patients. One way the patient can tell, apart from not getting well, is that the patient can't talk to the doctor. If he is unhappy, he can ask his doctor for a consultation. If the doctor is unwilling, I would raise an eyebrow.

Q. If you do switch doctors, how would you go about obtaining your medical records from your former doctor and making them available to your new doctor?

A. Easily. All you have to do is sign a request slip authorizing your former doctor to release information to your new doctor.

Q. Does he have to release that?

A. It is the customary procedure.

Q. With whom do you sign the release—the old or the new doctor?

A. The new doctor. This is very common; it happens all the time.

Personal Attention

Q. Do doctors nowadays have too many patients to be able to give them enough personal attention? This seems to be one of the major complaints of patients: that doctors just don't spend enough time with them.

A. This is partially true. This depends again on the doctor. One of the reasons that many patients wind up coming to see me is because the previous doctor has not given them enough time. I think that patients have to be able to talk honestly to the doctor and ask questions when they want to. When they arrange for their appointment they can let the secretary or nurse know that they would like a little bit of extra time. This is not unreasonable. At the same time many patients' demands are insatiable in this regard.

Q. In other words, a doctor like any other busy person has to learn to turn people off in a way?

A. Right.

Q. What do you think of doctors calling patients they've just met by their first names?

A. Terrible. This is not a social situation, and I prefer that patients be treated with a certain sense of respect and formality, and feel that this is much better for everybody. I don't like calling patients by their first names.

Fees

Q. Can you give any guidelines on "reasonable" medical fees?

A. No. This is an impossible question. There are guidelines, there are very real guidelines. In fact, most fees are set as a matter of custom, form, and what is "fair" in the area. And this is the kind of thing I cannot discuss in absolute terms and won't, but merely suggest that the patient has to discuss this with the doctor or his delegate, meaning his nurse or secretary.

Q. It's often said that doctors don't mind discussing fees before the examination. But many people have difficulty doing so. How do *you* respond to those who ask about fees?

A. My secretary informs all prospective patients exactly what the charges will be—if the patient asks.

Q. How many of your patients discuss fees with you before being treated? Is this commonplace or an exception?

A. It is common. This raises a very good question, because any time anything that is expensive has to be done I think the patient has to be informed not just that something has to be done, but that it is going to cost money. I also think that many patients have to understand that if something has to be done and is important for their health, even if they can't pay for it now, it has to be done. If they are reasonable people they will accept the necessity of a debt. This can be arranged in terms of any convenient method of payment, even to the extent of $1 to $2 a week. This is not the problem. The point is, I think, that the patient should be informed why something that costs a lot of money is important to him. If this has to be done and the patient can't afford it and you have been taking care of him, then I think it is your obligation to see that he gets into the hands of some facility that can give him either a reduced cost or no cost.

Q. Do doctors have difficulty collecting their fees? If so, who gives them the most trouble—the relatively poor, the middle-class, or the well-to-do?

A. I really don't think that there is any basis for predicting who will not pay. Frequently the very wealthy as well as the very poor don't pay.

Q. Don't pay at all?

A. Right. There is no way to get it. You can sue, but it is hardly worth the effort or trouble. There are a small percentage of people who will not meet their obligations, and I think you just have to write it off as an experience.

Q. When one physician refers a patient to a specialist, does he ever get a cut of the consultant's fee? Is fee-splitting of this sort common?

A. It exists. I have never done it. It is not illegal. It is considered unethical by the profession. My experience with this is zero.

Q. When you as an internist refer someone to a surgeon, do you take into consideration or indicate to the patient how expensive the surgeon is likely to be?

A. I usually mention to a patient that a procedure—especially, for example, open heart surgery—is going to be expensive. At this point, I advise him to discuss the specific fee with the surgeon. If there is a hardship situation I will discuss this with the surgeon myself, quietly and privately.

(This concludes the interview with Dr. Wagman.)

Drug abuse

Q. Why do some addicts give up their habit in their mid-30s?

A. No one knows why, but if addicts manage to survive to their thirties, their need for drugs often moderates or disappears entirely, and they become good subjects for detoxification programs. Some spontaneously give up their addiction at this age without treatment.

Q. Is this true of alcoholics, too?

A. A common pattern of alcoholism is one in which the drug is spontaneously given up for periods of up to several months, but the alcoholic then resumes his former drinking habits with the same compulsion he had before. An alcoholic who "gives up" drinking is by no means cured. Such a period is comparable to a remission in a chronic disease, not a cure.

Ear discomfort

Q. After disembarking from an airplane after flight, some people experience a stuffy feeling in the ears and a temporary loss of hearing. What causes this?

A. Although modern commercial airplanes have pressurized interiors that compensate for changes in atmospheric pressure as the plane lands, some individuals are still sensitive enough to experience the sensations described. The air in the Eustachian tube is forced into the middle ear by the increased external pressure, and is replaced by body fluids. Similar symptoms can be caused by allergy, infection, or enlarged adenoids.

Enteritis, regional

Q. What are the symptoms of regional enteritis?

A. Regional enteritis—inflammation of the intestine—is a chronic disease characterized by abdominal cramps, diarrhea, loss of appetite, fever, lethargy, and sometimes a drop in weight. However, in some cases none of these symptoms appears until the disease has progressed considerably, and most patients experience periods of remission at various times during the course of the illness.

Epilepsy

Q. Is epilepsy ever cured?

A. Drugs can effectively control or reduce the frequency of seizures of the great majority of people with this disease. For unknown reasons, some epileptics eventually become and remain free of seizures while requiring no further medication; these people can be called cured.

Q. In addition to trying to create new medicines for the treatment of epilepsy, what are some of the other areas of epilepsy research?

A. Investigations are under way concerning the surgical removal of the particular brain cells responsible for triggering the convulsive seizures, and the implantation of a brain pacemaker that could act as a circuit breaker in preventing the electrical discharges that precipitate the seizures.

Eye disease/corneal transplant

Q. What is a corneal transplant?

A. A corneal transplant is the procedure in which a clear, healthy cornea provided by an eye bank replaces a cloudy or otherwise damaged one. Approximately 90 percent of such operations are successful in restoring vision.

Q. Does a corneal transplant correct all types of blindness?

A. No. A corneal transplant can correct only those disorders of vision that result from corneal defects caused by injury or disease.

Eye disease/diabetic retinopathy

Q. What is diabetic retinopathy?

A. Diabetic retinopathy, which is one of the leading causes of blindness in the U.S., is a disease of diabetics marked by the formation of new, abnormal blood vessels on the surface of the retina, sometimes protruding into the interior of the eye. They may also bleed.

Q. What causes diabetic retinopathy? Can it be treated successfully?

A. The precise cause of diabetic retinopathy is unknown, but the chance of its occurrence increases with the duration of a patient's diabetes. Current treatment is by a process called *photocoagulation,* in which beams of intense light are flashed into the eye to cause minute burns on the retina. This procedure has reduced the risk of blindness in some diabetics by preventing the proliferation of retinal blood vessels.

Foot care

Q. What is the difference between trench foot and chilblain?

A. Both are caused by prolonged exposure of the feet to cold, short of freezing. But trench foot is more serious, with possible neuromuscular damage. Chilblain is marked by a burning, itching sensation of the skin.

Q. Is it safe to remove corns or calluses with a sharp knife or razor blade?

A. No. The best home remedies are foot baths and corn plasters which soften these horny skin formations on the feet.

Frozen section

See TESTS AND DIAGNOSTIC PROCEDURES/FROZEN SECTION.

Funnel chest

Q. Can someone with "funnel chest" engage in normal physical activities? Is surgery recommended?

A. "Funnel chest," known technically as *pectus excavatum,* is a congenital deformity in which the sternum (the bone to which the ribs are attached, forming the chest wall) is depressed, so that the chest looks hollowed out. It is the opposite of "pigeon breast," in which the chest protrudes. So long as funnel chest does not impair the functioning of the lungs, there is no need to curtail normal physical activity, and no need for surgery. The main problem is usually psychological and social, especially for young people.

Gallstones

Q. Can some gallstones be dissolved medically?

A. Yes. The result of many years of research at the Mayo Clinic and elsewhere is an oral medicine containing a bile acid that dissolves cholesterol gallstones. This new therapy eliminates the need for surgical removal in a large number of cases.

Another alternative to surgery is CDCA (chenodeoxycholic acid) an oral medicine that effectively reduces cholesterol gallstones so that the need for surgery is eliminated in many cases.

Gout

Q. Is there a relationship between gout sufferers and intelligence?

A. Legend has it that gout afflicts the famous more often than ordinary folk. Certainly many gout sufferers have been famous—for example, Benjamin Franklin—but gout can strike anybody, and there does not seem to be any scientific basis for the popular association of gout and fame. Some research suggests, however, a connection between IQ and uric acid, the level of which is elevated in gout patients.

Q. Are men or women more subject to attacks of gout?

A. Men, by an almost ten to one ratio.

Q. Is gout hereditary?

A. Primary gout—that is, gout that is not caused by another disease—is hereditary.

Q. Are attacks of acute gout, as of the big toe, likely to go away without treatment?

A. Yes, usually in one or two weeks, but without treatment you are likely to have recurrences which will eventually cause degeneration of cartilage and deformity. This form of gout, incidentally, is called *acute gouty arthritis*.

Q. Are any other diseases often associated with gout?

A. Kidney stones are a frequent complication of gout. The excess of uric acid that causes gout can also result in uric acid stones occurring in the kidneys.

Growth, stunted

Q. Do stunted children show an abnormal growth pattern in their early years?

A. Yes. Stunted children can usually be identified even at an early age because instead of growing a normal two or three inches each year, their stature increases by only about one inch.

Q. When a stunted growth pattern becomes apparent, is there any possible treatment for it?

A. Yes. If the cause of the child's stunted stature is determined to be a deficiency of growth hormone, the child may be given injections of pituitary hormone. This treatment is called pituitary replacement therapy.

Guthrie test

See TESTS AND DIAGNOSTIC PROCEDURES/GUTHRIE TEST.

Hair

See UNWANTED HAIR.

Handedness

Q. What percentage of people are left-handed?

A. An estimated seven percent are left-handed. See also BRAIN/SPEECH.

Hansen's disease

Q. What is Hansen's disease?

A. Hansen's disease is the preferred designation for leprosy. G. H. A. Hansen was a Norwegian physician and scientist who was the first to identify the bacterial organism that causes the disease.

Hardening of the arteries (atherosclerosis)

See HEART DISEASE.

Headache

Q. Can emotional tension lead to a migraine headache?

A. In those subject to migraine headaches, emotional stress may precipitate a migraine episode.

Q. Should migraine sufferers avoid certain foods, such as chocolate?

A. Chocolate is a common offender in migraine headaches. Some individuals also suffer headaches due to allergies to milk, eggs, corn, legumes, cinnamon, and cola drinks.

Q. Does reading under a dim light cause headaches?

A. You are more likely to get a headache from reading under a light that is too bright and glaring than under one that is not bright enough. Of course, if you are tired to begin with, reading under a dim light may cause headache from general fatigue. The eyes, however, operate like a camera, and are not strained or otherwise damaged by use under a dim light.

Q. Can air or noise pollution cause headaches?

A. Some people apparently are sensitive to air pollutants and develop headaches after traveling from rural to industrialized urban areas. Loud noises can be painful; they also can aggravate headaches caused by stress.

Q. What is a "caffeine-withdrawal" headache?

A. Caffeine causes a constriction of the blood vessels in the head, an effect that inhibits headaches. When a person who drinks large amounts of coffee or other caffeine beverages suddenly stops using the beverage, the arteries become dilated. This stretches nerve endings in the arteries, causing a headache.

Heart attack

Q. Are heart attacks the leading cause of death?

A. In western society, among the 30-to-65-year-old age group, yes. They are more common among men than women, and are by far the commonest cause of sudden death; about 90 percent of sudden deaths are caused by heart attack.

Q. Are both left and right halves of the heart equally vulnerable to heart attack?

A. Myocardial infarction, the medical term for the death of heart tissue, usually strikes the left ventricle, the most muscular portion of the heart, which pumps the blood through the arteries to blood vessels throughout the body. Infarction of the right ventricle or atrium is much less common.

Heartburn

Q. What happens to cause heartburn?

A. Heartburn is a burning sensation in the lower esophagus—the tube that conducts swallowed food from mouth to stomach. It is caused by a flow of gastric juices from the stomach back into the esophagus. It can be caused from eating or drinking too much; it is also common in the aftermath of gastric surgery and in the later stages of pregnancy. It has nothing to do with the heart, but the burning sensation may be felt in the region of the heart.

Q. What can be done to relieve heartburn at night?

A. Avoid spicy or other foods that may irritate the digestive system, especially during the evening meal, and learn to sleep with the upper part of the body elevated.

Heart disease

Q. Can emotional stress trigger an attack of angina?

A. Yes, angina is often precipitated by extreme emotional excitement. Physical exertion and cold weather are also common precipitating factors, especially in combination.

Q. What causes angina?

A. The most common cause is atherosclerosis, a narrowing and hardening of the blood vessels that supply blood and oxygen to the heart. Thus, when the supply is inadequate to meet stepped-up needs, such as after a heavy meal or during strenuous activity, an angina attack may result.

Q. What is the relationship between atherosclerosis and heart disease?

A. Atherosclerosis describes a condition in which the interior of the blood vessel walls hardens and in which a deposit of various substances builds up, thus narrowing the opening in the vessel. Blood flow is therefore slowed. If it is slowed too much, angina may develop. If the

flow of blood is blocked entirely, a clot may break off and be carried by the bloodstream to the heart, where a blockage could trigger a heart attack. See also CHOLESTEROL.

Q. How common is congenital heart disease?

A. About two to five percent of all heart disease after infancy is congenital—that is, it existed at birth.

Q. What do heart valves do and what can go wrong with them?

A. The purpose of heart valves is to permit a free flow of blood in one direction only, either from the atria (or auricles) to the ventricles during diastole, or from the ventricles to the great vessels during systole. Essentially, two problems can develop:

(1) The valve can narrow, a condition known as *stenosis,* thus permitting an insufficient flow of blood; or

(2) The valve can close imperfectly or too slowly—i.e., it leaks—thus permitting a backward flow of blood, called valvular *regurgitation, insufficiency,* or *incompetence.*

Q. Can both stenosis and regurgitation exist in the same valve at the same level?

A. Yes, they can and frequently do.

Q. What is mitral stenosis?

A. A narrowing and hardening of the mitral heart valve, which regulates the flow of blood from the left atrium to the left ventricle.

Q. Does mitral stenosis occur equally often in men and women?

A. No, it is much more common in women. The reasons for this are obscure.

See also ADAMS-STOKES DISEASE.

Heart pacemaker

Q. How many people use pacemakers to control the rate of heartbeat?

A. In 1976, there were about 45,000 persons in North America wearing permanently implanted heart pacemakers.

Q. What is the purpose of a heart pacemaker that is implanted in the body?

A. The artificial pacemaker replaces or supplements a natural pacemaker in the heart that normally generates electric signals to make the heart muscles contract. In some diseases, the natural pacemaker fails to produce a proper series of signals needed to make the heart pump blood at a normal pace. Unless corrected, as with an artificial pacemaker, ·the patient faces disability or death.

Q. Where is a permanent pacemaker implanted in a patient's body?

A. A pacemaker generally is implanted under the skin in an area below the collarbone. It is connected to the heart tissue by a wire running through a vein from the heart to the shoulder area.

Q. Is an operation for implanting a heart pacemaker dangerous?

A. Permanent pacemaker implantation is a very safe operation, even in elderly patients, and generally results in relieving symptoms of heart distress.

Q. Is a general anesthetic used during implanting of a heart pacemaker?

A. A general anesthetic is required if the wires for a pacemaker are connected directly to the heart muscle. However, pacemaker wires sometimes can be inserted via a catheter in a vein, in which case a local anesthetic may be used.

Q. Is a heart pacemaker heavy?

A. The average heart pacemaker, including power source, transistors, and other components, weighs about six ounces.

Q. Can the pacemaker generator malfunction after it is implanted?

A. Failure of pacemaker components, except for batteries, is rare. But some electrical equipment such as electric razors, microwave ovens, and even automobile ignitions can interfere with pacemaker activity.

Q. How long do batteries for heart pacemakers last?

A. Pacemaker batteries usually last from three to five years before they must be replaced.

Q. How can a doctor check up on a heart pacemaker after it is implanted in the body?

A. By studying X-ray pictures which will show if wires are in place, if the batteries are still good, etc. Newer model pacemakers have special markings designed to reveal important information on X-ray pictures. Wires have a special coating to make them show up better on X-ray film.

Q. Can pacemakers be powered by nuclear energy without harm to the patient?

A. Since 1970, more than 1,600 nuclear-powered pacemakers have been implanted. They have an expected life of 20 years but are still being studied for possible complications before wider use is approved.

Hernia, hiatus

Q. What is hiatus hernia?

A. It is hernia, or "rupture" of the muscle barrier between the stomach and esophagus that permits a backflow of the stomach's gastric acid into the esophagus.

Q. What is the treatment for hiatus hernia?

A. The best results can be

achieved by following a careful diet, wearing loose-fitting clothing around the abdominal area, and sleeping with the upper part of the body elevated. Surgery may be recommended if conservative measures fail to improve the condition.

Herpes

Q. Is the herpes virus that causes "cold sores" responsible for any other disorders?

A. Yes. The most serious disorder caused by the herpes simplex virus is an infection of the cornea that may result in scar tissue and impairment of sight. The infection is called *herpes simplex keratitis*.

Hirschsprung's Disease

Q. What is Hirschsprung's disease?

A. Hirschsprung's disease is a congenital disorder of childhood in which the colon becomes enlarged as a result of a defect in part of the nervous system that controls bowel movement. In this disorder, the colon never completely evacuates its contents into the rectum. Cases that do not respond to medical treatment may require surgical correction.

Hirsutism

See UNWANTED HAIR.

Hospitalization/ambulation

Q. Why do hospitals have people out of bed and walking about so soon after an operation?

A. Primarily to prevent the development of blood clots that might spread to the lungs. This therapy actually began by necessity during World War II when an acute doctor-and-hospital-bed shortage made it necessary to get patients physically out of the hospital earlier. The results convinced doctors that early ambulation was more effective than traditional confinement to bed. It presented fewer complications.

Hypertension

Q. What is meant by "essential hypertension"?

A. "Essential" means without a known cause. Essential hypertension refers to a group of symptoms including elevated blood pressure and progressive damage to the blood vessels.

Immunization

Q. Are there some parts of the U.S. where immunization requirements must be complied with before a child can enter a public school?

A. Yes. In many parts of the United States, local city and county departments of health require immunization against diphtheria, polio, measles, and rubella (German measles) before a child is permitted to attend school.

Immunology/SCID

Q. What is the meaning of SCID?

A. SCID stands for Severe Combined Immune Deficiency. It is a congenital disease in which a child is born with an inability to fight off infectious organisms and other foreign cells or substances that enter the body.

Q. What happens to a child diagnosed as having SCID?

A. Until recently, the condition has been fatal if untreated unless the child was kept in an isolation room which is germfree. Such rooms do exist in some hospitals.

Q. Is there any possible treatment for SCID?

A. The ideal treatment for SCID is transplantation of bone marrow from a sibling whose tissues are compatible with those of the patient. Such a donor is available in only about 15 percent of all cases.

Q. Is any progress being made in treating SCID?

A. Recent research indicates that the disorder in some patients is due to a lack of a crucial enzyme called adenosine deaminase which is found in normal red blood cells and is essential for the manufacture of antibodies. Periodic transfusions of small amounts of washed and irradiated red blood cells have corrected the SCID syndrome in a few cases.

Indigestion

Q. Is it all right to take a laxative to get rid of a stomach pain?

A. No. In fact, if the pain continues for more than an hour or so, and if it is severe, it would be wise to call your doctor. The cause could be appendicitis or another serious condition.

Q. What is the cause of stomach gas following a meal?

A. Most of the "gas" in the stomach is caused by swallowing air during a meal.

Q. Can indigestion be caused by a lack of gastric acid in the stomach?

A. Yes. There is a wide range of acid levels in normal individuals, and while some people are troubled by too much gastric acid, others can suffer from too little stomach acid.

Infectious and contagious diseases

Q. What is the difference between "infectious" disease and "contagious" disease?

A. Contagious in general means "spread by contact from one person to another person." An infectious disease involves an invading organism, whether it be bacteria or virus. In general, there is more of a tendency to think of infection in an isolated setting within the individual himself as opposed to someone else.

Q. But are most infectious diseases also contagious?

A. Not necessarily. Cystitis is a bacterial infection of the bladder. This is infectious within the given individual but not contagious, meaning that others are not going to catch it because they are in the same room.

Ingrown toenails

Q. How can you avoid ingrown toenails?

A. By wearing shoes that provide enough room for toes and nails, and by trimming the nails carefully—not too short—and by rounding them only slightly at the corners. See also NAILS.

Injury

Q. Why do some persons experience a severe chill after an injury?

A. Some people react to a painful injury or cramp with a brief chill of several minutes. The effect seems to be a reaction to pain.

Jet lag

Q. Is jet lag a serious health problem?

A. Jet lag is a popular term used to describe a disturbance in a person's normal day-night cycle caused by rapidly moving into a different time zone. It is not serious, but the human body usually needs two to four days to adjust to a new schedule for eating and sleeping. See also AIR TRAVEL.

Lipids

Q. What are lipids?

A. Lipids are fatty substances that are essential to living cells. An excess of some lipids, especially cholesterol, is believed to be a factor in contributing to heart disease. Other lipids which are the products of normal metabolism accumulate in the bodies of people who are the victims of rare hereditary disorders grouped together as "lipid storage diseases."

Q. What are the lipid storage diseases?

A. Among the lipid storage diseases are Tay-Sachs disease, Gaucher's disease, fucosidosis, and metachromatic leukodystrophy. All are at present incurable.

Q. Is the cause of lipid storage diseases known?

A. In each case, the particular lipid storage disease is caused by the lack of a single enzyme among the many thousands of enzymes produced by the body for the normal chemical processes of metabolism.

Q. Do all lipids storage diseases have the same symptoms?

A. No. Symptoms vary from disease to disease. Some cause mental retardation, one causes blindness, another results in kidney failure. Practically all of the inherited lipid storage diseases result in early death.

Q. Is there any way of finding out whether an unborn child may inherit one of the lipid storage diseases?

A. Yes. Through genetic counseling, it is possible to identify carriers of the faulty genes that transmit some of these diseases.

Liver spots

See SKIN CARE.

Medical insurance

Q. Does medical insurance ever provide coverage for a second or third expert opinion on whether to have elective surgery?

A. Yes. In an attempt to curb some unnecessary nonemergency surgery, some health insurance plans provide compensation for charges incurred for a second and sometimes a third consultation.

Mg.%

See TESTS AND DIAGNOSTIC PROCEDURES.

Migraine

See HEADACHE.

MLNS

Q. What do the initials MLNS stand for?

A. A children's disease known as mucocutaneous lymph node syndrome in which the symptoms of fever, rash, swollen hands and feet, and bright "strawberry" tongue are self-limiting. However, in about two percent of all cases, a heart involvement occurs that is fatal.

Moles

See SKIN CARE.

Munchausen's syndrome

Q. What kind of disease is Munchausen's syndrome?

A. This is not a real disease but an assortment of make-believe complaints used by some people, otherwise normal, who want to obtain medical care or hospitalization.

Nails

Q. What causes a fingernail to loosen or fall off?

A. A number of things, among them fungus infections, bacterial or yeast infections, psoriasis, or hemorrhage such as that caused by hitting a finger with a hammer.

Q. Does nail polish injure the nail?

A. Nail polish protects the nails except in rare cases of allergic reaction. Nail polish remover can injure the nails if too much is applied, because the drying effect of polish removers can split the nails.

Narcolepsy

Q. What is narcolepsy?

A. Narcolepsy is a neurological syndrome in which an abnormality of the brain results in the disorganization of sleep and the components of sleep. It is estimated that this chronic and disabling sleep disorder affects about 250,000 Americans of all ages.

Q. What are the symptoms of narcolepsy?

A. There are four main symptoms of narcolepsy; a narcoleptic can have one of the symptoms, all four of them, or any combination. The first symptom is known as sleep attacks —falling asleep at unsuitable times and having an exhausted feeling most of the time. The second symptom is catalepsy—a total collapse of muscle tone usually triggered by some strong emotion, particularly surprise, anger, or great pleasure. The third is hallucinating immediately before sleep, and the fourth is a feeling of paralysis or immobility immediately after waking up or just as one falls asleep.

Q. How is true narcolepsy diagnosed?

A. Narcolepsy is diagnosed by observation of the symptoms described and by measurements of the patient's sleep patterns.

Neuropharmacology

Q. What is neuropharmacology?

A. Neuropharmacology is the study of the effects of drugs such as amphetamines, barbiturates and the like on the chemistry of the brain. Compare PSYCHOPHARMACOLOGY.

Nevus, junction

See SKIN CARE.

Newborns

Q. Is there a kind of doctor who specializes in the care of newborn babies?

A. Yes, a perinatologist is a pediatrician who specializes in providing intensive care before, during, and after birth to the newborn baby, especially to one born prematurely or with congenital defects requiring surgery.

Nurse-Midwife

Q. Why aren't nurse-midwives considered as respectable in the United States nowadays as they are in Europe?

A. They are. In 1971, the American College of Obstetricians and Gynecologists officially stated that "in medically directed teams, qualified nurse-midwives may assume responsibility for the complete care and management of uncomplicated maternity patients."

Q. How do nurse-midwives qualify for their profession?

A. A nurse-midwife begins her training by attending a three- or four-year nursing school and becoming a registered nurse. She then affiliates with a hospital in order to get one year of experience in obstetrical nursing. Student nurse-midwives must also observe and assist at about 50 labors and deliveries, and under supervision they are required to manage a minimum of 20 deliveries on their own.

Osgood-Schlatter disease

Q. What is Osgood-Schlatter disease?

A. Degeneration of the protuberant upper end of the tibia just below the knee joint. It usually occurs in adolescents during periods of rapid growth. In most cases the affected bone tissue eventually regenerates.

Osteoarthritis

See ARTHRITIS.

Pacemaker, artificial

See HEART PACEMAKER.

Perspiration

Q. Is there really such a thing as breaking out in a "cold sweat"?

A. Yes. Normally, the eccrine glands that secrete sweat respond only to exercise or heat—except for those on the palms and soles and under the arm, which also respond to emotional excitement, such as fear, sexual stimulation, etc. But under extreme conditions, emotional stimulation can make the eccrine glands over the whole body respond, even when the body has not been warmed from physical effort. The evaporation of this sweat results in a chill, or "cold sweat."

Q. What causes body odor?

A. The aprocrine glands, much less numerous than the eccrine glands which secrete sweat, respond to emotional stimulation by secreting a fluid that acts on the sweat, especially under the arms, where perspiration cannot easily evaporate, to multiply bacteria already present on the skin; the proliferation of such bacteria produces body odor.

Q. What is the purpose of the apocrine glands?

A. They have no known purpose. One theory suggests that, since these glands develop only with sexual maturity and decline with age—which is why children and the elderly do not have the characteristic body odor—the odor once served as a sexual attraction to the opposite sex. Many other animals utilize body scents in this way.

Q. What's the difference between a deodorant and an antiperspirant?

A. A deodorant is designed to suppress or mask body odor. Many deodorants therefore contain antibacterial ingredients and are also pleasantly scented. An antiperspirant is designed to reduce perspiration, although many antiperspirants also have antibacterial properties.

Q. Isn't stopping sweating unhealthy?

A. No antiperspirant can suppress all perspiration; at most it is reduced by about half. Sweating is not, as commonly believed, a way to dispose of body waste. The purpose of sweating is to help regulate body temperature.

Q. Won't one build up an immunity to deodorants or antiperspirants and have to switch?

A. No, this is a misconception. You do not build up an immunity to deodorants or antiperspirants. On some occasions they may not seem to work well enough, but they have not lost their effectiveness; you have just lost your confidence in them.

Q. Why do men need a stronger deodorant than women do? Do they sweat more?

A. Men don't need a stronger deodorant than women do. The secretion from the body-odor-causing apocrine glands is about the same for both sexes. However, the fact that most women shave under their arms probably gives them an advantage, since hair serves to encourage bacteria growth.

Q. Are allergic responses to underarm deodorants very common?

A. You certainly may be allergic to a deodorant, but you should also suspect other causes, such as irritation from clothing or, in the case of women, from shaving. When drying under the arms, you should pat the area gently; hard rubbing can cause irritation to the sensitive skin there.

Physical fitness

Q. Can someone who has had a heart attack ever engage in strenuous physical activity, such as tennis?

A. Every case is different. There are many former heart patients who have, under a doctor's care, resumed their physical activities in sports such as tennis. However, it is imperative to resume such activities only after consulting your physician, and then in gradual stages of increased participation.

Pigeon breast

Q. Can pigeon-breasted people engage in normal physical activities?

A. "Pigeon breast," known technically as *pectus carinatum,* is a congenital deformity in which the sternum (the bone to which the ribs are attached, forming the chest wall) protrudes. It is the opposite of "funnel chest," in which the chest is depressed. There is usually no need to curtail normal physical activity. The chief problem is usually a cosmetic one, i.e., the psychological effect on one's social life and self-image, which can be very severe, especially for young people. Corrective surgery, however, would be extensive and complicated, and is not usually recommended in the absence of physical problems.

Prader-Willi syndrome

Q. What is Prader-Willi syndrome?

A. Prader-Willi syndrome refers to a bizarre eating disturbance whose victims, chiefly children between the ages of two and five, are afflicted with an insatiable desire for food. The disorder, which is named for the two doctors who first described it in 1956, is not inherited, nor does it appear to be related to emotional stress. Present studies indicate that it is the result of a neurological disturbance caused by malfunction of the hypothalamus of the brain.

Psoriasis

Q. How common is psoriasis?

A. About two percent of people in the United States have psoriasis.

Q. Does it affect one sex more than the other?

A. No, it affects men and women equally.

Q. At what age does it first appear?

A. Usually between the ages of 15 and 30.

Q. Is psoriasis contagious?

A. No, not at all. It is probably an inherited disorder.

Psychological counseling

Q. How does group therapy work?

A. Group therapy is the general term for a wide variety of therapeutic situations in which the participants try to find more satisfactory ways of living their lives through honest self-examination and the expression of their authentic feelings. Mutual respect, support, and trust are the principles on which the effectiveness of group therapy is based. The group may be led by a professional psychiatrist, a lay analyst, or a psychiatric social worker, or the leadership of each session may rotate among the participants.

Q. What are encounter groups?

A. An encounter group is a form of group therapy in which people are encouraged by each other and by a trained counselor to get in touch with their suppressed feelings of fear, rage, anger, shame, etc., by means of unrestrained verbalization and physical contact.

Psychopharmacology

Q. What kind of research is done by psychopharmacologists?

A. Psychopharmacologists are scientific specialists who study the actions of drugs such as LSD or tranquilizers on the mind. Compare NEUROPHARMACOLOGY.

Puberty

Q. Are middle-class American girls reaching sexual maturity at a younger age with each succeeding decade?

A. No. The average age at which girls begin to menstruate is 12.8 years, and this figure has remained the same over the last 30 years.

Raynaud's disease

Q. What is Raynaud's disease?

A. Raynaud's disease is a condition in which the arteries in the fingers and toes experience spasms, usually after exposure to cold. The tips of fingers and toes become bluish (cyanotic) or ashen, then sometimes red.

Q. What causes this condition?

A. It can be a complication of rheumatoid arthritis, a connective tissue disease, neurological disease, etc. It can also result from piano playing or other occupations in which the fingertips are struck or jarred repeatedly. (In such cases, the condition is usually known as *Raynaud's phenomenon.*) But Raynaud's disease is frequently not secondary to any known underlying condition. Its cause in such cases is unknown. It is known that emotional states can trigger an attack of finger and/or toe spasms, but this certainly does not preclude physiological causes.

Q. Who is most likely to get Raynaud's disease?

A. Women, by a five to one ratio, are more commonly afflicted than men.

Q. How is it treated?

A. In most cases, the condition will stay the same or improve with age (usually at about age 40). Patients subject to Raynaud's disease should definitely not smoke and should take care to avoid exposure to cold. Mild sedatives may be prescribed by a physician if spasm episodes are frequent or severe.

Reye's syndrome

Q. What is Reye's syndrome?

A. Reye's syndrome is a complication that may follow a number of different kinds of viral infections, including influenza and chicken pox. The disorder, which is extremely rare, affects mainly children and involves primarily the liver, interfering with that organ's ability to help remove poisonous substances from the bloodstream. The resulting buildup of toxic wastes in the blood results in damage to the liver, the brain, and the kidneys. Symptoms include mental confusion, severe nausea and vomiting, hyperactivity and excitability, followed by convulsions and finally coma. Because the disorder frequently is fatal if not treated at an early stage, immediate medical attention is required.

Q. How is it treated?

A. The patient is closely watched on an around-the-clock basis so that any serious complication, such as a buildup of pressure on the brain, can be immediately counteracted with drugs or by other means. Treatment may include transfusions of fresh blood to replace the patient's blood containing the toxic agent.

Q. Is there a cure for Reye's syndrome?

A. No, but the disease is believed to be self-limiting. Treatment is directed at enabling the patient to survive during the critical period in which the disease is running its course.

Rickettsial diseases

Q. What causes typhus and is there a "shot" you can get as protection against typhus?

A. Typhus is a debilitating, frequently fatal disease caused by a tiny organism called a rickettsia. The rickettsia usually is transmitted to humans through the bite of a body louse. A vaccine is available and is recommended for travelers to some underdeveloped countries of the world.

Q. Is Rocky Mountain spotted fever a disease you can get only in the Rocky Mountains?

A. No, this rickettsial disease was discovered in the Rocky Mountains but occurs in other areas as well, particularly in the eastern U.S. It is transmitted by wood ticks.

SCID
See IMMUNOLOGY.

Serum sickness

Q. What is serum sickness?

A. Serum sickness is an immunological reaction to the introduction of serum (the clear fluid portion of the blood), as an animal serum used as an antitoxin, into the body. The reaction may be acute and severe. It is a form of allergic shock or anaphylaxis, and can be avoided by always having a skin test to check for reaction before a serum is introduced into the body.

SGOT
See TESTS AND DIAGNOSTIC PROCEDURES/BLOOD.

Shaving
See UNWANTED HAIR.

Skin cancer

Q. Is skin cancer more common in the South than in the North?

A. Yes, skin cancer is about ten times more common in the South than the North because of increased exposure to sunlight in the South.

Q. Are dark-skinned people less likely to develop skin cancer than fair-skinned people?

A. Yes, blonds and redheads are more subject to skin cancer than dark-skinned people.

Skin care

Q. What is the cause of "liver spots" on the skin?

A. The brownish areas of discoloration that may appear on the skin in later life have nothing to do with the liver but sometimes indicate a minor systemic disorder. A general physical examination usually is needed to pinpoint the exact cause.

Q. Please explain why dark circles sometimes appear under the eyes.

A. Because the skin of eyelids is thin, blood in veins beneath the skin may make the area seem darker and bluer than surrounding skin. During menstruation or illness, this discoloration may become more obvious.

Q. What causes "bags" under the eyes?

A. As a person ages, tissues that normally hold the skin of the eyelids firmly become weak, and subcutaneous fat pushes the skin outward. Plastic surgery is the only cure for this effect. Puffiness of the eyelids may be a sign of fluid accumulation due to kidney or heart disease.

Q. What is a junction nevus?

A. A junction nevus is a darkly pigmented tumor, resembling a common mole, that develops at the junction of the two layers of the skin, the dermis and epidermis.

Q. Can a mole or junction nevus become a skin cancer?

A. While unusual, a mole or junction nevus can darken and enlarge into a precancerous tumor. It is wise to have a physician remove the growth before the change can occur.

Q. What is the difference between a boil and a carbuncle?

A. The main difference is that a carbuncle is bigger than a boil and involves two or more hair follicles.

Q. What is dermabrasion and will it remove acne scars?

A. Dermabrasion is a technique of rubbing away the outer layer of skin to get rid of scars. The skin is covered with bandages to control bleeding and infection and a new skin layer replaces the old in about a month.

Q. Are warts contagious?

A. Yes. They are caused by a virus and are likely to develop on moist areas of the skin or areas that have been injured.

Q. What are the medical treatments for warts?

A. Some warts can be removed by freezing them with supercooled liquids. Warts also are treated with X rays, medicines applied to the skin, and by surgical excision.

Q. Can warts be "charmed" away by suggestion?

A. There is no scientific basis for this notion; when warts disappear after hexing, the wart is regressing because of other factors and the apparent "charm" effect is coincidental.

Q. What is the cause of skin wrinkling?

A. It is not completely known why skin wrinkles, although heredity apparently is one factor. Others are loss of weight, exposure to wind and sun, and loss of supporting tissue beneath the skin as a part of aging.

Sleep

Q. During the onset of sleep, one occasionally has the sensation of falling or floating. Is this effect a symptom of a serious disorder?

A. No. The sensation of falling or floating while drifting off to sleep is a not unusual hypnagogic illusion, or hallucination. It occurs in a semi-dreamlike state but is not a true dream. Some people experience visual illusions—faces, landscapes, or geometric shapes—while falling asleep.

Q. Sometimes while sleeping the entire body may jerk for no apparent reason. Is this normal?

A. The sudden incoordinate jerking of a part or the whole body, called nocturnal jerking, is a natural occurrence during light sleep. The phenomenon is believed to result from a sudden release of muscle tension by a nervous system impulse in the cerebral cortex of the brain. Usually no harm is done and the event is quickly forgotten. Pet owners are well aware that this phenomenon is not restricted to humans. Dogs and cats also jerk reflexively during light sleep.

Q. What is REM sleep?

A. REM sleep is a phase of sleep during which there are bursts of rapid eye movements—abbreviated REM. This phenomenon, originally reported in 1953, coincides with a state of intense physiological activity. In addition to the rapid eye movements, the heartbeat quickens, blood pressure rises, and the rate of electrical impulses in the brain increases. The rapid eye movements are also associated with dreaming.

Q. What is NREM sleep?

A. NREM sleep (non-REM sleep) is qualitatively different from REM sleep. It seems to be a restful and recuperative state. Approximately 75 percent of all sleep time is spent in NREM sleep.

Q. Does the sleeper first experience one kind of sleep and then the other, and then wake up?

A. No. Sleep occurs in cycles: a period of about 90 minutes of NREM sleep precedes the onset of the first REM period, which lasts from 5 to 15 minutes. This alternation occurs throughout the night, with the REM phases getting somewhat longer toward waking. The NREM-REM alternation is sometimes called the *sleep-dream cycle* because dreams occur more often and more dramatically in REM sleep than they do in NREM sleep.

Speech

See BRAIN/SPEECH.

Stimulant drugs

Q. Can stimulant drugs affect the growth of children?

A. It has been found that two types of drugs (Dexedrine and Ritalin) used to treat hyperactive children seem to retard the normal gains in height and weight when administered in large doses over long periods of time.

Stitch

Q. What causes a stitch in the side?

A. A stitch—or sudden ache in the upper left or right part of the abdomen—is associated with vigorous activity, often occurs after eating, and is aggravated by cold weather. Its cause is not known, but it is believed to be linked to a decreased supply of oxygen in the blood circulating to the diaphragm.

Suicide

Q. What are the two main causes of death among young people in the United States?

A. Accidents are the leading cause of death among young people in the United States. The second leading cause is suicide.

Q. Are young people in the highest risk age group for suicide?

A. No. The highest risk age group is the elderly, who account for one-fourth of all suicides in the United States.

Sweat

See PERSPIRATION.

Tests and diagnostic procedures

Q. On some laboratory reports, test results are written as numbers followed by mg.%. Please explain.

A. Mg.% is a scientific notation that means the number of milligrams of a substance found in 100 milliliters of blood. See below under BLOOD.

Q. On your physical exam sheet, you may see something like "BP 130/74." What does this mean?

A. It means your blood pressure (BP) was 130 (systolic) over 74 (diastolic) as measured in millimeters of mercury. See also BLOOD PRESSURE.

Biopsy

Q. What is a biopsy?

A. A microscopic examination of the tissue cells from a lump, nodule, ulcer, or hard mass. The procedure is commonly used to determine if an abnormal growth may be cancer.

Q. What is meant by needle biopsy?

A. A sample of tissue cells from an organ is taken through a long needle inserted into the body—an alternative to using surgery to examine tissue from the liver, kidney, or other organs.

Blood

Q. What does BUN on a laboratory report mean?

A. BUN is an abbreviation for blood urea nitrogen; it is a measure of the health of the kidneys. The normal range is 10–20 mg.%

Q. Why is cholesterol measured in blood tests?

A. The cholesterol level of the blood indicates possible premature hardening of the arteries. A normal level is 150–300 mg.%

Q. On a copy of a blood test from the laboratory there may be a reference to SGOT. What does this mean?

A. This is medical shorthand for serum glutamic oxaloacetic transaminase; sometimes it is called simply transaminase. It is an enzyme which in abnormal quantities could indicate liver disease or coronary heart disease.

Q. Is there a blood test for diabetes?

A. Yes. An abnormally high level of sugar in the blood suggests diabetes.

Q. What is bilirubin and what does its presence in the blood tell a doctor?

A. Bilirubin is a pigment that colors the bile. An abnormally high level in the blood could mean the patient has liver or gall bladder disease.

Q. What does it mean if one's blood sugar is below normal?

A. It could indicate a tumor of the pancreas or an overactive production of insulin.

Cough Plate

Q. What is a cough plate?

A. It is a sterile plate used to collect bacteria from a patient for study. The patient coughs onto the plate. The test may be used, for example, in the diagnosis of whooping cough.

Frozen Section

Q. What is a frozen section?

A. A suspicious lump of tissue is frozen quickly with carbon dioxide gas, and a thin slice cut from the tissue is stained with a dye for study under a microscope. The test usually is done during surgery in order to determine quickly if the tissue should be removed or if it is relatively harmless.

Guthrie Test

Q. What is a Guthrie test?

A. This is a special method of examining a urine sample in order to determine if a patient may have phenylketonuria (PKU), an inherited metabolic disease.

Urine

Q. Does sugar in the urine mean one has diabetes?

A. Generally, yes. It is one test for diabetes. However, it is possible to have the disease without a significant level of sugar in the urine.

Q. Why is a urine sample tested for albumin?

A. The presence of albumin in urine would suggest an abnormal functioning of the kidneys, perhaps due to a disease such as nephritis.

Q. Why does the lab technician check the color of a urine sample?

A. Normal urine is clear or amber in color. If it is tinged with red, the cause could be bleeding in the urethra, bladder, kidneys, prostate (in men), or elsewhere in the urinary tract. A brown coloration could indicate liver disease.

Tetanus

Q. How often should you get a tetanus booster?

A. Every ten years, assuming that you haven't sustained a wound, especially a puncture-type wound, that might be infected with tetanus germs. In that event, you should have a booster if you haven't had one in a year's time.

Q. What should someone who is not immunized do when he sustains a wound that may be infected with tetanus germs?

A. He should seek medical assistance immediately. He will be given tetanus toxoid and may also be given an antitoxin—either a human antitoxin or one from a horse or cow.

Tic douloureux

Q. Can a young person have "tic douloureux," or trigeminal neuralgia?

A. These severe facial pains can occur at any age after puberty, but usually do not begin to appear before the age of 50.

Tourette's disease

Q. What is Tourette's disease?

A. Named for the French neurologist, Gilles de la Tourette, this disease is marked by violent muscular jerking of the head and shoulders, as well as of the extremities, along with grunting, explosive obscenities uttered by the victim.

Toxoplasmosis/cats

Q. Can people catch diseases from cats?

A. Yes. Cats are the chief source of a disease called toxoplasmosis, which is caused by a parasite to which cats as well as other animals are the host.

Q. Is toxoplasmosis a serious disease?

A. Not in most cases. Animals themselves may harbor the infectious organism without showing symptoms, and probably half the adult population has been infected by the "toxo" parasite at one time or other without knowing it. In some people, the infection runs a course similar to mononucleosis; in others, it may cause inflammation of the retina. However, the disease is very dangerous if contracted by a pregnant woman. While symptoms usually bypass the mother, prenatal infection of the fetus can cause irreversible brain damage, blindness, or death.

Typhus
See RICKETTSIAL DISEASES.

Ulcers

Q. Are peptic ulcers caused by too much stomach acid?

A. Not necessarily; some individuals have high levels of stomach acid but never develop ulcers. However, oversecretion of stomach acid can aggravate an existing ulcer.

Q. What are some of the signs of a bleeding ulcer?

A. The patient may vomit blood or, more commonly, the blood will travel through the intestine and cause the patient's stools to be colored black.

Q. Will a stomach ulcer eventually become a stomach cancer?

A. A stomach ulcer may occasionally develop into a cancerous growth. A person with a peptic ulcer should be examined regularly by a doctor who can watch for possible precancerous changes.

Unwanted hair

Q. Is excessive hair in women caused by too much male hormone production?

A. Women with excessive facial hair are entirely feminine, and tests usually do not indicate an elevated production of the male hormone. It is normal for those of each sex to produce both male and female hormones; women normally produce about two-thirds as much of the male hormone as do men.

Q. Does shaving make hair grow faster than before?

A. No. Shaving has no effect on the rate of growth of hair. However, since short hair is thicker and less flexible than long hair, a trimmed beard may give a denser appearance than untrimmed facial hair.

Q. Why is it better to shave hair when it is wet?

A. Hair can absorb a great deal of water, making it softer and much easier to cut. The best time to shave body hair is after a bath or shower.

Urine & urinalysis
See TESTS AND DIAGNOSTIC PROCEDURES/URINE.

Warts
See SKIN CARE.

Weight problems

Q. Is exercising a good way to lose weight?

A. No. Exercising is beneficial for other reasons, such as maintaining good muscle tone, but it is not an efficient way to lose weight. The only way to lose weight is to diet so that your body is taking in fewer calories than it is consuming.

Wrinkling
See SKIN CARE.

X Rays

Q. How often should a dentist take a full set of X rays?

A. Unless there is some special problem, a full set of X rays—16 to 18 pictures of an adult patient's teeth—need not be conducted more often than every three to five years. Some authorities feel that a full set of dental X rays need not be made more than every six to ten years.

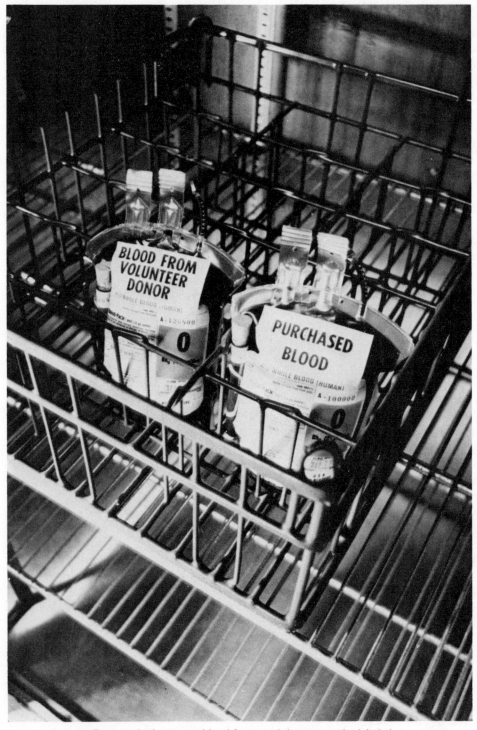

In Illinois and other states, blood from paid donors must be labeled as such—to distinguish it from the safer blood from volunteer donors.

CHAPTER 6

Voluntary Health Agencies

The establishment of over 100 voluntary health agencies since the beginning of this century has been a major factor in the growth of health services to the American public. These agencies, whose activities are made possible by donations of time and money from the public, occasionally augmented by government grants for special projects, have the following objectives: spreading information about various diseases to the professional and lay public; sponsoring research; promoting legislation, and operating referral services on the community level to patients in need of diagnosis, treatment, and financial aid.

Some of these agencies, such as the American Diabetes Association or the Arthritis Foundation, focus on a particular disease; others deal with problems arising from related disorders, such as the National Association for Mental Health and the American Heart Association. Still others, such as Planned Parenthood and the American Social Health Association, have programs vital not only to individuals, but to society as a whole.

To coordinate the activities of these many groups, to promote better health facilities, and to establish standards for the organization and conduct of these agencies, the National Health Council was founded in 1920. Its membership includes government, professional, and community associations, as well as the 19 voluntary health agencies described below, which command a total budget of almost $300 million and involve the services of almost 9 million volunteers.

All of these organizations function on the national, state, and community level. Information and literature may be obtained through local chapters or by writing to the national

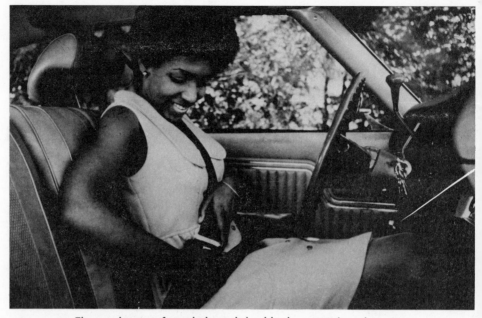

The regular use of seat belts and shoulder harnesses is an important factor in reducing the risk of serious injury in automobile accidents.

office of the organization. Volunteers may offer their services in a variety of ways: as office workers, fund raisers, speakers, and community coordinators.

On the following pages, voluntary health agencies are discussed under the subjects with which they are concerned; the subjects are arranged alphabetically. Other voluntary health agencies are discussed briefly beginning on p. 324. Due to limitations of space, however, many worthwhile organizations have had to be omitted.

A special subsection deals with hospices, nursing homes, hospital and other social service offices and agencies, and the visiting nurse.

Accident Prevention

The National Safety Council, 444 North Michigan Avenue, Chicago, Illinois 60611, was founded in 1913 to improve factory safety but soon broadened its activities to preventing every type of accident. The Council is now composed of groups and individuals from every part of the population: business, industry, government, education, religion, labor, and law. Its main efforts are devoted to building strong support for official safety programs at the national, state, and community level in specific areas, such as traffic, labor, and home.

The Council believes that practically all accidents can be prevented with the application of the right safeguards. These safeguards include public education and awareness of danger, enforcement of safety laws and regulations, and improved design standards for machines, farm equipment, and motor vehicles.

It maintains the world's largest library of accident prevention materials, distributes a wide variety of safety literature, and issues awards for outstanding safety achievements. It also serves as a national and international clearing house of information about the causes of accidents and how they can be prevented.

In addition to campaigning for increased safety legislation on the national and state level, the Council's current programs include a defensive driving course, which provides effective adult driver training on a mass scale; a safety training institute; and, in cooperation with the American Medical Association, a new approach to the alcohol and driving problem.

Its publication, *Family Safety*, has a record circulation of almost 2 million readers, and its manual called *Fundamentals of Industrial Hygiene* provides more than 1,000 pages of material essential to the safety of factory workers.

For the last few years, the organization has been engaged in a factfinding project, the Home Safety Inventory, designed to improve building standards and other hazardous environmental factors that contribute to making accidents the fourth leading cause of death in the United States.

Alcoholism

The National Council on Alcoholism, 733 Third Avenue, New York, New York 10017, is the only national voluntary health agency founded to combat alcoholism as a disease by an extensive program on the professional and community level. The Council is completely independent of Alcoholics Anonymous, although the two organizations cooperate fully.

In the more than 70 cities where the Council has branches, alcoholism information centers have been established that provide referral services for alcoholics and their families as well as educational materials for all segments of the community, including doctors and nurses, the clergy, the courts, social workers, and welfare agencies. Local affiliates also help to develop labor-management programs that provide help for employees who suffer from the disease.

The NCA also sponsors research, professional training, legislative action, and treatment centers on the national and local level.

As its national headquarters in New York, the Council maintains the only library in the country devoted exclusively to the subject and study of alcoholism. The collection was begun in 1957 and now consists of over 1,500 books, periodicals, and technical documents on the subject. Its publications department distributes more than 100 different books and pamphlets divided into special categories. Information on this literature as well as on all aspects of the Council's programs is available to anyone who writes to the national headquarters or contacts the nearest local affiliate.

Arthritis

The Arthritis Foundation, 475 Riverside Drive, New York, New York 10027, was established to help arthritis sufferers and their doctors through programs of research, patient services, public health information, and education on the professional and popular level. Its long-term goal is to find the cause,

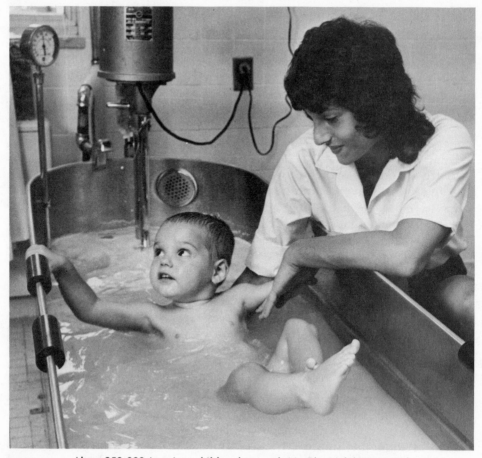

About 250,000 American children have arthritis. Physical therapy and other forms of treatment offer promise of effective rehabilitation.

prevention, and cure for the nation's number one crippling disease.

Two special groups work within the organization: the American Rheumatism Association Section, which governs medical and scientific programs, and the Allied Health Professions Section, which devotes itself to overcoming the shortage of specialized health workers in the field.

The Foundation operates local chapters throughout the United States whose chief concern is the patient who has or might have arthritis. These chapters are centers for in-formation about the disease itself and also serve as referral centers for treatment facilities. In addition, they distribute literature and sponsor forums on the latest developments in research and patient care.

Some chapters support arthritis clinics and home care programs; others provide mobile treatment units that travel to rural communities and work with local doctors and their patients.

A major part of the Foundation's program consists of a network of arthritis clinical research centers which specialize in experiments with new medicines and treatment procedures. The publications distributed by this organization include a wide variety of pamphlets and brochures for the professional reader as well as the interested public.

Cancer

The American Cancer Society, 777 Third Avenue, New York, New York 10017, was established in 1913 by a small group of doctors and volun-

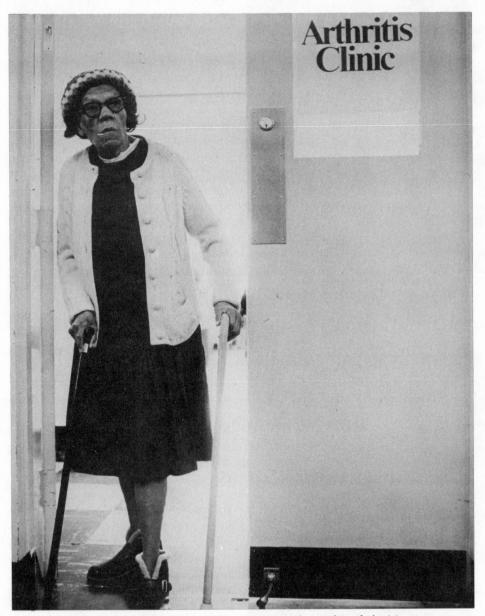

The Arthritis Foundation is working to increase the number of physicians qualified to give the special treatment needed by arthritis patients.

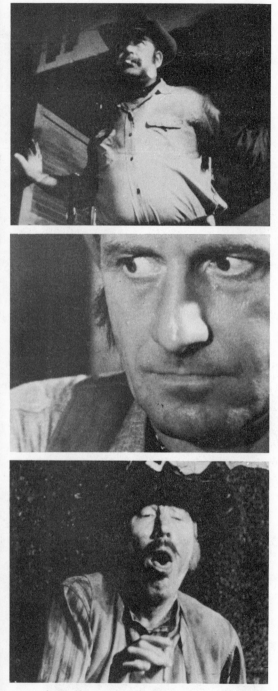

In waging war against cigarette smoking, the American Cancer Society showed a TV commerical in which typical western "bad guys" couldn't draw their six-shooters because smoking doubled them up in fits of coughing.

teer workers to inform the public about the possibility of saving lives through the early diagnosis and treatment of cancer. The Society now has 58 incorporated divisions, one in each state plus one in the District of Columbia and seven other metropolitan areas, devoted to the control and eradication of cancer. In addition to the doctors, research scientists, and other professional workers engaged in the Society's activities, over two million volunteers are connected with its many programs.

The ACS conducts widespread campaigns to educate the public in the importance of annual medical checkups so that cancerous symptoms can be detected while they are still curable. Such checkups should include an examination of the rectum and colon and, for women, examination of the breasts and a Pap test for the detection of uterine cancer.

In another of its campaigns, the Society emphasizes the link between cigarette smoking and lung cancer. It also sponsors an extensive program to persuade teen-agers not to start smoking. During its annual April Crusade Against Cancer, the Society distributes approximately 40 million copies of the leaflet listing the seven warning signals of the disease.

On the professional level, the major objective of ACS is to make every doctor's office a cancer-detection center. To achieve this goal, it publishes a variety of literature, offers refresher courses, sponsors seminars, and cooperates closely with local and state medical societies and health departments on the diagnosis and treatment of

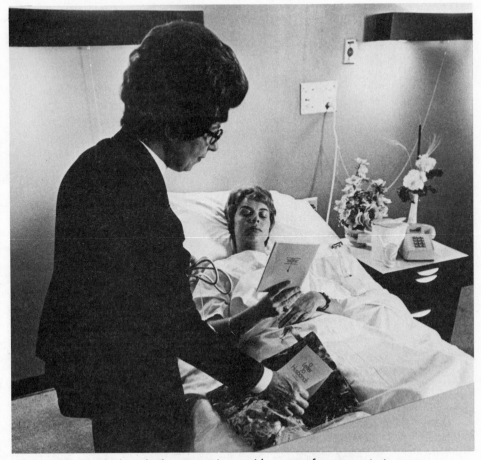

Women who have had mastectomies provide support for new mastectomy patients in the American Cancer Society's volunteer Reach to Recovery program.

cancer. It also arranges national and international conferences for the exchange of information on the newest cancer-fighting techniques, and finances a million-dollar-a-year clinical fellowship program for young physicians.

Among its special services to patients are sponsorship of the International Association of Laryngectomees, for people who have lost their voices to cancer; and Reach to Recovery, a program for women who have had radical mastectomies (breast removal) and who need support and guidance in order to return to normal living. On the community level, ACS operates a counseling service for cancer patients and their families, referring them to the proper medical facilities and social agencies for treatment and care. Through its "loan closets," it provides sickroom necessities, hospital beds, medical dressings, and so on.

Some local divisions of ACS also offer home care programs through the services of the Visiting Nurse Association or a similar agency. Although the Society does not operate medical facilities, treat patients, or pay doctors' fees, some of the chap-

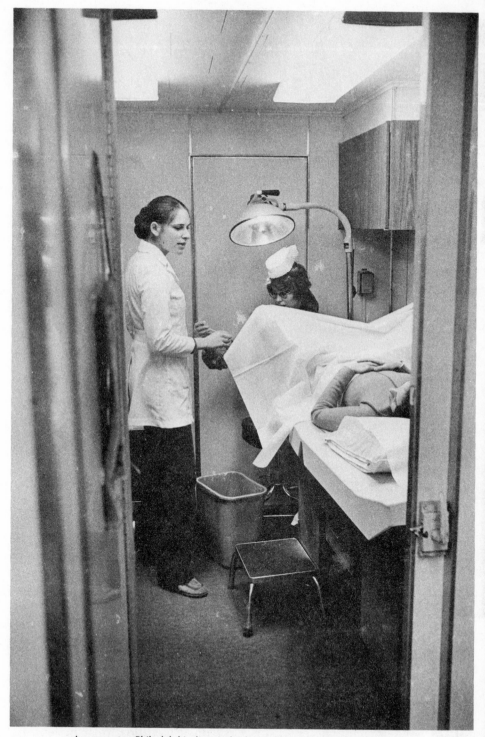

A nurse at a Philadelphia hospital takes a Pap smear from a patient in a "Community Outreach" program sponsored by American Cancer Society.

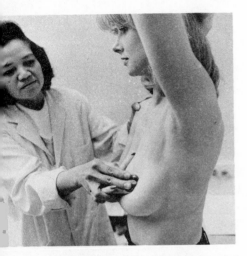

A woman learns Breast Self-Examination at the Guttman Institute in New York City so she can check regularly herself for possible symptoms of breast cancer.

A scene from "Cancer Chemotherapy (Solid Tumors)," a professional education film for medical students, demonstrates the technique for injecting chemotherapy drugs.

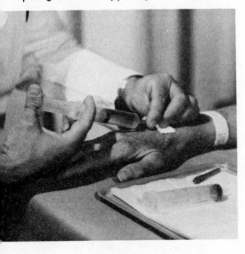

ters support cancer detection programs and professionally supervised rehabilitation services.

Cerebral Palsy

The United Cerebral Palsy Associa-

tions, Inc., 66 East 34th Street, New York, New York 10016, founded in 1949 by a small group of concerned parents, now has 301 affiliates across the country where those who are afflicted with the disorder may obtain treatment referral, therapy, and education. The Associations also play an important role in vocational training, job placement programs, and recreational services.

The Research and Educational Foundation of this organization supported the studies that led ultimately to the development of a safe vaccine against rubella, the disease which is responsible for a significant number of birth defects if it occurs during the early months of pregnancy. It is also investigating other possible causes of cerebral palsy in the newborn, such as the misuse of drugs during pregnancy, and oxygen deprivation during labor and delivery. Grants are also given to universities and medical schools for research into the causes of cerebral palsy and new methods of therapy for treatment of cerebral palsied patients, and also for training medical personnel to deal with this disease.

Cystic Fibrosis

The National Cystic Fibrosis Research Foundation, 3379 Peachtree Road, N.E., Atlanta, Georgia 30326, was organized in 1955 by a group of concerned parents whose children were born with this lung disease. The Foundation now concerns itself with all serious lung ailments of children regardless of their medical names, and it engages in a broad program of research, medical education, public information, and the sponsorship of diagnostic and treatment centers.

The Foundation's 135 local chapters offer advice and information to parents of children with severe lung disease, and have direct connections with the 110 Cystic Fibrosis Centers throughout the country. They refer patients to sources of financial aid, make arrangements for the purchase of drugs at a discount, and lend home treatment equipment to families who cannot afford to buy it.

The national organization makes grants for research activities, conducts professional conferences, and publishes literature for doctors and the general public on various aspects of childhood lung diseases.

Diabetes

The American Diabetes Association, 1 West 48th Street, New York, New York 10020, which was established as a professional society in 1940, has in recent years enlarged its scope so that it currently has 53 affiliated chapters throughout the country which promote the creation of better understanding of diabetes among patients and their families; the exchange of knowledge among physicians and other scientists; the spreading of accurate information to the general public about early recognition and supervision of the disease; and the sponsorship of basic research.

Since 1948, the ADA has conducted an annual Diabetes Detection Drive supported by widespread publicity in all news media. During this drive, approximately three million testing kits are provided to state and county medical societies to facilitate the early detection and prompt treatment of the disorder. This annual activity hopes to find the estimated 1,600,000 people who are unaware that they have diabetes.

Among the Association's publications of special interest to diabetics and their families are the *ADA Forecast,* a national magazine that presents news items on research and treatment; *Meal Planning with Ex-*

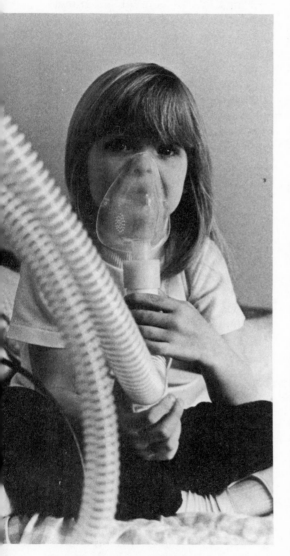

This girl, who has cystic fibrosis, inhales aerosol medications three times a day to liquefy the sticky mucus that blocks the airways of her lungs.

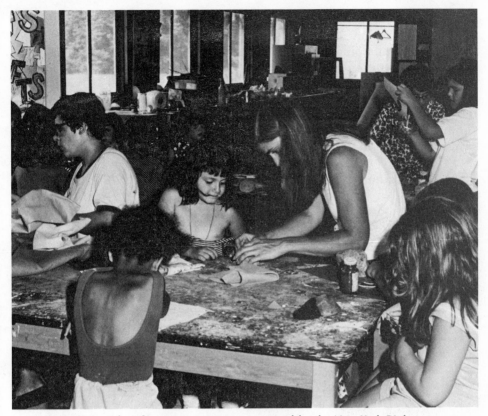

An arts and crafts group at a camp sponsored by the New York Diabetes Association. Such camps are tailored to meet the needs of diabetic children.

change Lists, prepared with the cooperation of the American Dietetic Association and the U.S. Public Health Service; and *A Cookbook for Diabetics,* which contains attractive recipes for meals that can be served to diabetics.

Other activities of the ADA include encouraging the employment of diabetics, and providing special groups such as teachers, police, and social agencies with information on the condition. It has also established a classification of the disease according to its severity. Guidelines on emergency medical care and the scientific journal *Diabetes* are available to doctors.

Drug Abuse

The American Social Health Association, which was organized originally to combat the spread of venereal disease, expanded its program in 1960 to include drug abuse education. For information about its activities in this field, see below under *Venereal Disease.*

Eye Diseases

The National Society for the Prevention of Blindness, 79 Madison Avenue, New York, New York 10016, was founded in 1908 to reduce the number of infants born with impaired sight. In subsequent years, it merged with the American Association for the Conservation of Vision and the Ophthalmological Foundation. The Society is now concerned with investigating all causes of blindness and supports measures and community services that will eliminate them. It also distributes information on the proper care and use of the eyes.

The organization's first and most significant victory was the adoption of laws by almost all states requiring that silver nitrate solution be routinely dropped into the eyes of all newborn babies to counteract the possibility of congenital blindness. This resulted in a dramatic drop in the number of children suffering from eye impairment dating from birth.

For almost half a century, the Society has actively campaigned to reduce the number of people suffering from glaucoma, the second leading cause of blindness in the United States. It has also conducted a national program to educate the elderly in the ease, safety, and advantages of surgery for cataracts, the leading cause of blindness among the aged.

Since 1926, the Society has been conducting preschool vision screening programs administered by teams that travel from big cities to isolated rural communities. Current activities also include research into the cause, treatment, and prevention of eye diseases leading to blindness; assembling data and publishing reports; cooperating with community agencies to improve eye health; promoting conditions in schools and industry to safeguard vision; and advocating eye examinations in early childhood so that disorders can be properly and promptly corrected.

The education division of the Society produces pamphlets, films, and circulating exhibits on all aspects of eye safety and sight preservation. This material is available on request.

Family Planning

Planned Parenthood Federation of America, 810 Seventh Avenue, New York, New York 10019, established in 1961, is the direct result of the birth control clinics originally founded by Margaret Sanger in 1916. The comparatively young organization has quickly grown from a single center in Brooklyn to a nation-wide network of 181 affiliates, with a total of 620 clinics operating in 350 cities. It also assists national family planning organizations in more than 100 countries throughout the world.

Planned Parenthood has five principal goals: to help make information and effective means of family planning—including contraception, voluntary sterilization and abortion—available and easily accessible to all; to educate all American parents in the advantages of limiting the size of their families; to stimulate medical and sociological research; to combat the world population crisis; and to support the efforts of others to achieve these goals in the United States and throughout the world.

Each year, through its clinics, the organization offers family planning information, education, and medically supervised services to over 400,000 men and women of varied social and economic backgrounds at little or no cost. In addition, it conducts clinical research, furnishes and directs professional training of medical and health personnel, and assists city, county, and state governments in developing their own family planning programs.

To meet the increased demand on the part of men for voluntary sterilization, Planned Parenthood has opened 13 vasectomy clinics in various parts of the country. It is also providing migrant workers in more than 20 states with a unique referral program of family planning services. Films and publications on all aspects of the organization's activities are distributed to individuals, community agencies, citizen action groups, schools, and hospitals.

Heart Disease

The American Heart Association, 7320 Greenville Avenue, Dallas, Texas 75231, was founded in 1924 as

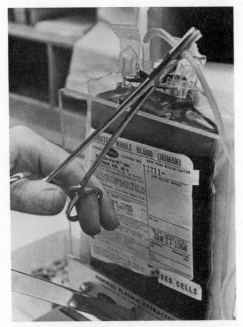

Modern blood bank techniques make quantities of whole blood available to hemophiliacs. Blood can also be fractionated (separated into components).

a professional organization of cardiologists. It was reorganized in 1948 as a national voluntary health agency to promote a program of education, research, and community service in the interests of reducing premature death and disability caused by diseases of the heart and blood vessels. The complex of heart disorders, including atherosclerosis, stroke, high blood pressure, kidney diseases, rheumatic fever, and congenital heart disturbances, is by far the leading cause of death in the United States.

Since its first Annual Heart Fund Campaign in 1949, the Association has contributed more than 150 million dollars to research and has been a major factor in the reduction of cardiovascular mortality statistics. It has spent over two million dollars since 1959 studying human heart transplantation procedures, and has contributed to the development of an artificial heart, plastic heart valves, and synthetic arteries.

Public and professional education programs designed to reduce the risk of heart attack through avoidance of cigarette smoking, obesity, and foods high in cholesterol are conducted on a nation-wide and community level by the Association's affiliates throughout the country. The local chapters are also engaged in service programs for rheumatic fever prevention, stroke rehabilitation, school health, cardiopulmonary resuscitation, and industrial health. In addition, they conduct information and referral services for patients and their families.

The AHA publishes many technical and professional journals as well as material designed for the general public.

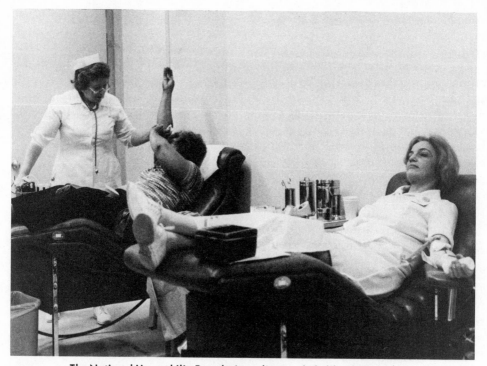

The National Hemophilia Foundation relies on whole blood from donors such as these to supply the clotting factor needed by hemophiliacs.

Hemophilia

The National Hemophilia Foundation, 25 West 39th Street, New York, New York 10018, was established in 1948 to serve the needs of hemophiliacs and their families by insuring the availability of treatment and rehabilitation facilities. It is estimated that there are as many as 100,000 males suffering from what is popularly known as "bleeder's disease," an inherited condition passed from mothers to sons.

The long-term goal of the foundation is to develop a national program of research and clinical study that will provide new information about early diagnosis and effective treatment of the disorder as well as trained professional personnel to administer patient care.

The development in recent years of blood-clotting concentrates is the most important advance to date in the treatment of the disease. This development, supported in part by the Foundation's 53 chapters, makes it possible for patients to have elective surgery and dental work, and to eliminate much of the pain, crippling, and hospitalization of those suffering from hemophilia.

The need for blood supplies from which to extract the clotting factor caused the Foundation to embark on an extensive campaign for blood donations. For this purpose, it has been working closely since 1968 with the American Red Cross and the American Association of Blood Banks. It also maintains close ties with various laboratories and research groups in the development of more powerful concentrates that can be manufactured and sold at the lowest possible cost.

The organization's activities include a national network of facilities with blood banks, clinics, and treatment centers as well as referral services. It has also established a Behavioral Science Department to explore the nonmedical aspects of hemophiliacs' problems, such as education, vocational guidance, and psychological needs.

Kidney Disease

The National Kidney Foundation, 116 East 27th Street, New York, New York 10016, formerly the National Nephrosis Foundation, was organized in 1950 to work toward improved care and treatment for those afflicted with kidney disease through improved methods and services in research, prevention, detection, and diagnosis.

Although the Foundation is growing rapidly, it has scarcely begun to meet the needs of the nearly eight million people who suffer from kidney disorders. However, since its establishment, the number of deaths from nephrosis has been drastically reduced by the use of transplantation from matched donors and the technique of hemodialysis.

Through its 40 affiliates in 35 states, the NKF endorses the wider application of these procedures and supports research, training of professional personnel, construction of facilities, and programs that help to defray the high cost of treatment.

Emphasis is currently being placed on the establishment of screening and diagnostic centers to detect kidney disease as early as possible and to educate the public in recognizing its symptoms. The Foundation distributes many publications on kidney-related subjects to the professional and general public. For the general reader, there are leaflets explaining kidney function and disease, the role of hypertension, and recognition of symptoms of disorder.

Mental Health

The National Association for Mental Health, 1800 N. Kent Street, Rosslyn, Virginia 22209, had its beginnings in 1909, when an ex-mental patient founded the National Committee for Mental Hygiene. In 1950, this group merged with the National Mental Health Foundation and the Psychiatric Foundation to create the organization as it now stands. The purpose of the NAMH is to improve attitudes toward and services for the mentally ill, to work for the prevention of mental illness, and to promote mental health.

Since 1960, the Association's national research program has invested more than one million dollars in studies aimed at finding out more about the causes, treatment, and new ways of preventing mental illness. It has played a significant and pioneering role in the study of schizophrenia.

The NAMH implements its service programs through its chapters in some 1,000 cities, counties, and metropolitan areas throughout the country, and its divisions, which are state associations. In the past few decades, its watchdog efforts have resulted in improved care and treatment in state hospitals, the upgrading of old hospitals and clinics, and

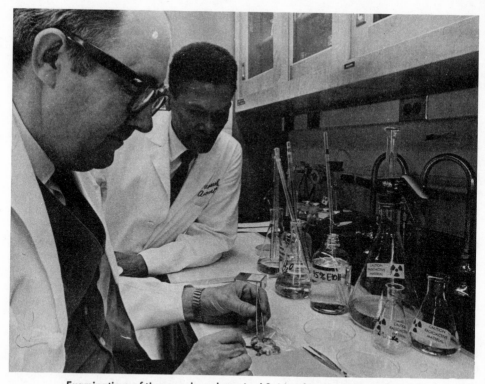

Examinations of tissue and cerebrospinal fluid aid in diagnosing multiple sclerosis. Here a neurologist and his assistant study a tissue specimen.

the erection of better treatment facilities. It constantly provides lawmakers with information about mental illness and the need for a greater number of government-funded resources.

Through widespread campaigning, the Association has helped to focus attention on childhood mental illness and the importance of providing better diagnostic and treatment facilities for young people with serious mental disturbances.

To reduce the number of patients who return to mental hospitals because of inadequate rehabilitation services in their communities, the NAMH has activated local agencies in their effort to help such patients return to normal life and find suitable employment.

Multiple Sclerosis

The National Multiple Sclerosis Society, 205 East 42nd Street, New York, New York 10017, was organized in 1946 with the initial goal of supporting research into the causes and possible cure for this baffling disease of the central nervous system. One of the earliest efforts of the Society was to increase professional and public awareness of the symptoms of multiple sclerosis and the large number of people suffering from it. In addition, a campaign was launched in 1949 for the creation of a new branch of the U.S. Public Health Service to foster and subsidize studies of the disorder. By 1950, the National Institute for Neurological Diseases and Stroke was founded

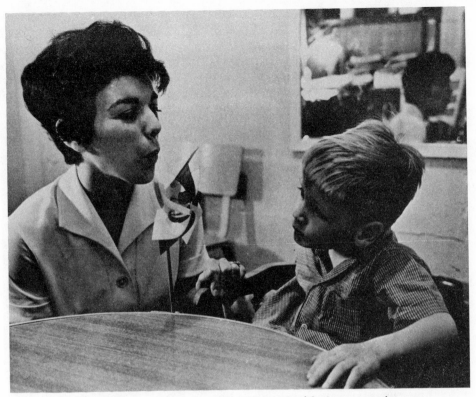

A speech therapist for the National Easter Seal Society uses a pin-wheel as a visual aid in improving her patient's breath control.

as an official government agency. It now spends upwards of three million dollars annually on multiple sclerosis research alone.

Through its more than 200 chapters and affiliated units, the NMSS engages in home and hospital visits, distributes aids to daily living, organizes recreational programs, and supports diagnostic clinics. The local units also arrange educational programs for doctors and rehabilitation and social workers, as well as for patients and their families.

The national office distributes publications for medical personnel and for the interested public, and issues guides for the development of patient services and a quarterly newsletter on research and treatment developments. A medical film and two public information films as well as speakers are available for community programs.

Physical Handicaps

The National Easter Seal Society for Crippled Children and Adults, 2023 West Ogden Avenue, Chicago, Illinois 60612, has grown from its pioneering origins in 1919 to a national organization that serves hundreds of thousands of physically handicapped people of all ages. Among its network of over 3,000 facilities are 83 comprehensive rehabilitation centers in 25 states; 131 treatment and diagnostic centers in 28 states; and vocational training workshops, residential camps, special education programs, and transportation services in many different parts of the country.

Because many crippled children and adults in rural areas and small communities are unaware of the services available to them, the Society gives top priority to publicizing its information, referral, and follow-up activities. In recent years, it has also established mobile treatment units in hospitals and nursing homes in rural areas.

Other innovative activities include screening and testing programs to detect hearing loss in newborns and learning disabilities in preschool children, and providing treatment and referral for those who are disabled by respiratory diseases.

The Society collaborates with federal and professional agencies in all programs designed to eliminate architectural barriers to the disabled, and was instrumental in the enactment of legislation making it mandatory that all buildings constructed with government funds be fully and easily accessible to the handicapped. It also initiates and supports significant studies in rehabilitation procedures as well as scientific research in bone transplant techniques.

Extensive literature is distributed to professionals, the public, to parents, and employers. It also assembles special educational packets for parents of the handicapped.

Tuberculosis and Respiratory Diseases

The American Lung Association, 1740 Broadway, New York, New York 10019, is the direct descendant of the first voluntary health organization to be formed in the United States. In 1904, when the National Association for the Study and Prevention of Tuberculosis was organized, this disease was the country's leading cause of death. Since 1975, with the sharp increase in the problems relating to smoking and air pollution, the Association has been known by its present name, which was adopted to reflect the broader scope of its activities.

It now concerns itself not only with the elimination of tuberculosis but with chronic and disabling conditions, such as emphysema, and with acute diseases of the respiratory system, such as influenza. Through its 1,500 affiliates and nation-wide state organizations, it is actively engaged in campaigns against smoking and air pollution.

The early endeavor of the Association to have tuberculosis included among the reportable diseases was accomplished state by state, and since the 1920s, all states have required that every case in the country be brought to the attention of local health officials.

Public awareness of better care and the development of effective drugs have dramatically reduced the number of TB patients, but the Association continues to concern itself with the fact that there are still more than 45,000 new cases each year.

Through its local affiliates, the ALA initiates special campaigns to combat smoking and air pollution, using radio and television announcements, car stickers, posters, and pamphlets, as well as films and exhibits. Educational materials on respiratory diseases are regularly distributed by the national office to

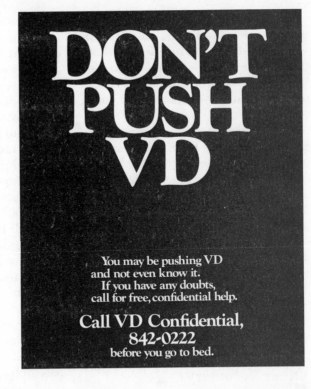

An advertisement for a VD hotline stresses the importance of seeking help if there is any possibility of venereal disease.

doctors, patients, and the general public. Funds raised by the annual Christmas Seal drive also support research and medical education fellowships.

Venereal Disease

The American Social Health Association, 260 Sheridan Avenue, Suite 307, Palo Alto, California 94306, was organized in 1912 to promote the control of venereal disease and to combat prostitution. Since 1960, it has also concerned itself with problems relating to drug dependence and abuse. Although it has no local units, it appoints regional staff members to work with private and public community organizations on special programs related to special health and family life education. For such programs, it provides research and

statistical information, educational materials, professional consultation, and plans for voluntary citizen action.

The Association is in close touch with government agencies such as the Public Health Service, the National Institutes of Health, and the various branches of the Armed Forces, as well as the Federal Bureau of Narcotics, the Children's Bureau, and the Office of Education. Through these channels, it promotes its program for VD education in the schools and for research toward the discovery of an immunizing vaccine against syphilis and gonorrhea.

In the drug field, the ASHA is the major national voluntary repository for information and consultation, and maintains the world's most comprehensive collection of source materials on the misuse of narcotics, barbiturates, and the like. It constantly helps communities in diagnosing their problems and produces a number of publications for teachers, guidance counselors, and youth workers.

The agency's original sex education program has been broadened to include all aspects of family life. In literature, lectures, and conferences, it stresses the importance of introducing family life education into the curriculum of elementary and secondary schools and of establishing training programs on this subject in teachers' colleges. These efforts have resulted in the inclusion of family life education in an increasing number of school systems throughout the United States.

Other Voluntary Health Agencies

In addition to those voluntary health agencies which are members of the National Health Council, there are many other organizations which function on a national scale and offer specialized services as well as literature and guidance to professionals, patients, parents, and concerned families. The following is a partial list:

Alcoholics Anonymous, Box 459, Grand Central Annex, New York, New York 10017, is a fellowship of men and women who share their experience and give each other support in overcoming the problem of alcoholism. Chapters exist throughout the country and offer referral services, literature, and information about special hospital programs.

Al-Anon Family Groups, P.O. Box 182, Madison Square Station, New York, New York 10010, is unaffiliated with Alcoholics Anonymous but cooperates closely with it. This organization serves the families and friends of alcoholics, organizing groups for supportive therapy, providing speakers, distributing literature, and offering referral services. There are more than 5,500 such groups in the United States.

Allergy Foundation of America, 801 Second Avenue, New York, New York 10017, was established to help solve all health problems related to allergic diseases by sponsoring research and treatment facilities. It also grants scholarships to medical students specializing in the study of allergy.

American Foundation for the Blind, 15 West 16th Street, New York, New York 10011, is a national research and information center that coordinates the activities of local and regional agencies serving the blind and the deaf-blind. It also records over two million books and magazines each year. Known as The Talking Books, they are produced in cooperation with the Library of Congress and are made available to the blind and other handicapped people free of charge through special libraries throughout the United States.

The Association for Voluntary Sterilization, 708 Third Avenue, New York, New York 10017, was founded in 1937 to inform professionals and the public about the nature and merits of voluntary sterilization as a method of birth control; to encourage family counseling services to include advice on this procedure; and to encourage physicians and hospitals to establish policies that will make this type of surgery

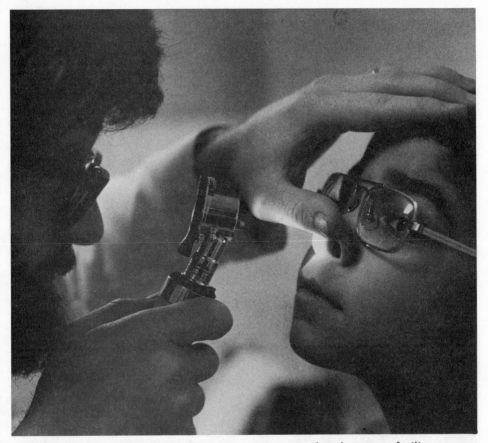

The Allergy Foundation of America sponsors research and treatment facilities for allergic diseases. This patient is being examined for a skin allergy.

available to properly screened applicants. The organization has a roster of 1,600 cooperating physicians in all parts of the United States who accept referrals and perform sterilizations.

The Epilepsy Foundation of America, 1828 L Street, N.W., Washington, D.C. 20036, is the result of a merger in 1967 of two similar organizations. At present, the Foundation has 78 local affiliates which provide information, referral services, and counseling. It conducts a research grant program for medical and psychosocial investigation and distributes a wide variety of literature on request to doctors, teachers,

employers, and the interested public on such subjects as anticonvulsant drugs, insurance, driving laws, and emergency treatment. The national office also maintains an extensive research library and a speakers' bureau.

The Leukemia Society of America, 211 East 43rd Street, New York, New York 10017, was organized in 1950 and now has 69 chapters in 21 states. It supports research in the causes, control, and eventual eradication of the disease which, though commonly thought of as a disorder of the blood, is in fact a disorder of the bone marrow, lymph nodes, and spleen, which manufacture blood. The Society has a continuing program of education through special publications directed to doctors, nurses, and the public. Through its local affiliates, it conducts patient-aid services which provide counseling, transportation, and—to those who need financial assistance—drugs, blood transfusions, and laboratory facilities.

Muscular Dystrophy Associations of America, 810 Seventh Avenue, New York, New York 10019, has as its goal the scientific conquest of muscular dystrophy and all related neuromuscular diseases. Through its 325 chapter affiliates in the United States, the MDAA offers a large number of patient and community services, all of them free. Diagnostic

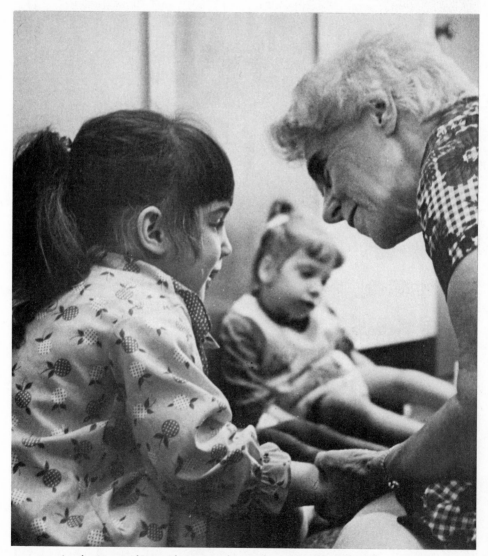

A volunteer working with a young hospital patient. Many service organizations use older volunteers to work with hospitalized or handicapped children.

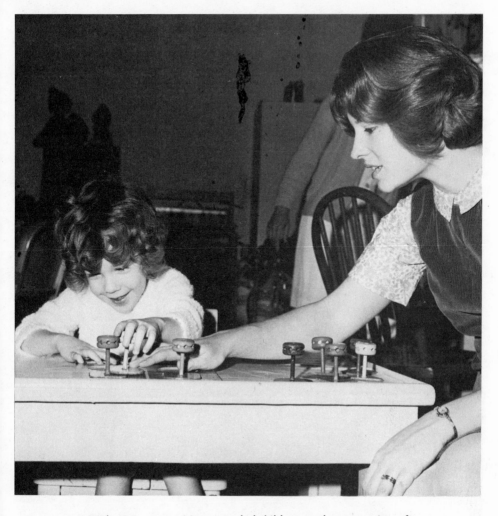

With proper supervision, retarded children can learn a variety of
skills that can be developed into occupational goals in adulthood.

workups and tests are available to all those who may, in the opinion of their physician, be suffering from neuromuscular ailments. The local chapters assist in the purchase and repair of such items as walkers and crutches, braces, wheelchairs, and hospital beds when they are prescribed by a doctor.

Other activities include work with elementary and secondary schools for the inclusion of disabled children in existing educational programs and providing recreational programs for these children. Chapters also maintain patient service committees which serve as clearinghouses for information and referral.

The National Association for Retarded Citizens, 2709 Avenue E East, Arlington, Texas 76011, established in 1950, is the only national voluntary agency specifically devoted to promoting the welfare of the mentally retarded of all ages, of whom it is estimated that there are approximately six million in the United States. Through its 1,300 affiliates, it conducts sheltered workshops, encourages employment, supports research, and works for better diagnostic and treatment facilities. Counseling and referral services, as well as extensive literature for professionals and concerned families, are available on request.

The National Foundation-March of Dimes, P.O. Box 2000, White Plains, New York 10602, founded in

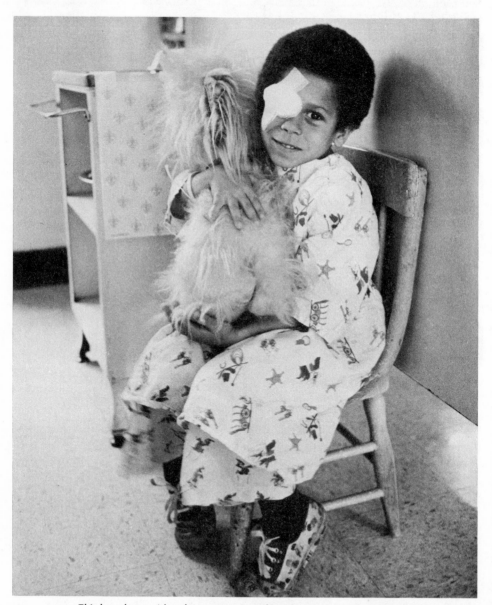

This boy, born with only one eye, is undergoing a series of operations to provide him with an eye socket so that he can wear an artificial eye.

1938 to combat infantile paralysis, is now chiefly concerned with birth defects: finding their causes, most effective treatments, and ways to prevent their occurrence. The Foundation supports 87 medical service centers and 17 research centers which focus on mental retardation of prenatal origin; congenital blindness, deafness, and heart disease; birth malformations such as club feet and cleft palates; and diseases such as diabetes, muscular dystrophy, and cystic fibrosis. The organization has also established the Salk Institute in California, directed by Dr. Jonas Salk, for the purpose of carrying on basic research in the life processes in order to discover what causes the abnormalities associated with birth defects. Since proper prenatal care plays a critical role in the normal development of the fetus, the Foundation enlists the support of every available community service in order to initiate prenatal care programs. Known as PNC clinics, these centers are set up in those parts of the country where they are most needed.

Special Health Services and Agencies

Many factors have contributed to the growth of the American system of health services. Specialists in various medical specialties have tried to meet needs for new types of health care. Medical care has become so effective that individual life expectancy has increased enormously; as one result, the number of Americans aged 65 and older tripled in the three-quarters of a century between 1900 and 1975.

As the population of the United States has grown older, in percentage terms, the problems of the aged have received more attention. New methods and devices have been developed for the care and assistance of the ill or disabled of any age.

Special health services and agencies help to fill such needs. Many older persons have utilized the services of trained individuals who make survival possible— sometimes at home—or slow down the rate of deterioration. Other institutions and agencies perform simple maintenance tasks for the aged or the seriously ill or handicapped, or help with rehabilitation. Social service agencies and groups with health roles, for example, provide adult day care, homemaker assistance, and home health services that may include the following:

• Part-time or occasional nursing care, often under the supervision of a registered nurse

• Physical, occupational, or speech therapy

• Medical social services that help the patient and his or her family to adjust to the social and emotional conditions accompanying illness or disability of any kind

• Assistance from a home health aide, including help with such tasks as bathing and going to the bathroom, taking medications, exercising, and getting into and out of bed

• Under some circumstances, medical attention from interns or residents in training

In this context *long-term care* has evolved as a special area of medical services. Used mainly by the aged or handicapped, long-term care may be provided as well for anyone of any age who needs continuing help because of recurring or long-lasting symptoms, disabilities, or sickness. Social service agencies and specialists are frequently called upon to provide preliminary or follow-up care or services.

Other factors have encouraged the creation of special health services and agencies. For example, *social work* as a profession has gained broad acceptance among educators and professional medical personnel. Young people in greater numbers have for that reason sought careers in social work. Awards of degrees in such specialties as psychiatric social work have underscored the trend.

The idea of service has played a key role. Efforts have been exerted steadily over recent years to answer the special needs of the socially, occupationally, or physically handicapped or disabled (see *"Social Workers,"* p. 1331). The social service concept has effected changes in both the hospital and the community. Thus most major hospitals have staff social workers, and forward-looking communities have health service groups and agencies of many different kinds.

Five such health agencies may be described. Four of these have for years played important roles in the community health picture. One, the hospice for terminally ill patients, has grown steadily in significance, and promises to become an integral part of the health scene.

The Hospice

In medieval times, weary travelers could halt along the road at a hospice to find refreshment and a night's rest. Today, that concept of a place of rest survives in the hospice, the special care setting or institution for the care of the dying.

The modern institution started with St. Christopher's Hospice at Sydenham, on the outskirts of London. St. Christopher's offered residents an informal, "freestanding" program. For the most part, private or smaller rooms gave way to larger wards. But each patient had his or her private space within a colorful curtain. The beds were low, ensuring easy transfer in and out, and could be wheeled as freely as a wheelchair. Thus patients had maximum mobility. Within the curtained area, each patient had private belongings, comfortable chairs, flowers, and paintings.

The Sydenham program has provided an example for the hospices now operating in the United States, notably New Haven, Connecticut, and Tucson, Arizona. But programs vary from one institution to another. Typically, visiting hours cover the entire day from 8 A.M. to 8 P.M. Children are allowed to visit, and birthdays and other events are celebrated with parties. Family members may bring food and other refreshments when visiting.

The Sydenham-type program permits "polypharmacy," a term indicating that drugs may be used broadly to control pain. Heroin may be administered orally at four-hour intervals. Scheduled administration of such drugs has been found to eliminate pain more thoroughly because the sensations of pain cannot develop fully. While patients may become dependent on drugs, that has not been considered a problem among the terminally ill.

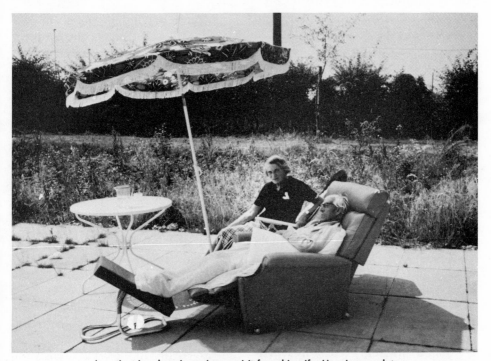

A patient in a hospice enjoys a visit from his wife. Hospices work to provide a friendly, supportive environment for their patients.

Hospice programs in the United States appear to share some common characteristics. These include:

• In making the patient as comfortable as possible, stress is placed more on the quality of life than on its quantity

• The staff views the patient in a family context—to the point where the dying person's entire family becomes the "patient"

• Rules of care emphasize pain alleviation and control, maintenance of normal life styles, and continuity

• Home care, even to the moment of death, is stressed; where the terminally ill have to enter the hospice, the institutional aspects of the arrangement are minimized

• Mechanical life-support systems are not used.

A modified type of hospice program functions in some hospitals in the United States. Usually, the hospice unit operates under the hospital's regular inpatient program. A special hospice team including, possibly, a full-time nurse, two part-time clinical nurse specialists, three or four part-time physicians, a social worker, and a chaplain may visit the patient daily. The team discusses symptom control, gives support, and provides other services for the patient.

The Nursing Home

Along the spectrum of special health services and agencies in the United States, nursing homes probably rank as the most important. The reasons are simple. Nursing homes exist in greater numbers than

332 VOLUNTARY HEALTH AGENCIES

other extended-care institutions and take care of more people. In the late 1970s the U.S. Department of Health, Education, and Welfare estimated that nearly 20,000 American nursing homes were providing accommodations and care for as many as 1.3 million persons.

The quality level of nursing home care has caused great concern in recent years. Efforts to establish standards for nursing homes have resulted in various sets of questions against which nursing home services can be measured (see pp. 678–679). Such standards usually point to at least four characteristics of "good" nursing homes:

• Beds are available for residents in greater numbers

• Occupancy rates are higher

• Good nursing homes are certified for more levels of care than others

From a health point of view, it has proved difficult to define *quality of care*. A generally accepted rule indicates that the phrase refers mainly to the quantity of interaction between patients and staff or other residents.

Judging the quality of care delivered by a nursing home may involve still other considerations (see "Nursing Homes," pp. 677–679). Those investigating such homes may, for example, try to determine the degree of accountability borne by the director and staff. The key question to ask: Are there persons or agencies in the community that care about the patient and can act in his or her behalf? The researcher can also ask whether the nursing home has direct community, church, civic organization, or other sponsorship. Another rule of thumb holds that

the good nursing home is not isolated; rather, it welcomes volunteers, suppliers, inspectors, relatives and friends of patients, and other community representatives. In many cases the nursing home administrator or director invites participation by relatives in home activities. Also, community groups may become involved in operations and events and the federal nursing home ombudsman program has a solid foundation.

Social Service Agencies

Social service agencies share so many different characteristics and take part in so many activities, both medical and nonmedical, that they are difficult to classify. Agencies providing social services have, however, been differentiated from *social action* groups or organizations that stress community involvement for specific improvement goals.

In medical settings social services have evolved for various purposes. In hospitals, they have served to bring a personal, helping element to the patient's bedside. They have also grown to keep pace with elaborations on purely medical services. In the community, social service agencies have increasingly become the instruments bringing the reality of comprehensive medical care to the man in the street. That means, most importantly, that the individual in need of medical care can obtain it when and where it is needed and at the time of need. Social service care of a medical nature may thus be provided in such facilities as the physician's office, the group-practice center, the patient's home, or a long-term care facility. Such services may be offered in many other types of settings.

To some extent, social service agencies function as extensions of the formal medical system that includes hospitals and other institutions, offices, and clinics. Social service agencies in effect add an essential element to the care continuum. Providing adult day care, agency employees or volunteers may drive elderly individuals to and from a center. The social worker may also help provide recreation, offer rehabilitative treatment or therapy, dispense meals, and take part in arts and crafts activities.

Home health services cover an extremely broad range. Some important types of services were enumerated in the introduction to this section. Most of these services—nursing care, physical, occupational, or speech therapy, and so on—are paid for by Medicare if a physician certifies that the patient needs them. But home care services reach into all areas of personal and social functioning; necessarily, many of them are not covered by Medicare.

What agency or individual services have been devised to help the disabled or elderly remain in their homes? Depending on the community, they range across this kind of spectrum:

• The meals-on-wheels program, under which a meal can be delivered daily to the person needing it

• A home visiting service

• A telephone reassurance program run by volunteers to guarantee to the home-bound at least one call a day

• An emergency aid or crisis intervention plan, often run in conjunction with the telephone reassurance program

• Congregate living arrangements, in facilities such as foster homes or retirement villages, that may or may not offer meals, housekeeping services, medical supervision, and social activities.

To ensure that elderly persons receiving part-time care at home run the fewest possible risks, many communities today have crisis intervention programs (CIPs). The persons assisting with such programs—usually social workers —go into action on receiving a report that an older person has a major problem. A landlord may believe that a tenant has fallen and cannot help himself. In another case, a relative calling from a distant city may be unable to reach the aged person—and may contact the CIP caseworker. Usually, CIP services are dovetailed with other forms of aid that may be provided by legal, medical, psychological-psychiatric, social, and other services.

Church-sponsored group homes have also sprung up in the United States. Most offer arrays of services and, often, the guarantee of lifelong support in exchange for an initial lump-sum payment or continuous monthly payments. The group homes have for the most part proved superior to urban hotels and boarding homes as an alternative to hospitalization or long-term care. For one thing, the group homes can provide social services on a professional level. As a second factor, the homes have avoided many of the problems of the boarding homes, among them inadequate dietary provisions, overcrowding, and structural deficiencies.

Social service agencies created to help the aged provide what has been called *open care:* various programs designed to make possible continued home residence. Open care has the general goal of forestalling institutionalization, or *closed care* inside a medical facility or old-age home. Care by relatives, friends, or other "natural networks" including community caretakers or irregular volunteers is referred to as *nonorganized care.*

Social Services in Hospitals

Aside from its role as a source of advice and assistance to the patient, the hospital social service department may work to solve family problems. Many of these arise as direct results of the hospitalization. With a father hospitalized, for example, a family may suffer severe economic dislocations. Problems centering on means of caring for a patient after discharge may require counseling, telephone calls, or direct assistance of one kind or another.

Standards for hospital social service departments are set by the National Association of Social Workers. The Association also certifies qualified workers through registry in the Academy of Certified Social Workers (ACSW).

Once qualified, the social worker in the hospital offers services that may deeply affect the patient's chances of achieving full recovery. Initially, the social worker may investigate the patient's situation, seeking facts that will help place the patient in the total economic and social environment in which he lives and works. The worker may then be qualified, in case of need, to counsel patients and their families.

Individual cases require individual solutions. A social worker may have to evaluate a patient's ability to cooperate with a program of medical or psychiatric treatment. Acting as a member of the hospital staff, the social worker may describe the patient's situation to a doctor to clarify special needs. More suitable plans of care and treatment often result. On the other side, the worker may have to explain details of treatment to the patient's family.

Medical and psychiatric social workers are in demand in a variety of institutions other than hospitals. These others include local, state, and federal health departments, voluntary health agencies, and public and private health centers. Many social workers have sought to raise their levels of professional skill by obtaining master's degrees in social work. In doing so, they are responding to needs that point to social work as a long-term, satisfying career.

Visiting Nurses

In most communities in the United States, a Visiting Nurse Association or similar agency provides liaison between professional nurses and potential patients. Rural areas generally have county public health nurses that give home assistance to those needing it.

The decision on whether the patient can recuperate or receive treatment at home may lie with the physician. Often, that decision depends on the availability of the visiting nurse. In a sense, the nurse then becomes the doctor's substitute. He or she nearly always receives advice from the doctor on what is to be done for the patient and who should do it. But the nurse maintains contact between doctor and patient in at least the following areas:

• The progress of medication; changes in medication; reactions observed when medication is administered

• Temperature checks, usually carried out on a schedule

• Special treatments, including enemas, massage, body rubs

• If the patient is confined to bed, the progress of exercises, steps toward mobility, meal service, amounts of food and liquid to be ingested, and so on

• Adherence to special diets

• Circumstances under which the doctor should be called

• Precautions taken by other members of the family

The latter may be particularly important. The nurse works full-time in the patient's home only in the extreme case. In the typical situation, the visiting nurse assigns basic tasks to members, or a member, of the family. The nurse may also try to develop an organized care plan so that nothing important to the patient's well-being will be overlooked.

Before the patient arrives at home, the nurse may want to arrange the sickroom for the greatest convenience. Importantly, where records must be kept the nurse will make certain that the appropriate record-keeping necessities are available: chart or pad, pencil, and so on. But furniture may require rearrangement as well; and factors of home geography may have to be considered. Among these are proximity to a bathroom or kitchen.

The goal of all the work done by the visiting nurse is to help the patient get well or become more comfortable. In pursuing those goals, the nurse tries to establish a calm, pleasant atmosphere. It may prove possible to encourage some distractions such as television or reading. Quiet games geared to the patient's tastes and age may be appropriate.

On the physician's instructions, the nurse may carry out basic treatment procedures. Treatments may be designed to prevent additional problems, such as infections that spread from one part of the body to another. Hot and cold applications may serve to relax muscles, relieve pain, and help the patient in other ways. Cold applications may be used to reduce body temperatures, stop bleeding, or relieve pain or inflammation.

The nurse encounters special challenges as well as routine chores. At times he or she may be called on to dress wounds or give shots. In caring for the handicappped, the nurse tries to eliminate or reduce emotional and other problems, including despondency, along with physical difficulties such as bedsores and lack of mobility.

The aged present the nurse with special problems. In addition to the normal ones of physical weakness and reduced mobility, the aged person may also suffer from emotional or psychological problems. Senility may cut off the older person from those who want to love or help him or her. Deep understanding of the difficulties that age brings may be required to maintain a professional level of care and to ensure that all steps necessary or appropriate are taken—and taken on time.